Pharmaceutical Drug Development

Pharmaceutical Drug Development

Edited by Sean Boyd

hayle
medical

New York

Hayle Medical,
750 Third Avenue, 9th Floor,
New York, NY 10017, USA

Visit us on the World Wide Web at:
www.haylemedical.com

ISBN: 978-1-63241-468-7

The publisher's policy is to use permanent paper from mills that operate a sustainable forestry policy. Furthermore, the publisher ensures that the text paper and cover boards used have met acceptable environmental accreditation standards.

Printed in the United States of America.

Cataloging-in-Publication Data

Pharmaceutical drug development / edited by Sean Boyd.
    p. cm.
Includes bibliographical references and index.
ISBN 978-1-63241-468-7
1. Drug development. 2. Pharmacology. 3. Pharmacy. 4. Drugs. I. Boyd, Sean.
RM301.25 .P43 2017
615.19--dc23

Table of Contents

Preface..IX

Chapter 1   **Development of a validated UPLC-qTOF-MS Method for the determination of curcuminoids and their pharmacokinetic study in mice**... 1
Mahendra K Verma, Ishtiyaq A Najar, Manoj K Tikoo, Gurdarshan Singh, Devinder K Gupta, Rajneesh Anand, Ravi K Khajuria, Subhash C Sharma and Rakesh K Johri

Chapter 2   **Binary Solvents Dispersive Liquid—Liquid Microextraction (BS-DLLME) Method for Determination of Tramadol in Urine using High-Performance Liquid Chromatography**.................................... 10
Vahid Kiarostami, Mohamad-Reza Rouini, Razieh Mohammadian, Hoda Lavasani and Mehri Ghazaghi

Chapter 3   **Novel 9-(alkylthio)-Acenaphtho[1,2-e]-1,2,4-triazine derivatives: synthesis, cytotoxic activity and molecular docking studies on B-cell lymphoma 2 (Bcl-2)**......................... 18
Mohammad K Mohammadi, Omidreza Firuzi, Mehdi Khoshneviszadeh, Nima Razzaghi-Asl, Saghi Sepehri and Ramin Miri

Chapter 4   **A case report of hearing loss post use of hydroxychloroquine in a HIV-infected patient**... 29
Hossein Khalili, Farzaneh Dastan and Seyed Ali Dehghan Manshadi

Chapter 5   **Synthesis, analgesic and anti-inflammatory activities of new methyl-imidazolyl-1,3,4-oxadiazoles and 1,2,4-triazoles**... 33
Ali Almasirad, Zahra Mousavi, Mohammad Tajik, Mohammad Javad Assarzadeh and Abbas Shafiee

Chapter 6   **Quantitative analysis of piroxicam using temperature-controlled ionic liquid dispersive liquid phase microextraction followed by stopped-flow injection spectrofluorimetry**........................ 41
Mohsen Zeeb, Parisa Tayebi Jamil, Ali Berenjian, Mohammad Reza Ganjali and Mohamad Reza Talei Bavil Olyai

Chapter 7   **Effects of rutin on acrylamide-induced neurotoxicity**.................................. 49
Vahideh Sadat Motamedshariaty, Sara Amel Farzad, Marjan Nassiri-Asl and Hossein Hosseinzadeh

Chapter 8   **Amitriptyline, clomipramine, and doxepin adsorption onto sodium polystyrene sulfonate**.. 58
Akram Jamshidzadeh, Fatemeh Vahedi, Omid Farshad, Hassan Seradj, Asma Najibi and Gholamreza Dehghanzadeh

Chapter 9   Beneficial effects of pioglitazone and metformin in murine model of
             polycystic ovaries via improvement of chemerin gene up-regulation...................... 64
             Nahid Kabiri, Mohammad Reza Tabandeh and
             Seyed Reza Fatemi Tabatabaie

Chapter 10   Unraveling the cytotoxic potential of Temozolomide loaded into
             PLGA nanoparticles.. 74
             Darshana S Jain, Rajani B Athawale, Amrita N Bajaj, Shruti S Shrikhande,
             Peeyush N Goel, Yuvraj Nikam and Rajiv P Gude

Chapter 11   Study of the pharmacokinetic changes of Tramadol in diabetic rats........................ 83
             Hoda Lavasani, Behjat Sheikholeslami, Yalda H Ardakani,
             Mohammad Abdollahi, Lida Hakemi and Mohammad-Reza Rouini

Chapter 12   Formulation and optimization of itraconazole polymeric lipid
             hybrid nanoparticles (Lipomer) using box behnken design.. 92
             Balaram Gajra, Chintan Dalwadi and Ravi Patel

Chapter 13   The hypoglycemic effect of *Juglans regia* leaves aqueous extract in
             diabetic patients... 107
             Saeed Hosseini, Hasan Fallah Huseini, Bagher Larijani, Kazem Mohammad,
             Alireza Najmizadeh, Keramt Nourijelyani and Leila Jamshidi

Chapter 14   Synthesis and biological evaluation of novel benzyl piperazine
             derivatives of 5-(5-nitroaryl)- 1,3,4-thiadiazoles as
             Anti-*Helicobacter pylori* agents... 112
             Negar Mohammadhosseini, Parastoo Saniee, Ameneh Ghamaripour,
             Hassan Aryapour, Farzaneh Afshar, Najmeh Edraki, Farideh Siavoshi,
             Alireza Foroumadi and Abbas Shafiee

Chapter 15   Silymarin effect on amyloid-β plaque accumulation and gene
             expression of APP in an Alzheimer's disease rat model... 120
             Parichehreh Yaghmaei, Katia Azarfar, Mehrooz Dezfulian and
             Azadeh Ebrahim-Habibi

Chapter 16   Introduction of a mathematical model for optimizing the drug
             release in the patient's body.. 127
             Mohammad Reza Nabatchian, Hamid Shahriari and Mona Shahriari

Chapter 17   Factors affecting viability of *Bifidobacteriumbifidum* during
             spray drying.. 139
             Zahra Shokri, Mohammad Reza Fazeli, Mehdi Ardjmand,
             Seyyed Mohammad Mousavi and Kambiz Gilani

Chapter 18   Cardanol isolated from Thai Apis mellifera propolis induces cell
             cycle arrest and apoptosis of BT-474 breast cancer cells via p21
             upregulation... 148
             Sureerat Buahorm, Songchan Puthong, Tanapat Palaga,
             Kriengsak Lirdprapamongkol, Preecha Phuwapraisirisan,
             Jisnuson Svasti and Chanpen Chanchao

Chapter 19   **Clinical results with two different pharmaceutical preparations of riboflavin in corneal cross-linking: an 18-month follow up**.................................. 159
Hassan Hashemi, Mohammad Amin Seyedian, Mohammad Miraftab, Hooman Bahrmandy, Araz Sabzevari and Soheila Asgari

Chapter 20   **Carum induced hypothyroidism: an interesting observation and an experiment**... 164
Seyede Maryam Naghibi, Mohamad Ramezani, Narjess Ayati and Seyed Rasoul Zakavi

Chapter 21   **Statistical optimization of tretinoin-loaded penetration-enhancer vesicles (PEV) for topical delivery**.. 168
Neda Bavarsad, Abbas Akhgari, Somayeh Seifmanesh, Anayatollah Salimi and Annahita Rezaie

Chapter 22   **Physico-chemical characterization and pharmacological evaluation of sulfated polysaccharides from three species of Mediterranean brown algae of the genus *Cystoseira***.................................. 180
Hiba Hadj Ammar, Sirine Lajili, Rafik Ben Said, Didier Le Cerf, Abderrahman Bouraoui and Hatem Majdoub

Chapter 23   **Blessings in disguise: a review of phytochemical composition and antimicrobial activity of plants belonging to the genus *Eryngium***.. 188
Sinem Aslan Erdem, Seyed Fazel Nabavi, Ilkay Erdogan Orhan, Maria Daglia, Morteza Izadi and Seyed Mohammad Nabavi

Chapter 24   **Metabolic effects of newly synthesized phosphodiesterase-3 inhibitor 6-[4-(4- methylpiperidin-1-yl)-4-oxobutoxy]-4-methylquinolin-2(1H)-one on rat adipocytes**.. 210
Bagher Alinejad, Reza Shafiee-Nick, Hamid Sadeghian and Ahmad Ghorbani

Chapter 25   **Does pharmacist-supervised intervention through pharmaceutical care program influence direct healthcare cost burden of newly diagnosed diabetics in a tertiary care teaching hospital in Nepal: a non-clinical randomised controlled trial approach**.................................. 219
Dinesh Kumar Upadhyay, Mohamed Izham Mohamed Ibrahim, Pranaya Mishra, Vijay M. Alurkar and Mukhtar Ansari

Permissions

List of Contributors

Index

Preface

Over the recent decade, advancements and applications have progressed exponentially. This has led to the increased interest in this field and projects are being conducted to enhance knowledge. The main objective of this book is to present some of the critical challenges and provide insights into possible solutions. This book will answer the varied questions that arise in the field and also provide an increased scope for furthering studies.

Pharmaceuticals can be defined as drugs that prevent and cure disease. This book on pharmaceutical drug development encompasses an interdisciplinary study of the field that discusses the medicine industry, drug manufacturing processes. This book provides significant information of this discipline to help develop a good understanding of this discipline and related fields. It includes some of the vital pieces of work being conducted across the world, on various topics related to pharmaceutical drug development. For students and researchers in the fields of pharmacology, hospital management, public health policy and pharmaceutical sciences, this book would prove to be very helpful.

I hope that this book, with its visionary approach, will be a valuable addition and will promote interest among readers. Each of the authors has provided their extraordinary competence in their specific fields by providing different perspectives as they come from diverse nations and regions. I thank them for their contributions.

Editor

Development of a validated UPLC-qTOF-MS Method for the determination of curcuminoids and their pharmacokinetic study in mice

Mahendra K Verma[2*†], Ishtiyaq A Najar[1], Manoj K Tikoo[1†], Gurdarshan Singh[1†], Devinder K Gupta[3†], Rajneesh Anand[2†], Ravi K Khajuria[2†], Subhash C Sharma[1*†] and Rakesh K Johri[1*†]

Abstract

Background: A specific and sensitive UPLC-qTOF-MS/MS method has been developed for the simultaneous determination of curcuminoids. These Curcuminoids comprises of curcumin, a principal curcuminoid and other two namely, demethoxycurcumin, and bisdemethoxycurcumin obtained from rhizomes of *Curcuma longa* an ancient Indian curry spice turmeric, family (*Zingiberaceae*).

Methods: These analytes were separated on a reverse phase C18 column by using a mobile phase of acetonitrile: 5% acetonitrile in water with 0.07% acetic acid (75:25 v/v), flow rate of 100 μL/min was maintained. The qTOF-MS was operated under multiple reaction monitoring (MRM) mode using electro-spray ionization (ESI) technique with positive ion polarity. The major product ions in the positive mode for curcuminoids were at m/z 369.1066, 339.1023 and 309.0214 respectively. The recovery of the analytes from mouse plasma was optimized using solid phase extraction technique.

Results: The total run time was 5 min and the peaks of the compounds, bisdemethoxycurcumin, demethoxycurcumin and curcumin occurred at 2.06, 2.23 and 2.40 min respectively. The calibration curves of bisdemethoxycurcumin, demethoxycurcumin and curcumin were linear over the concentration range of 2–1000 ng/mL (r2, 0.9951), 2–1000 ng/mL (r2, 0.9970) and 2-1000 ng/mL (r2, 0.9906) respectively.
Intra-assay and inter-assay accuracy in terms of % bias for curcumin was in between −7.95to +6.21, and −7.03 to + 6.34; for demethoxycurcumin was −6.72 to +6.34, and −7.86 to +6.74 and for bisdesmetoxycurcumin was −8.23 to +6.37 and −8.47 to +7.81. The lower limit of quantitation for curcumin, demethoxycurcumin and bisdemethoxycurcumin was 2.0 ng/mL. Analytes were stable under various conditions (in autosampler, during freeze-thaw, at room temperature, and under deep-freeze conditions). This validated method was used during pharmacokinetic studies of curcumin in the mouse plasma.

Conclusions: A specific, accurate and precise UPLC-qTOF-MS/MS method for the determination of curcumin, demethoxycurcumin and bisdemethoxycurcumin both individually and simultaneously was optimized.

Background

Curcuma longa L. (*Zingiberaceae*) is a coloring agent, has been found to be a rich source of phenolic compounds, namely, curcuminoids (2-5%) [1]. *C. longa* consists of a mixture of three naturally occurring curcuminoids. Curcumin the principal curcuminoid (about 80%) and other two curcuminoids are demethoxycurcumin (about 12%) and bisdemethoxycurcumin (about 8%).

Curcuminoids are recognized for their broad spectrum biological activities and have been generally regarded as safe (GRAS) in foods or pharmaceuticals. Curcumin is widely used for coloring of foods like pickles and snacks.

Many pharmacological properties have been attributed to curcuminoids including anti-inflammatory and hepatoprotective activities [2], antioxidant and cholekinetic activities [3,4] and anti-protease activity [5,6]. In addition, apoptosis have been shown to induce in human

* Correspondence: mkvermadr@yahoo.com; scsharma@iiim.ac.in; rkjohri@iiim.ac.in
†Equal contributors
[2]Analytical Chemistry Division (Instrumentation), CSIR-Indian Institute of Integrative Medicine, Canal Road, Jammu, India
[1]PK/PD and Toxicology Division, CSIR-Indian Institute of Integrative Medicine, Canal Road, Jammu, India
Full list of author information is available at the end of the article

cancer cells by the curcuminoids [7] and act as a chemo-preventive agents for major types of cancer, including the stomach, lung, breast, prostate, colon and duodenal cancers, as well as leukemias [8-12] and display neuro-protective effects [13]. Curcumin has also been reported a more potent free radical scavenger than vitamin E [14].

It is also known for its potential use of curcumin in the treatment of infections such as human immunodefi-ciency virus (HIV) is also reported [15].

Quantification of the active metabolite, THC in plasma and urine by HPLC method has also been reported [16] and simultaneous quantification of diferuloylmethane and its metabolites in biological matrices has been reported by LC/MS/MS [17].

Hence, due to the immense biological importance [18] of curcumin and its analogues, there is a need for effect-ive, rapid and more sensitive methods to monitor cur-cuminoids. Various HPLC methods are available in literature for determination of curcuminoids [19-29]. HPLC-MS methods also reported to provide quantitation of curcuminoids [30-32].

In recent times UPLC with qTof-MS is widely consid-ered analytical technique for better quality data in terms of increased detection limits, and chromatographic reso-lution with greater sensitivity. This paper presents (i) a method for the simultaneous determination of curcumi-noids by UPLC–qTOF-MS, and (ii) a pharmacokinetic study of curcumin in mice.

Methods
Material and methods
Curcumin, demethoxycurcumin and bis-demethoxycur-cumin used as standards were isolated from the rhi-zomes of C. longa by the method already reported in literature. The isolated curcuminoids were identified on the basis of NMR and Mass spectral data. The purity of standards was >99%. All solvents/chemicals used were of HPLC grade and obtained from E-Merck, Mumbai, India. The HPLC grade water was obtained from a Water Purifi-cation System (Synergy UV, Millipore, USA).

Instrumentation
A UPLC-qTOF-MS system (Synapt, Waters, USA, equipped with MassLynx acquisition software, version 4.1) was used. Experimental conditions were column, C-18 (50×2.1 mm); particle size, 1.7 μm; (Acquity, BEH); flow rate, 100 μL/min; mobile phase, acetonitrile: 5% aceto-nitrile in water with 0.07% acetic acid (75: 25 v/v), injection volume, 5 μL. The analyte infusion experiments were per-formed using an in-built syringe pump. A mass spectro-meter with ESI interface was used for MS/MS analysis. ESI parameters were as follows: capillary voltage, 2.7 kV for positive mode; source temperature, 83°C; desolvation temperature, 200°C; cone gas flow, 50 L/h and desolvation

gas flow, 550 L/h. The multiple reaction monitoring (MRM) mode was used to monitor the transition of curcumin m/z 391.0864 [M+Na], 369.1066 (M+H) to 285.0912, demethoxycurcumin at 339.1023 (M+H) to 255.0848 and of bisdemethoxycurcumin at m/z 309.0968 [M+H] to 225.0790.

Preparation of reference, standard and quality control solutions
Reference solutions of curcumin (C) (stock I), demethoxy-curcumin (DMC), (stock II) and bisdemethoxycurcumin (BDMC) (stock III) were prepared by weighing 5 mg of each compound. The quantities were transferred to 5 mL volumetric flasks, dissolved and diluted suitably with HPLC grade methanol. All the reference solutions (1 mg/mL) were covered with aluminium foil and sealed with paraffin film to avoid photodegradation and loss due to evaporation. Stock I, stock II and stoke III were mixed together, and diluted suitably with methanol. A 50-uL of this solution was used to spike blank mouse plasma samples (450 uL) to achieve 8 calibration standards (CAL STD) containing curcuminoids combination. CAL STD-1: curcuminoids, 2 ng/mL; CAL STD-2: 5 ng/mL each; CAL STD-3: 10 ng/mL each; CAL STD-4: 50 ng/mL each; CAL STD-5: 100 ng/mL each; CAL STD-6: 200 ng/mL each; CAL STD-7: 500 ng/mL each; and CAL STD-8: 1000 ng/mL each. Three quality control (QC) standards (LQC: 2 ng/mL; MQC: 450 ng/mL; HQC 900 ng/mL each of curcuminoids) were prepared and used to spike blank mouse plasma.

Method validation procedures
The analytical method was validated to meet the accept-ance criteria as per guidelines of the International Confer-ence on Harmonization of Technical Requirements for Registration of Pharmaceuticals for Human Use (ICH). The specificity of the method was established by comparing blank plasma samples with those spiked with the analytes to find out interference from endogenous components. The CAL STD solutions were utilized for establishment of linearity and range (linear least-squares regression with a weighting index of 1/x). The precision and accuracy para-meters were ascertained in LLOQ, LQC, MQC, and HQC samples (7 replicates each in 3 sets) on the same day and on 3 consecutive days. The intra-assay and inter-assay ac-curacy (% bias) of the method was determined from mean measured concentrations and nominal concentrations as follows: % bias = [(mean measured conc.–nominal conc.)/ nominal conc.]×100. The intra-assay and inter-assay precision (% relative standard deviation or RSD) of the method was calculated from mean measured concentra-tions as follows: % RSD = (SD of mean measured conc./ mean measured conc.)×100. The stability of analytes in plasma was investigated under following conditions:

(a) 1 month storage at deep freeze (−80°C); (b) 3 consecutive freeze–thaw cycles from −20°C to room temperature; (c) 24 h storage at room temperature; and (d) short-term stability (of processed samples) at 10°C for 24 h in autosampler. After specified storage conditions, samples were processed and analyzed. The matrix effect was investigated by post extraction spike method. Peak area (A) of the analyte in spiked blank plasma with a known concentration (MQC) was compared with the corresponding peak area (B) obtained by direct injection of standard in the mobile phase. The ratio (A/B×100) is defined as the matrix effect.

Sample preparation

The curcumin (C), demethoxycurcumin (DMC), and bis-demethoxycurcumin (BDMC) were recovered simultaneously from plasma using solid phase extraction (SPE) technique involving semi-automated vacuum chamber and vacuum pump (Supelco, USA). The various steps involved in the recovery procedure were: (a) conditioning of SPE cartridge (C18, 3 mL capacity, 100 mg bed, Samprep-Ranbaxy, Mumbai, India) with 1.0mLmethanol, followed by 1.0 mL water, (b) loading of diluted (1:4, v/v) plasma samples (1.0 mL) onto cartridge and drying under positive pressure, and (c) samples were washed with 2 mL of water followed by elution with 2 mL of methanol. The eluants were carefully collected in 2.0 mL capacity glass vials for direct analysis in UPLC–qTOF-MS system.

Experimental animals

Swiss mice (22–30 g) were obtained from the Animal House of this Institute, and kept in regulated environmental conditions (temperature: $25 \pm 2°C$, humidity: $60 \pm 5\%$, 12 h dark/light cycle). Animals were fed on standard pelleted diet (Ashirwad Industries, Chandigarh, India) and water was provided ad libitum. Animal experiments were approved by Institutional Ethics Committee. Animals were fasted overnight before the experiment and segregated into different groups for the sample collections at different time intervals. All these animals were administered with curcumin (100 mg/kg, p.o.). Blood samples were collected in pre-heparinized glass tubes at different time intervals post dosing (0–24 hr). Blood samples were centrifuged (5000 rpm; 10 min at 20°C) to separate the plasma.

Pharmacokinetics

Concentration-time curves for Concentration–time curves were established for curcumin from the treated mice and used for the determination of pharmacokinetic parameters such as peak plasma concentration (Cmax), peak time (Tmax), extent of absorption (AUC), half-life (t1/2), clearance (Cl), and volume of distribution (Vd) by a non-

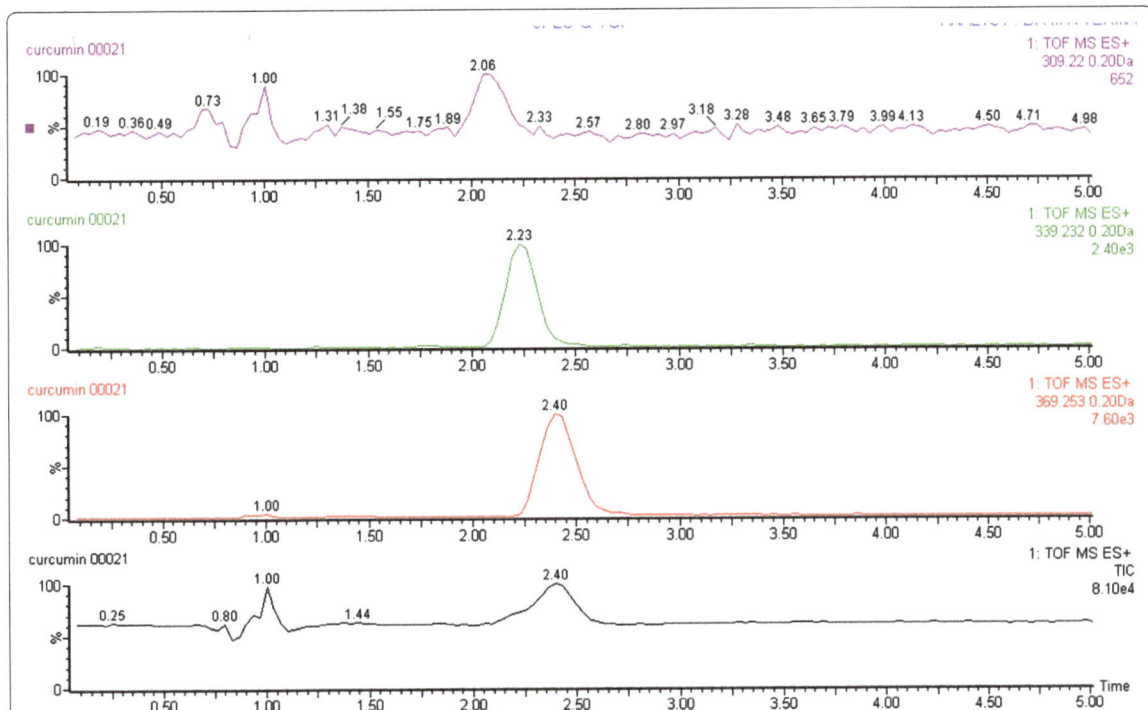

Figure 1 Typical UPLC-qTOF-MS/MS chromatograms showing Curcuminoids. 1 **A**. Extracted ion chromatogram (EIC) of bisdemethoxycurcumin. 1 **B**. Extracted ion chromatogram (EIC) of demethoxycurcumin. 1 **C**. Extracted ion chromatogram (EIC) of curcumin. 1 **D**. Total ion chromatogram (TIC) of Curcuminoids.

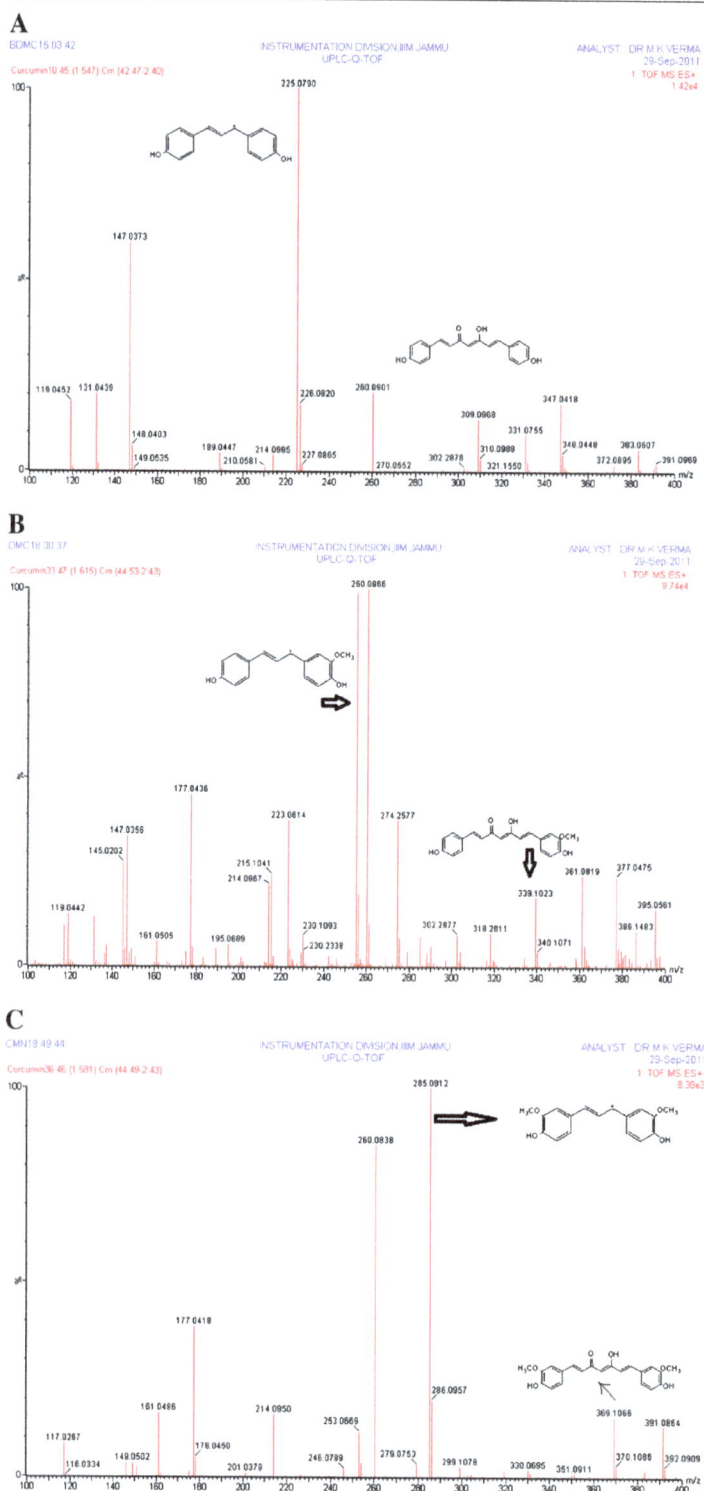

Figure 2 2 **A** - **Product ion spectra of bisdemethoxrcurcumin showing fragmentation transitions.** 2 **B** - Product ion spectra of demethoxrcurcumin showing fragmentation transitions. 2 **C** - Product ion spectra of curcumin showing fragmentation transitions.

compartmental analysis using PK Solutions Version 2.0; Summit Research Services, USA.

Results

UPLC–qTOF-MS/MS analysis

Optimum chromatographic separation of curcuminoids was achieved by acetonitrile: 5% acetonitrile in water with 0.07% acetic acid (75:25 v/v). Flow rate of 100 µL/min was maintained. All the analytes were added simultaneously in the samples and the resulting chromatograms showed a retention time of 2.06, 2.23 and 2.40 min for bisdemethoxycurcumin, demethoxycurcumin and curcumin respectively (Figure 1A, B & C). A full scan in positive ion mode was used for all the analytes. During direct infusion, the mass spectra of the major product ions in the positive mode for bisdemethoxycurcumin m/z 309.0968 $[M+H]^+$ to the product ion 225.0790 (Figure 2A) demethoxycurcumin m/z 339.1023 (M+H) to 255.0848 (Figure 2B) and of curcumin m/z 391.0864 [M+Na], 369.1066 (M+H) to 285.0912 (Figure 2C).

Method validation

Specificity

The method was found to be specific: Extracted blank plasma when compared with plasma samples spiked with curcuminoids did not show any interference at the respective retention times of each analyte.

Linearity and range

The calibration curves of bisdemethoxycurcumin, demethoxycurcumin and curcumin were linear over the concentration range of 2–1000 ng/mL (r2, 0.9951), 2–1000 ng/mL (r2, 0.9970) and 2-1000 ng/mL (r2, 0.9906) respectively.

Accuracy and precision

The combined recovery of curcumin, demethoxycurcumin and bisdemethoxycurcumin was carried out in LLQC, LQC, MQC and HQC samples. The recovery (mean ± S.E.) of curcumin was 93.2% ± 4.1 (from LLQC), 95.6% ± 3.9 (from LQC), 96.2% ± 3.2 (from MQC), and 93.4% ± 2.9 (from HQC). The recovery (mean ± S.E.) of demethoxycurcumin was 92.8% ± 4.3 (from LLQC) 94.3% ± 3.8 (from LQC), 91.7% ± 3.3 (from MQC), and 91.5% ± 2.7 (from HQC). The recovery (mean ± S.E.) of bisdemethoxycurcumin was 89.9% ± 6.2 (from LLQC), 93.3% ± 5.2 (from LQC), 91.6% ± 3.2 (from MQC), and 90.5% ± 2.6 (from HQC). The intra-assay and inter-assay accuracy in terms of % bias were given in Table 1.

Intra- assay and inter-assay precision (% RSD) were presented in Table 2.

The accuracy and precision of the method were within the acceptable limits of ±15%.

Table 1 Accuracy (% bias) data

Compound	Nominal conc. (ng/mL)	Intra -assay			Inter-assay		
		Set 1	Set 2	Set 3	Set 1	Set 2	Set 3
Curcumin	2	+5.81	−7.95	−7.02	+6.34	+5.38	−5.86
	6	+5.98	−6.29	+6.21	−7.03	+4.39	+5.39
	450	−4.23	+5.09	− 3.86	−5.61	+5.94	4.79
	900	+3.84	−4.72	−5.37	+4.67	−5.38	−5.01
DMC	2	+6.34	−5.81	−6.62	+6.74	+5.89	−5.06
	6	+5.68	−6.72	+6.04	−7.86	+4.95	+6.21
	450	−4.73	+5.89	− 5.31	−5.88	+5.04	−5.86
	900	+5.09	−4.38	−5.66	+5.17	−6.72	−4.71
BDMC	2	+6.37	−8.23	−7.91	+6.73	+7.81	−6.54
	6	+ 5.28	−6.98	+7.41	−8.47	+6.39	+5.86
	450	−6.29	+5.73	− 6.06	−6.80	+5.68	− 6.89
	900	+5.87	−6.32	−6.98	+5.69	−4.63	− 7.08

Lower limit of quantitation (LLOQ)

The LLOQ for curcumin, demethoxycurcumin and bisdemethoxycurcumin were 2.0 ng/mL.

Stability

The stability of the analytes in plasma was investigated in LQC and HQC samples. The recoveries of the analytes after one month (storage stability), after 1, 2 and 3 cycles of freeze–thaw and after 24 h (stability at room temp.) relative to that at time zero are summarized in Table 3.

Matrix effect

The matrix effect (A/B×100) for Curcumin was 96.78% (% RSD: 3.14; n = 5), and for DMC it was 97.31% (% RSD: 4.05; n = 5) and for BDMC it was 96.13% (% RSD: 3.89;

Table 2 Precision (% RSD) data

Compound	Nominal conc. (ng/mL)	Intra -assay			Inter-assay		
		Set 1	Set 2	Set 3	Set 1	Set 2	Set 3
Curcumin	2	8.31	7.34	7.93	8.59	6.57	7.81
	6	6.38	7.51	8.76	7.77	8.32	6.68
	450	4.68	6.39	5.51	5.31	6.07	5.85
	900	2.94	3.89	4.79	5.28	4.79	5.53
DMC	2	9.27	8.86	9.65	9.85	8.89	9.41
	6	7.41	6.09	7.38	7.05	6.59	9.77
	450	5.24	4.84	6.07	6.18	7.04	6.17
	900	4.41	4.79	6.06	4.69	5.31	4.99
BDMC	2	11.37	9.98	10.57	9.23	10.88	10.54
	6	8.68	7.98	9.07	9.35	8.47	9.86
	450	5.86	7.79	8.95	6.32	5.89	5.49
	900	4.46	5.32	5.48	3.69	4.79	6.24

Table 3 Stability data

Condition	CMN		DMC		BDMC	
	LQC	HQC	LQC	HQC	LQC	HQC
Recovery (ng) after storage (−80°C) 0 month	5.92 ±0.141	888.974 ± 1.876	5.90 ±0.161	885±1.948	5.71±0.209	874 ±2.375
1 month	5.81±0.165 (98.14%)	853.41 ± 1.451 (95.99%)	5.78±0.178 (97.97%)	861±1.381 (97.29%)	5.57±0.393 (97.55%)	845 ±3.058 (96.68%)
Recovery (ng) after freeze thaw cycles	5.92 ± 0.141	888.974 ± 1.876	5.90± 0.161	885±1.948	5.71±0.209	874 ±2.375
Cycle 0	5.82±0.186	878.413±	5.84±0.181	869±1.768	5.65±0.219	870 ±2.435
Cycle 1	(98.31%)	1.381 (98.81%)	(98.98%)	(98.19%)	(98.94%)	(99.54%)
Cycle 2	**5.76**±0.314 (97.29%)	871.274± 1.576 (98.00%)	5.81± 0.173 (98.47%)	865±1.549 (97.74%)	5.63±0.179 (98.59%)	864 ±2.021 (98.85%)
Cycle 3	**5.62** ±0.372 (94.93%)	852.560± 1.732 (95.90%)	5.78± 0.196 (97.96%)	861±1.598 (97.28%)	5.60±0.247 (98.07%)	859 ±2.564 (98.28%)
Recovery (ng) after storage at room temp.	5.92 ± 0.141	888.974 ± 1.876	5.90± 0.161	885±1.948	5.71±0.209	874 ±2.375
0 h	5.62± 0.198	832.231 ±	5.77± 0.293	829±1.321	5.37±0.901	821 ±1.967
24 h	(94.93%)	1.451 (93.61%)	(97.79%)	(93.67%)	(94.04%)	(93.93%)
Recovery (ng) after storage in auto sampler	5.92 ± 0.141	888.974 ± 1.876	5.90± 0.161	885±1.948	5.71±0.209	874 ±2.375
0 h	5.80± 0.219	872.136 ±	5.77± 0.293	858±1.973	5.56±0.214	854 ±3.057
24 h	(97.97%)	2.151 (98.10%)	(97.79%)	(96.95%)	(97.37%)	(97.71%)

n=5) Percent RSD < 5 suggested that the method was free from matrix effect.

Pharmacokinetics

Concentration vs. time profile of Curcumin and pharmacokinetic parameters (Figure 3, Table 4). Each time point is mean±SE (n = 6). For details refer Section 1.6.

Discussion

Three curcuminoids were used as a standard in the present study showed separate peaks in the extracted ion chromatogram (EIC) at 2.06, 2.23 and 2.40 min for bisdemethoxycurcumin demethoxycurcumin and Curcumin respectively. The bisdemethoxycurcumin demethoxycurcumin and Curcumin, were also appeared in the

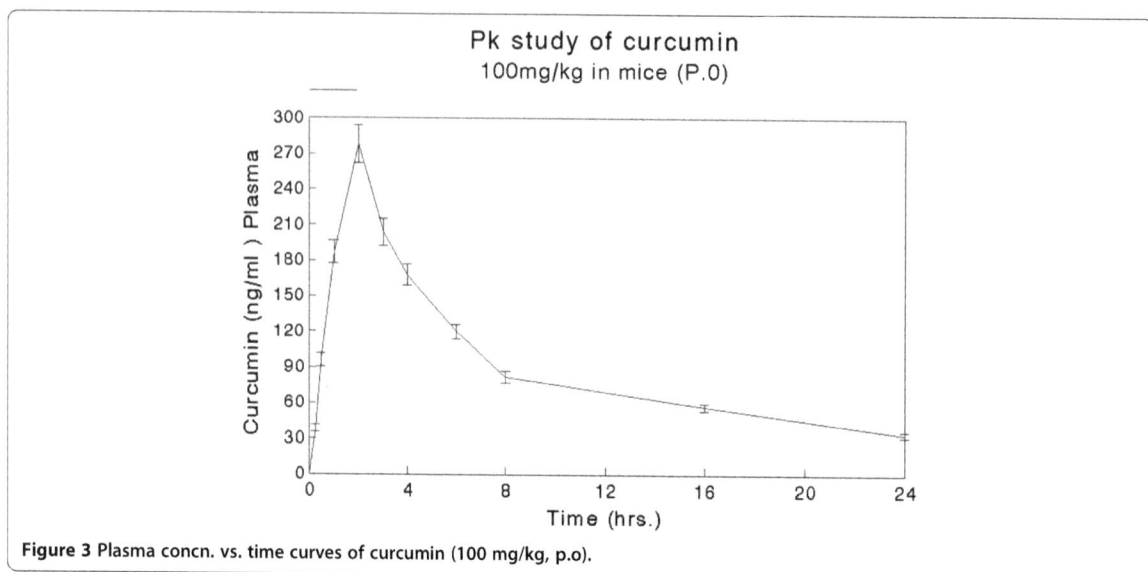

Figure 3 Plasma concn. vs. time curves of curcumin (100 mg/kg, p.o).

Table 4 Pharmacokinetic parameters (curcumin)

$AUC_{0-\infty}$ (ng*hr/ml)	2650.9± 13.2
C_{max} (ng/ml)	278.0± 18.6
T_{max} (hr)	2.0
Half Life (hr.)	10.1±0.96
Clearance (L/hr)	46.125±2.39
Vd (L/kg)	502.06±23.2
MRT (hr.)	18.3±1.21

total ion chromatogram TIC. These three curcuminods were also shown together in the ESI spectra (Figure 4).

A method for the determination of curcumin, demethoxycurcumin and bisdemethoxycurcumin by UPLC-qTOF-MS/MS has not been reported, prior to this investigation, in which curcuminoids have been quantified on the basis of their major fragment. The major product ions observed in the positive ion ESI spectra curcumin m/z 391.0864 [M+Na], 369.1066 (M+H) to 285.0912, demethoxycurcumin at 339.1023 (M+H) to 255.0848 and of bisdemethoxycurcumin at m/z 309.0214 $[M+H]^{+}$ to the production 225.0790. The quantification of the analytes was achieved by using MRM which makes the proposed method most acceptable.

Previously reported HPLC-UV methods for the quantification and determination of curcuminoids have several disadvantages, such as unsatisfactory separation times (needs more analysis time), poor resolution and complicated solvent mixtures with gradient elution. These methods are not selective, rapid, so a time-consuming pretreatment of a sample, or complicate gradient elution is required.

We have developed a simple, reliable and an isocratic UPLC-qTOF-MS/MS method which require only binary solvent system containing water and acetonitrile. This method has shown high degree of simplicity, accuracy, sensitivity, reproducibility and also provides short analysis time (5 min.). In the proposed method the linearity was in the range between 2 ng/mL to 1000 ng/mL which makes the method most suitable for the trace quantification of analytes. This method can also be used for the quantification of individual curcuminoids for routine analysis.

The method was validated in terms of specificity, accuracy, precision, sensitivity and stability of the analytes, and utilized for the determination of curcumin, demethoxycurcumin and bisdemethoxrcurcumin either individually or simultaneously in plasma (mice). After oral administration curcumin could be quantified only up to 24 h of sampling time. A pharmacokinetic parameters from plasma concentration-time data usually involves the maximum

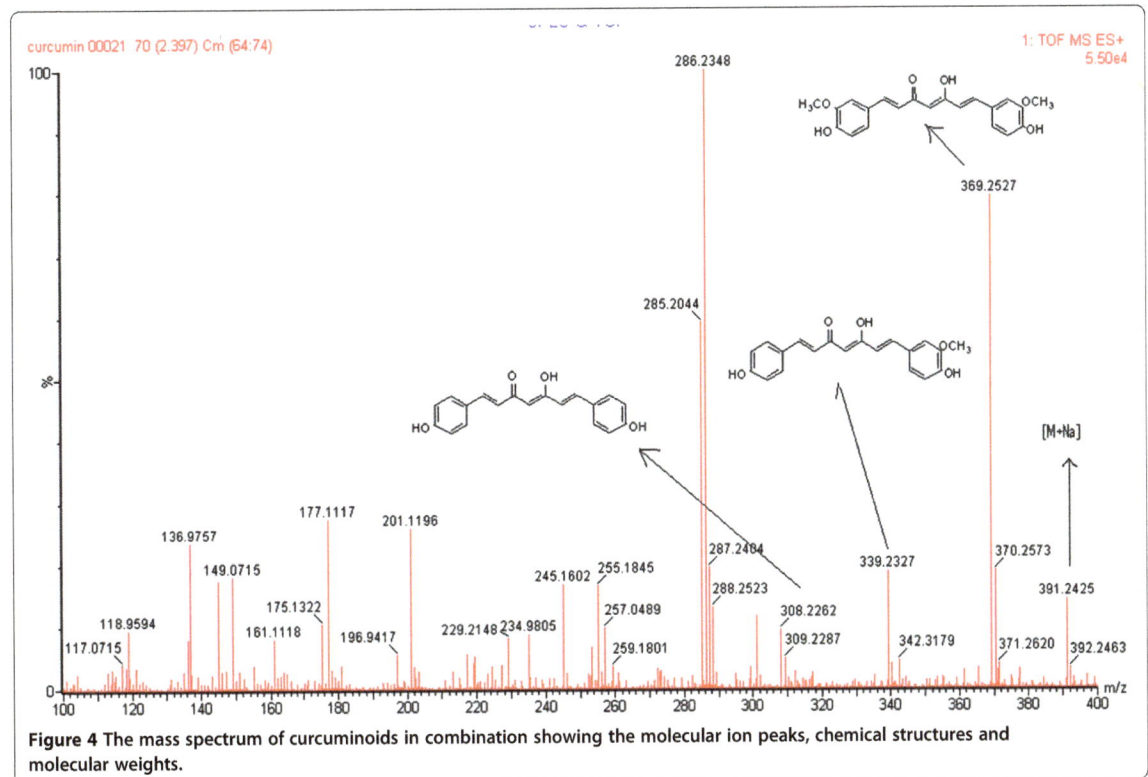

Figure 4 The mass spectrum of curcuminoids in combination showing the molecular ion peaks, chemical structures and molecular weights.

(peak) plasma drug concentrations (C_{max}) and the area under the plasma concentration –time curve (AUC). The plasma drug concentration increases with the rate of absorption; therefore the most widely used general index of absorption is C_{max}. AUC is another reliable measure for the extent of absorption. It is directly proportional to the total amount of unchanged drug that reaches systemic circulation.

Conclusions

A specific, accurate and precise UPLC-qTOF-MS/MS method for the determination of curcumin, demethoxycurcumin and bisdemethoxycurcumin both individually and simultaneously was optimized. Pharmacokinetic study of curcumin was carried out by using this validated method.

Competing interests
The authors declare that they have no competing interests.

Authors' contributions
MK, SC and RK conceived and designed the study and prepared the manuscript. MK, SC, IA, GD and MT carried out all the experimental work and statistical analysis and helped to draft the manuscript. MK carried out the UPLC –Q-TOF-MS studies, DK isolated the compounds by using column chromatography studies and compounds were characterized by MK, DK, RA and RKK. All authors read and approved the final manuscript.

Acknowledgements
Authors are thankful to the Director, CSIR-IIIM, Jammu for providing necessary facility for the work.

Author details
[1]PK/PD and Toxicology Division, CSIR-Indian Institute of Integrative Medicine, Canal Road, Jammu, India. [2]Analytical Chemistry Division (Instrumentation), CSIR-Indian Institute of Integrative Medicine, Canal Road, Jammu, India. [3]Biorganic Chemistry Division, CSIR-Indian Institute of Integrative Medicine, Canal Road, Jammu, India.

References
1. Inoue K, Nomura C, Ito S, Nagatsu A, Hino T, Oka H: Purification of curcumin, demethoxycurcumin, and bisdemethoxycurcumin by high-speed countercurrent chromatography. *J Agric Food Chem* 2008, 56:9328–9336.
2. Lukita-Atmadja W, Ito Y, Baker GL, McCuskey RS: Effect of curcuminoids as anti-inflammatory agents on the hepatic microvascular response to endotoxin. *Shock* 2002, 17:399–403.
3. Masuda T, Hidaka K, Shimohara A, Maekawa T, Takeda Y, Yamaguchi H: Chemical studies on antioxidant mechanism of curcuminoid: analysis of radical reaction products from curcumin. *J Agric Food Chem* 1999, 47:71–77.
4. Rasyid A, Rahman AR, Jaalam K, Lelo A: Effect of different curcumin dosages on human gall bladder. *Asia Pac J Clin Nutr* 2002, 11:314–318.
5. Nishigaki I, Kuttan R, Oku H, Ashoori F, Abe H, Yagi K: Suppressive effect of curcumin on lipid peroxidation induced in rats by carbon tetrachloride or 60Co-irradiation. *J Clin Biochem Nutr* 1992, 13:23–29.
6. Sui Z, Salto R, Li J, Craik C, De Montellano PRO: Inhibition of the HIV-1 and HIV-2 proteases by curcumin and curcumin boron complexes. *Bioorg Med Chem* 1993, 1:415–422.
7. Choudhuri T, Pal S, Agwarwal ML, Das T, Sa G: Curcumin induces apoptosis in human breast cancer cells through p53-dependent Bax induction. *FEBS Lett* 2002, 512:334–340.
8. Kelloff GJ, Crowell JA, Steele VE, Lubet RA, Malone WA, Boone CW, Kopelovich L, Hawk ET, Lieberman R, Lawrence JA, Ali I, Viner JL, Sigman CC: Progress in cancer chemoprevention: development of diet-derived chemopreventive agents. *J Nutr* 2000, 130:467S–471S.
9. Shao ZM, Shen ZZ, Liu CH, Sartippour MR, Go VL, Heber D, Nguyen M: Curcumin exerts multiple suppressive effects on human breast carcinoma cells. *Int J Cancer* 2002, 98:234–240.
10. Duvoix A, Blasius R, Delhalle S, Schnekenburger M, Morceau F, Henry E, Dicato M, Diederich M: Chemopreventive and therapeutic effects of curcumin. *Cancer Lett* 2005, 223:181–190.
11. Kawamori T, Lubet R, Steele VE, Kelloff GJ, Kaskey RB, Rao CV, Reddy BS: Chemopreventive effect of curcumin, a naturally occurring anti-inflammatory agent, during the promotion/progression stages of colon cancer. *Cancer Res* 1999, 59:597–601.
12. Kanai M, Imaizumi A, Otsuka Y, Sasaki H, Hashiguchi M, Tsujiko K, Matsumoto S, Ishiguro H, Chiba T: Dose-escalation and pharmacokinetic study of nanoparticle curcumin, a potential anticancer agent with improved bioavailability, in healthy human volunteers. *Cancer Chemother Pharmacol* 2012, 69:65–70.
13. Lee HS, Jung KK, Cho JY, Rhee MH, Hong S, Kwon M, Kim SH, Kang SY: Neuroprotective effect of curcumin is mainly mediated by blockade of microglial cell activation. *Pharmazie* 2007, 62:937–942.
14. Zhao BL, Li XJ, He RG, Cheng SJ, Xin WJ: Scavenging effect of extracts of green tea and natural antioxidants on active oxygen radicals. *Cell Biophys* 1989, 14:175–185.
15. Ammon HP, Wahl MA: Pharmacology of *Curcuma longa. Planta Med* 1991, 57:1–7.
16. Pan MH, Huang TM, Lin JK: Biotransformation of curcumin through reduction and glucuronidation in mice. *Drug Metab Dispos* 1999, 27:486–494.
17. Heath DD, Pruitt MA, Brenner DE, Begum AN, Frautschy SA, Rock CL: Tetrahydrocurcumin in plasma and urine: Quantitation by high performance liquid Chromatography. *J Chromatogr B, Analyt Technol Biomed Life Sci* 2005, 824:206–212.
18. Esatbeyoglu T, Huebbe P, Ernst IMA, Chin D, Wagner AE, Rimbach G: Curcumin—from molecule to biological function. *Angew Chem Int Ed* 2012, 51:5308–5332.
19. Bos R, Windono T, Woerdenbag HJ, Boersma YL, Koulman A, Kayser O: HPLC-photodiode array detection analysis of curcuminoids in *Curcuma* species indigenous to Indonesia. *Phytochem Anal* 2007, 18:118–122.
20. Jadhav BK, Mahadik KR, Paradkar AR: Development and validation of improved reversed phase-HPLC method for simultaneous determination of curcumin, demethoxycurcumin and bis-demethoxycurcumin. *Chromatographia* 2007, 65:483–488.
21. Jayaprakasha GK, Rao LJM, Sakariah KK: Improve HPLC method for the determination of curcumin, demethoxycurcumin, and bisdemethoxycurcumin. *J Agric Food Chem* 2002, 50:3668–3672.
22. Khurana A, Ho CT: High-performance liquid chromatography analysis of curcuminoids and their photo-oxidative decomposition compound in *C. longa* L. *J Liq Chromatogr* 1998, 11:2295–2304.
23. Li R, Xiang C, Ye M, Li HF, Zhang X, Guo D: Qualitative and quantitative analysis of curcuminoids in herbal medicines derived from Curcuma species. *Food Chem* 1890, 2011:126.
24. Naidu MM, Shyamala BN, Manjunatha JR, Sulochanamma G, Srinivas P: Simple HPLC method for resolution of curcuminoids with antioxidant potential. *J Food Sci* 2009, 74:312–318.
25. Scotter MJ: Synthesis and chemical characterisation of curcuminoid colouring principles for their potential use as HPLC standards for the determination of curcumin colour in foods. *Food Sci Tech* 2009, 42:1345–1351.
26. Taylor SJ, McDowell IJ: Determination of the curcuminoid Pigments in turmeric *(Curcuma domestica* Val) by reversed-phase high performance liquid chromatography. *Chromatographia* 1992, 34:73–77.
27. Tonnesen HH, Karlsen J: High-performance liquid chromatography of curcumin and related compounds. *J Chromatogr* 1983, 259:367–371.
28. Wichitnithad W, Jongaroonngamsang N, Pummangura S, Rojsitthisak P: A simple isocratic HPLC method for the simultaneous determination of curcuminoids in commercial turmeric extracts. *Phytochem Anal* 2009, 20:314–319.
29. Xie Y, Jiang ZH, Zhou H, Cai X, Wong YF, Liu ZQ, Bian ZX, Xu HX, Liu L: Combinative method using HPLC quantitative and qualitative analysis for quality consistency assessment of a herbal medicinal preparation. *J Pharm Biomed Anal* 2007, 43:204–212.
30. He XG, Lin LZ, Lian LZ, Lindenmaier M: Liquid chromatography electrospray mass spectrometric analysis of curcuminoids and sesquiterpenoids in turmeric *(Curcuma longa). J Chromatogr A* 1998, 818:127–132.

Development of a validated UPLC-qTOF-MS Method for the determination of curcuminoids and their...

9

31. Liu R, Zhang J, Liang M, Zhang W, Yan S, Lin M: **Simultaneous analysis of eight bioactive compounds in Danning tablet by HPLC-ESI-MS and HPLC-UV.** *J Pharm Biomed Anal* 2007, **43**:1007–1012.

32. Jiang H, Timmermann BN, Gang DR: **Use of liquid chromatography–electrospray ionization tandem mass spectrometry to identify diarylheptanoids in turmeric (*C. longa* L.) rhizome.** *J Chromatogr A* 2006, **1111**:21–31.

Binary Solvents Dispersive Liquid—Liquid Microextraction (BS-DLLME) Method for Determination of Tramadol in Urine Using High-Performance Liquid Chromatography

Vahid Kiarostami[1*], Mohamad-Reza Rouini[2], Razieh Mohammadian[1], Hoda Lavasani[2] and Mehri Ghazaghi[3]

Abstract

Background: Tramadol is an opioid, synthetic analog of codeine and has been used for the treatment of acute or chronic pain may be abused. In this work, a developed Dispersive liquid liquid microextraction (DLLME) as binary solvents-based dispersive liquid-liquid microextraction (BS-DLLME) combined with high performance liquid chromatography (HPLC) with fluorescence detection (FD) was employed for determination of tramadol in the urine samples. This procedure involves the use of an appropriate mixture of binary extraction solvents (70 μL CHCl3 and 30 μL ethyl acetate) and disperser solvent (600 μL acetone) for the formation of cloudy solution in 5 ml urine sample comprising tramadol and NaCl (7.5%, w/v). After centrifuging, the small droplets of extraction solvents were precipitated. In the final step, the HPLC with fluorescence detection was used for determination of tramadol in the precipitated phase.

Results: Various factors on the efficiency of the proposed procedure were investigated and optimized. The detection limit (S/N = 3) and quantification limit (S/N = 10) were found 0.2 and 0.9 μg/L, respectively. The relative standard deviations (RSD) for the extraction of 30 μg L of tramadol was found 4.1% (n = 6). The relative recoveries of tramadol from urine samples at spiking levels of 10, 30 and 60 μg/L were in the range of 95.6 – 99.6%.

Conclusions: Compared with other methods, this method provides good figures of merit such as good repeatability, high extraction efficiency, short analysis time, simple procedure and can be used as microextraction technique for routine analysis in clinical laboratories.

Keywords: Dispersive liquid-liquid microextraction, Tramadol, HPLC, Urine

Background

Tramadol ((±) cis-2-[(dimethylamino) methyl]-1-(3meth-oxyphenyl) cyclohexanol hydrochloride) is an opioid, synthetic analog of codeine and is not currently classified as a controlled substance [1-3]. Tramadol has been used since 1977 like other narcotics applied for the treatment of acute or chronic pain may be abused [4]. In Iran, this drug is easily available for patient without prescription and according to annual reports of ministry of health; 350 million tramadol tablets (100 mg) were sold in 2006–2007

and recently, it has become one of the most widely dispensed analgesics in Iran's essential drugs list [5,6]. The extraction of tramadol from biological samples has usually been carried out by using liquid-liquid extraction (LLE) and solid phase extraction (SPE) [4,7-9]. However, LLE is time consuming and requires large amounts of organic solvent and SPE uses much less than LLE, but can be relatively expensive. Recently, other extraction methods as free solvent and miniaturized extractions, such as liquid phase microextraction (LPME) [10,11], solid phase microextraction (SPME) [12], solvent bar microextraction (SBME) [13], liquid phase microextraction with back extraction (LPME-BS) [14], three - phase hollow fiber liquid phase microextraction (HF-LPME) [15], have successfully been

* Correspondence: v_kiarostami@iau-tnb.ac.ir
[1]Department of Chemistry, North Tehran Branch, Islamic Azad University, P.O. Box 1913674711, Tehran, Iran
Full list of author information is available at the end of the article

developed for determination of tramadol from different matrices. Dispersive liquid-liquid microextraction (DLLME) is a miniaturized liquid extraction that was introduced in 2006 by Rezaee and coworkers [16]. However, in this method, the selection of extraction solvents is limited to one type of heavier or lighter extraction solvent than water.

In our previous work, a new method based on DLLME methodology as binary solvents–based dispersive liquid-liquid microextraction (BS-DLLME) was developed for determination of patulin from apple juice samples [17]. In this method, two kinds of extraction solvents (mixture of low and high density solvents) can be used simultaneously. In the present study, a rapid, sensitive and simple BS-DLLME and high performance liquid chromatography coupled with florescence detection has been carried out for the extraction and pre-concentration of tramadol in urine samples.

Methods

Reagent

HPLC-grade methanol, acetonitrile, acetone, chloroform, analytical grade ethyl acetate and deionized water were obtained from Merck chemical co (Darmstadt, Germany). Carbon tetrachloride (CCl_4) with grade of trace analysis was obtained from Merck. The pure substances of tramadol were kindly gifted by Grünenthal chemical co (Stolberg, Germany). Phosphoric acid, sodium hydroxide and sodium chloride were all of analytical grade from Merck and were used without further purification. All the glassware used in experiments first washed with HPLC grade water and acetone and then dried in an oven. For calibration studies, blank urine samples were kindly obtained from one female healthy volunteer in our lab which not exposed to the mentioned drug. The use of tramadol in healthy subjects has been approved in Tehran University of Medical Sciences ethics committee (Ethics board code 4233).

For recovery studies, fresh urine samples from three male volunteers with abuse of tramadol were kindly provided by the Loghman hospital (Tehran, Iran). The study of tramadol pharmacokinetics in drug abused subjects has been approved in Tehran University of Medical Sciences ethics committee (Ethics board code 20324).

Standard solution of tramadol in concentration of 1 mg/mL was prepared by dissolving 10 mg of this compound in 10 mL HPLC-grade water. Working standard solutions of tramadol were prepared by dilution of the stock solution using HPLC-grade water. Stock and standard solutions of this compound were stored at 4°C.

Instrumentation

For separating and analyzing the drug a WellChrom HPLC instrument from Knauer Company (Berlin, Germany) was applied. The chromatographic apparatus equipped with a fluorescence RF-10AXL detector (excitation wavelength of 200 nm and emission wavelengths of 301 nm). Gradient HPLC K-1001 pump and online K-5020 degasser. A Rheodyne model 7725i injector with a 20 µL loop was applied to inject the samples. Chromatographic data were acquired and analyzed using ChromGate Chromatography Software from Knauer Company. Separation was carried out on a ChromolithTM Performance RP-18e, 100 mm × 4.6 mm column (Merck, Darmstadt, Germany) protected by a ChromolithTM Guard Cartridge RP-18e 5 mm × 4.6 mm. A mixture of water and methanol (81:19 v/v) adjusted to pH 2.5 by phosphoric acid at a flow rate of 2 mL/min in isocratic elution mode was used as a mobile phase. Eppendorf centrifuge 4515c (Netheler-Hinz GMBH Germany) was used for sedimentation of the dispersive phase.

Sample preparation

Standard solutions containing 100 µg/mL of tramadol was prepared in HPLC grade water at (4°C) and brought to room temperature just prior to use. The pH of urine sample containing 100 µg/mL tramadol (spiked urine sample) at pH = 10 by addition of 5 M NaOH. Then 5 mL of this sample was placed in centrifuge tube, after centrifugation at 1133 × g for 10 min, upper solution was separated from sediment and was transferred to a 10 mL glass test tube [18].

BS-DLLME procedure A mixture of a disperser solvent and binary extraction solvents (ethyl acetate and chloroform) were injected rapidly into the mentioned pretreated urine solution (5 ml) by 1.00 mL syringe and immediately a cloudy solution was formed. After centrifuging the cloudy solution for 10 min at 1133 × g, the dispersed fine droplets of ethyl acetate and chloroform were settled in the bottom of conical test tube. The deposited phase was transferred to another glass tube and evaporated to dryness under a gentle air stream. The residue was dissolved in 70 µL mobile phase and 20 µL was injected into the HPLC with fluorescence detection system for analysis.

Results and Discussion

In order to optimize the BS-DLLME for determination of tramadol in urine samples, the effective parameters on extraction efficiency such as the type and volume of high density extraction solvent, the volume of ethyl acetate as low density extraction solvent, the type and volume of disperser solvent, salt addition and extraction time were studied. Statistical calculations (single factor analysis of variance and unpaired t-test) carried out with Microsoft® excel 2007 for comparing of data. Significant difference was pretended if the probability level (p) was less than of 0.05.

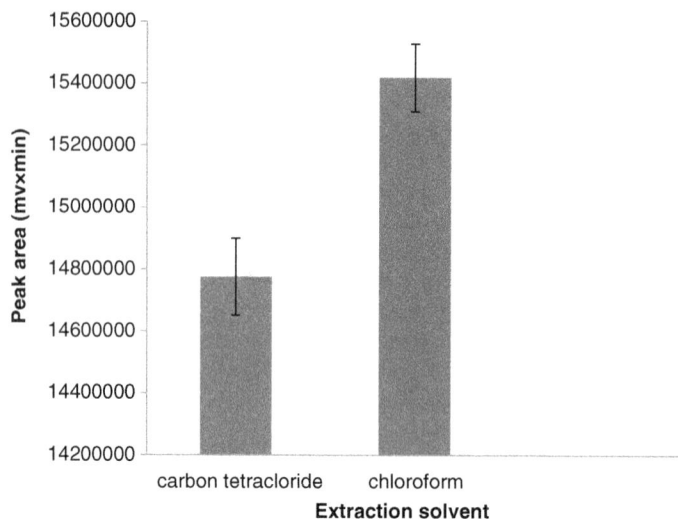

Figure 1 Effect of high density extraction solvent type on the extraction efficiency. Extraction condition: tramadol concentration, 100 μg/ L; volume of extraction solvent, 50 μL; disperser solvent and its volume, 0.6 mL acetonitrile; no salt addition.

Selection of high density extraction solvent

Selection of high density extraction solvent is very important in BS-DLLME procedure. For this purpose chloroform (CHCl$_3$, density 1.49 g/L), carbon tetrachloride (CCl$_4$, density 1.59 g/ml) and dichloromethane (CH$_2$Cl$_2$, density 1.32 gmL^{-1}) selected in this study. A series of urine samples were surveyed by using 0.6 mL of acetone (as disperser solvent) contains 70 μL of different high density extraction solvents. In the presence of dichloromethane as extraction solvent, no droplet was formed and therefore ignored as extraction solvent. As shown in Figure 1, chloroform has better extraction recovery with significant effect (unpaired t-test assuming unequal variances, $p < 0.05$) than the other tested solvents. Therefore, CHCl$_3$ was selected as the extraction solvent in subsequent experiments.

Effect of extraction solvent volume

To examine the effect of high density extraction solvent volume on performance of the presented BS-DLLME procedure, we used acetone with a constant volume (0.6 mL) and different volume of CHCl$_3$ (30–80 μL). As indicated in Figure 2, the extraction efficiency increases with CHCl$_3$ volume from 40 to 70 μL. Above 70 μL of chloroform, the recovery decreases probably due to decrease in the number of droplets available for extraction.

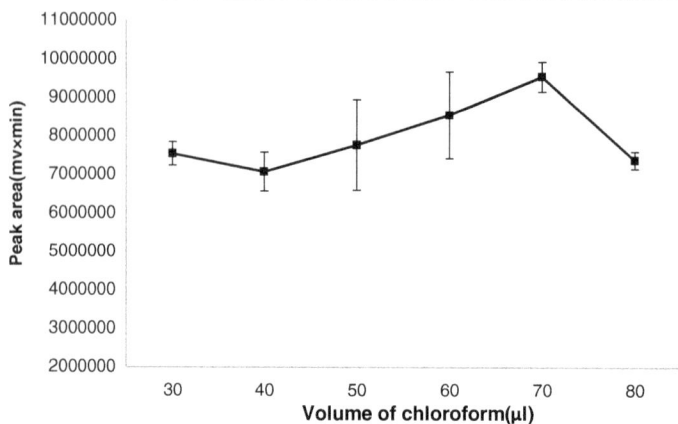

Figure 2 Effect of volume of chloroform on the extraction efficiency. Extraction condition: tramadol concentration, 100 μg/L; disperser solvent and its volume, 0.6 mL acetonitrile; extraction solvent, chloroform; no salt addition.

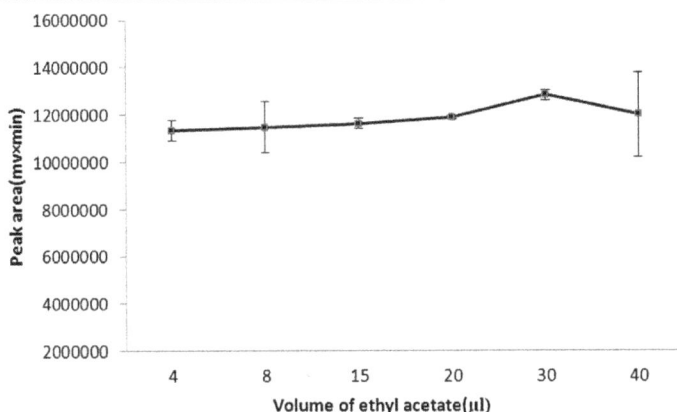

Figure 3 Effect of ethyl acetate volume on the extraction efficiency. Extraction condition: tramadol concentration, 100 µg/ L; extraction solvent and its volume, 70 µL chloroform; disperser solvent and its volume, 0.6 mL acetonitrile; no salt addition.

According to these results, 70 µL of chloroform with remarkable effect (single factor analysis of variance, $p < 0.05$) was selected as the optimal extraction solvent volume in the BS-DLLME procedure.

Effect of ethyl acetate and its volume

The effect of ethyl acetate ($C_4H_8O_2$, density 0.897 g /ml) as lighter extraction solvent in BS-DLLME of tramadol in urine samples was studied. For considering the influence of ethyl acetate volume on extraction efficiency, different volumes of ethyl acetate (0 – 40 µL), fixed volumes of chloroform (70 µL) and acetonitrile (600 µL) were used for BS-DLLME procedure. As can be seen in Figure 3, initially the extraction efficiency increased and then decreased by increasing the volume of ethyl acetate. Thus 30 µL of ethyl acetate as lighter density extraction solvent with lower error bar and 70 µL of chloroform as higher

density extraction solvent (100 µL of binary extraction solvents) were selected in the subsequent experiments.

Selection of disperser solvent

The most important factor affecting the selection on disperser solvent is relative miscibility of the disperser solvent with the binary extraction solvents and aqueous phase. Methanol, ethanol, acetonitrile and acetone exhibit adequate properties and were studied as disperser solvents. Then, the effect of these solvents on performance of BS-DLLME was investigated. For these purpose, 600 µL of disperser solvent and 100 µL of binary extraction solvents were used. In ethanol and methanol, whitish sediment was formed, which cannot be separated from supernatant. Thus, the sediment is interfered for analysis and therefore methanol and ethanol were ignored as disperser solvents. According to Figure 4,

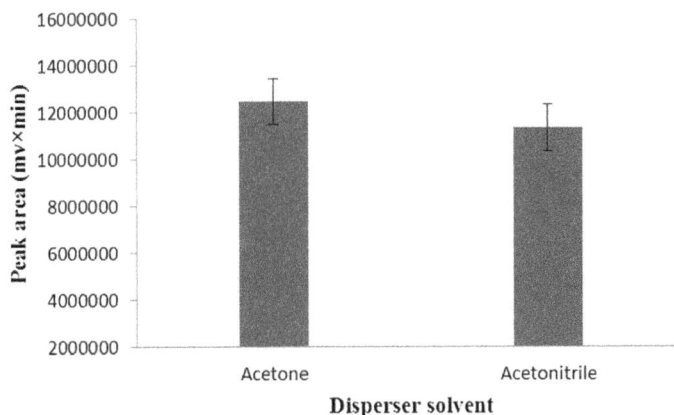

Figure 4 Effect of disperser solvent type on the extraction efficiency. Extraction condition: tramadol concentration, 100 µg/L; binary extraction solvents and their volume, 100 µL mixture of ethyl acetate and chloroform (3:7 v/v); disperser solvent volume, 0.6 mL; no salt addition.

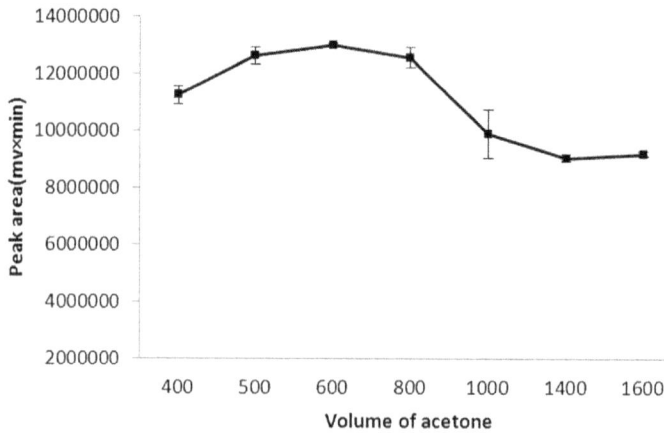

Figure 5 Effect of disperser solvent volume on the extraction efficiency. Extraction condition: tramadol concentration, 100 µg/ L; binary extraction solvents and their volume, 100 µL mixture of ethyl acetate and chloroform (3:7 v/v); disperser solvent, acetone; no salt addition.

acetone provided higher extraction efficiency with significant effect (one-tailed unpaired t-test, $p < 0.05$) and was chosen as disperser solvent in the following experiments.

Effect of disperser solvent volume

Effect of acetone (as disperser solvent) volume surveyed by using various volumes of acetone (400 – 1600 µL), while all experimental condition were kept constant (100 µL binary extraction solvents). As shown in Figure 5, the extraction efficiency increased by increasing the acetone volumes from 400 µL 600 µL. Above 600 µL of acetone the extraction efficiency decreased for tramadol, probably due to increase of tramadol solubility in the higher volume of acetone. Therefore 600 µL of acetone with significant effect (single factor analysis of

variance, $p < 0.05$) was selected as the optimal disperser solvent volume in BS-DLLME procedure.

Effect of salt addition

To evaluate the effect of salt addition on BS-DLLME performance, various experiments were performed by adding different amounts of NaCl (0 - 10%, w/v). Adding of salt may have different results in DLLME like increasing [19], reducing [20] and no impact on recovery [17]. In this study as indicated in Figure 6, by adding (0-10%, w/v) NaCl, initially, increasing the NaCl concentration to 7.5%, the extraction efficiency increased then decreased by increasing the NaCl concentration. Thus, 7.5% (w/v) NaCl with significant effect (single factor analysis of variance, $p < 0.05$) was selected for further experiments.

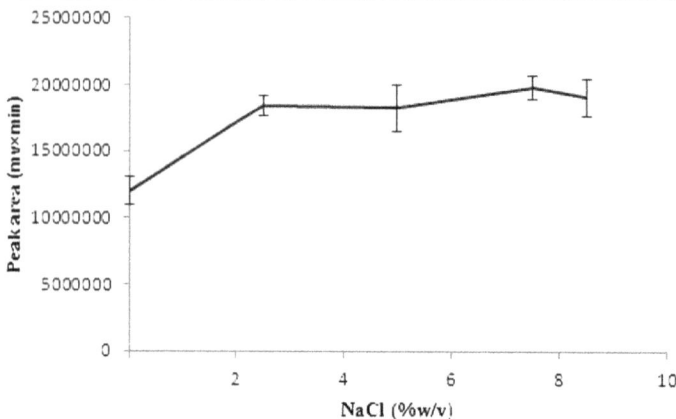

Figure 6 Effect of salt addition on the extraction efficiency. Extraction conditions: tramadol concentration, 100 µg/L; binary extraction solvents and their volume, 100 µL mixture of ethyl acetate and chloroform (3:7 v/v); disperser solvent and its volume, 0.6 mL acetone.

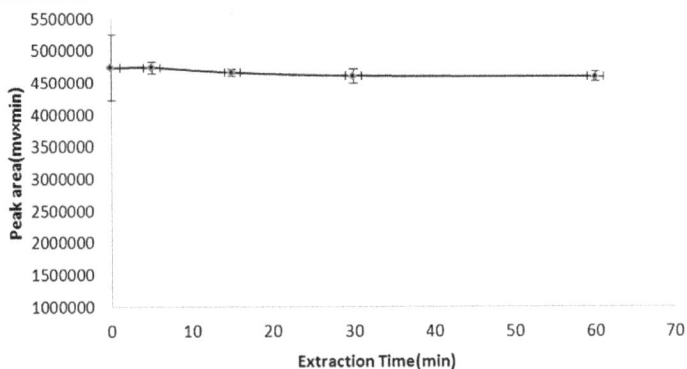

Figure 7 Effect of extraction time on the extraction efficiency. Extraction conditions: tramadol concentration, 100 µg/L; binary extraction solvents and their volume, 100 µL mixture of ethyl acetate and chloroform (3:7 v/v); disperser solvent and its volume, 0.6 mL acetone; 7.5% NaCl.

Effect of extraction time

In DLLME, extraction time is defined as the interval between injection of the mixture of organic solvents and centrifugation [21]. Generally extraction time has no impact on DLLME procedure [22]. As shown in Figure 7, the effect of extraction time on the extraction efficiency in the range of 0 – 60 min was investigated. The results showed that, the extraction time had no remarkable effect (single factor analysis of variance, $p > 0.05$) on BS-DLLME procedure.

Overall, according to optimum condition, the values of studied factors were as follows: 0.6 mL acetone as disperser solvent, 100 µL binary extraction solvents (70 µL of chloroform and 30 µL of ethyl acetate) and 7.5% (w/v) NaCl.

Analytical performance

Under optimization condition using blank urine samples spiked at various concentration of tramadol, the characteristic calibration data were obtained. As can be seen in Table 1, linearity was observed for tramadol in the range of 1–130 ng/ml with the determination coefficient (r^2) of 0.993. The enrichment factor for tramadol was obtained 71.42. The limit of quantification (LOQ, $S/N = 10$) and limit of detection (LOD, $S/N = 3$) were 0.9 and 0.2 ng/ml,

respectively. The relative standard deviation (RSD) determined by six replicate experiments was 4.1 at a concentration of 30 ng/ml.

Application in real sample

The applicability of proposed BS-DLLME method was evaluated for the analysis of different urine samples, which collected from the patient volunteers under treatment in Baharloo hospital (Tehran, Iran) without any dilution. The pH of urine samples was adjusted at 10 by dropwise addition of 5 M NaOH. The relative recoveries of tramadol from urine samples were determined at spiking level of 10, 30 and 60 ng/ml. As can be seen in Table 2, the results of six replicate experiments of each sample using the BS-DLLME method are in the range of 95.6 – 99.6%. Thus the proposed method can be applied for the determination of tramadol in urine samples.

Representative chromatograms with good resolution obtained for tramadol, from blank human urine sample (healthy volunteer) and urine sample (volunteer with abuse of tramadol) spiked with tramadol under the optimum BS-DLLME condition are shown in Figure 8.

Table 2 Relative recoveries of tramadol in urine samples

Sample	Initial concentration	Concentration added/µg/L	Concentration determined mean ± SD[b]/µg/ L	Relative recovery
Urine	nd[a]	10	9.96 ± 0.2	99.6
		30	28.67 ± 1.5	95.6
		60	59.03 ± 3.48	98.4

Extraction conditions: binary extraction solvents and their volume, 100 µL mixture of ethyl acetate and chloroform (3:7 v/v); disperser solvent and its volume, 0.6 mL acetone; 7.5% NaCl.
[a]Not detected.
[b]Standard deviation.

Table 1 Figures of merit in the BS-DLLME

Analyte	$r^{2,\,a}$	Regression equation	RSD, % (N = 6)	LOD[b]/ ng/ml	LOQ[c]/ ng/ml	LDR[d]/ ng/ml
Tramadol	0.993	Y = 78382x + 24663	4.1	0.2	0.9	1-130

[a]Determination coefficient.
[b]Limit of detection.
[c]Limit of quantification.
[d]Linear dynamic range.

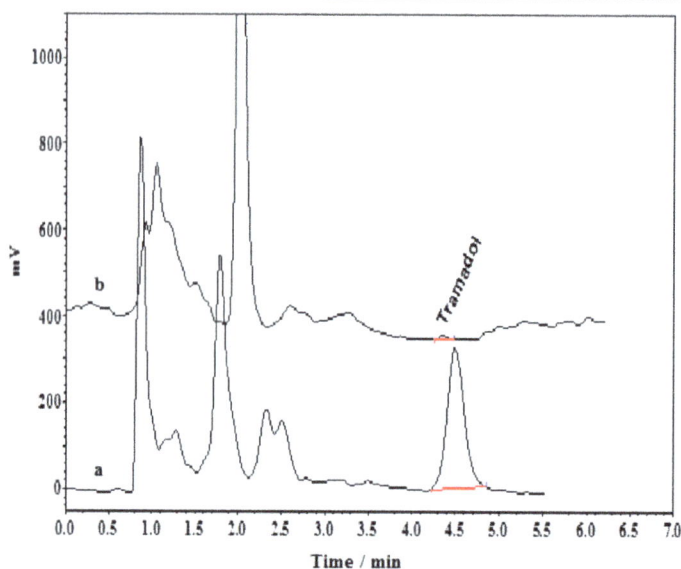

Figure 8 Chromatograms for the analysis of tramadol in urine samples. (a) HPLC chromatogram of the urine sample (volunteer with abuse of tramadol) spiked with tramadol at concentration level 60 μg/ Lafter employing BS-DLLME, **(b)** HPLC chromatogram of blank human urine sample (healthy volunteer) after performing BS-DLLME. Extraction conditions: tramadol concentration, 100 μg/L; binary extraction solvents and their volume, 100 μL mixture of ethyl acetate and chloroform (3:7 v/v); disperser solvent and its volume, 0.6 mL acetone; 7.5% NaCl.

Comparison of BS-DLLME with other methods

The figures of merit of BS-DLLME method for determination of tramadol in urine sample have been compared to earlier reported methods. As shown in Table 3, the proposed method has lower LOQ, good linear dynamic range (LDR) and higher relative recoveries in comparison to earlier methods. In addition, the extraction time in BS-DLLME is shorter and this method does not involve any labor-intensive and time consuming steps. Determination of tramadol at low levels in plasma is also important for the pharmacokinetic analysis [23] and therefore, DLLME procedure can be used as an alternative procedure for the previous analytical methods.

Conclusions

The present study has proposed a new method for determination of tramadol in urine samples using the BS-DLLME coupled with HPLC-fluorescence detection. BS-DLLME method provides good repeatability and higher recoveries within a short time. The comparison of this method with others demonstrated that BS-DLLME was very fast, simple and inexpensive with good figures of merit. In comparison to conventional DLLME, the selection of extraction solvents in BS-DLLME is not limited to high density solvents. In summary, the developed methodology shows good performance of analytical protocol, exhibits excellent recoveries for tramadol in urine samples.

Table 3 Comparison of the proposed method with other methods for the extraction of tramadol

Method	Sample matrix	RR[a], %	LDR/μg/ L	LOD/μg/ L	LOQ/μg/ L	r^2	Ref[e].
HPLC-FL[b], HPLC-MS/MS	Dog urine	82	1-1000	5	10	0.999	[24]
Liquid extraction HPLC	Human plasma	74.7-80.8	2.5-500	-	2.5	0.997	[25]
SPE[c]/GC-MS	Human oral fluid	87.7	10-100	-	10	0.999	[9]
MISPE[d]/HPLC-UV	Human plasma, urine	>91	2-300	1.2	3.5	-	[4]
LLE-ion pair formation	Urine	-	10000-50000	400	1200	0.997	[26]
BS-DLLME/HPLC-FL	Human urine	95.6-99.6	1-130	0.2	0.9	0.993	This work

[a]Relative recovery.
[b]High performance liquid chromatography with fluorescence Detection.
[c]Solid-phase extraction.
[d]Molecularly imprinted solid-phase extraction.
[e]Refferences.

Abbreviations

BS-DLLME: Binary solvents dispersive liquid liquid microextraction; SPE: Solid phase extraction; SPME: Solid phase microextraction; MISPE: Molecular imprinting solid phase extraction; FL: Fluorescence detection.

Competing interests

The authors declare that have no competing interests.

Authors' contributions

VK supervised the project and prepared the manuscript, MRR gave consultation on pharmaceutical analysis and final manuscript preparation and made substantial contribution for performing the project, RM carried out the data analysis and helped to draft the manuscript, HL gave consultation on HPLC assay and MGH performed the data analysis. All authors read and approved the final manuscript.

Author details

[1]Department of Chemistry, North Tehran Branch, Islamic Azad University, P.O. Box 1913674711, Tehran, Iran. [2]Biopharmaceutics and Pharmacokinetics Division, Department of Pharmaceutics, Faculty of Pharmacy, Tehran University of Medical Sciences, Tehran, Iran. [3]Department of Applied Chemistry, Faculty of Science, Semnan University, Semnan, Iran.

References

1. Küçük A, Kadıoğlu Y, Çelebi F: Investigation of the pharmacokinetics and determination of tramadol in rabbit plasma by a high-performance liquid chromatography–diode array detector method using liquid–liquid extraction. J Chromatogr B 2005, 816:203–208.
2. Rouini M, Ghazi-Khansari M, Ardakani Y, Dasian Z, Lavasani H: A Disposition Kinetic Study in Rat perfused Liver. Biopharm Drug Dispos 2008, 29:231–235.
3. Malana M, Zohra R: The release behavior and kinetic evaluation of tramadol HCl from chemically cross linked Ter polymeric hydrogels. DARU J Pharm Sci 2013, 21:10.
4. Javanbakht M, Attaran AM, Namjumanesh MH, Esfandyari-Manesh M, Akbari-adergani B: Solid-phase extraction of tramadol from plasma and urine samples using a novel water-compatible molecularly imprinted polymer. J Chromatogr B 2010, 878:1700–1706.
5. Report of tramadol consumption by officials [Persian Language]. [http://www.magiran.com/npview.asp?ID=1450199]
6. Hassanian-Moghaddam H, Kolahi A: Tramadol intoxication/abuse: a new issue on high-access population. In Sixth Annual Congress of Asia Pacific Association of Medical Toxicology. December, 12–14, 2007, Bangkok-Thailand, OP 56, http://www.asiatox.org/6thCongress2.html.
7. Gambaro V, Benvenuti C, Ferrari LD, Dell'Acqua L, Farè F: Validation of a GC/MS method for the determination of tramadol in human plasma after intravenous bolus. Il Farmaco 2003, 58:947–950.
8. Gan SH, Ismail R, Wan Adnan WA, Wan Z: Correlation of tramadol pharmacokinetics and CYP2D6*10 genotype in Malaysian subjects. J Pharm Biomed Anal 2002, 30:189–195.
9. Moore C, Rana S, Coulter C: Determination of meperidine, tramadol and oxycodone in human oral fluid using solid phase extraction and gas chromatography–mass spectrometry. J Chromatogr B 2007, 850:370–375.
10. Jeannot MA, Cantwell FF: Solvent Microextraction into a Single Drop. Anal Chem 1996, 68:2236–2240.
11. Jeannot MA, Cantwell FF: Mass Transfer Characteristics of Solvent Extraction into a Single Drop at the Tip of a Syringe Needle. Anal Chem 1997, 69:235–239.
12. Sha YF, Shen S, Duan GL: Rapid determination of tramadol in human plasma by headspace solid-phase microextraction and capillary gas chromatography–mass spectrometry. J Pharm Biomed Anal 2005, 37:143–147.
13. Ghasemi E: Optimization of solvent bar microextraction combined with gas chromatography mass spectrometry for preconcentration and determination of tramadol in biological samples. J Chromatogr A 2012, 1251:48–53.
14. Ebrahimzadeh H, Yamini Y, Sedighi A, Rouini MR: Determination of tramadol in human plasma and urine samples using liquid phase microextraction with back extraction combined with high performance liquid chromatography. J Chromatogr B 2008, 863:229–234.
15. Ghambarian M, Yamini Y, Esrafili A: Three-phase hollow fiber liquid-phase microextraction based on two immiscible organic solvents for determination of tramadol in urine and plasma samples. J Pharm Biomed Anal 2011, 56:1041–1045.
16. Rezaee M, Assadi Y, Milani Hosseini M-R, Aghaee E, Ahmadi F, Berijani S: Determination of organic compounds in water using dispersive liquid–liquid microextraction. J Chromatogr A 2006, 1116:1–9.
17. Maham M, Karami-Osboo R, Kiarostami V, Waqif-Husain S: Novel Binary Solvents-Dispersive Liquid—Liquid Microextraction (BS-DLLME) Method for Determination of Patulin in Apple Juice Using High-Performance Liquid Chromatography. Food Anal Methods 2013, 6:761–766.
18. Xiong C, Ruan J, Cai Y, Tang Y: Extraction and determination of some psychotropic drugs in urine samples using dispersive liquid–liquid microextraction followed by high-performance liquid chromatography. J Pharm Biomed Anal 2009, 49:572–578.
19. Melwanki MB, Chen W-S, Bai H-Y, Lin T-Y, Fuh M-R: Determination of 7-aminoflunitrazepam in urine by dispersive liquid–liquid microextraction with liquid chromatography–electrospray-tandem mass spectrometry. Talanta 2009, 78:618–622.
20. Saraji M, Bidgoli AAH: Dispersive liquid–liquid microextraction using a surfactant as disperser agent. Anal Bioanal Chem 2010, 397:3107–3115.
21. Li Y, Hu J, Liu X, Fu L, Zhang X, Wang X: Dispersive liquid–liquid microextraction followed by reversed phase HPLC for the determination of decabrominated diphenyl ether in natural water. J Sep Sci 2008, 31:2371–2376.
22. Daneshfar A, Khezeli T, Lotfi HJ: Determination of cholesterol in food samples using dispersive liquid–liquid microextraction followed by HPLC–UV. J Chromatogr B 2009, 877:456–460.
23. Lavasani H, Sheikholeslami B, Ardakani YH, Abdollahi M, Hakemi L, Rouini MR: Study of the pharmacokinetic changes of Tramadol in diabetic rats. Daru 2013, 21:17.
24. Saccomanni G, Del Carlo S, Giorgi M, Manera C, Saba A, Macchia M: Determination of tramadol and metabolites by HPLC-FL and HPLC–MS/MS in urine of dogs. J Pharm Biomed Anal 2010, 53:194–199.
25. Rouini M-R, Ardakani YH, Soltani F, Aboul-Enein HY, Foroumadi A: Development and validation of a rapid HPLC method for simultaneous determination of tramadol, and its two main metabolites in human plasma. J Chromatogr B 2006, 830:207–211.
26. Ismaiel OA, Hosny MM: Development and Validation of a Spectrophotometric Method for the Determination of Tramadol in Human Urine Using Liquid-Liquid Extraction and Ion Pair Formation. Int J Instrum Sci 2012, 1:34–40.

Novel 9-(alkylthio)-Acenaphtho[1,2-e]-1,2,4-triazine derivatives: synthesis, cytotoxic activity and molecular docking studies on B-cell lymphoma 2 (Bcl-2)

Mohammad K Mohammadi[1], Omidreza Firuzi[2], Mehdi Khoshneviszadeh[2], Nima Razzaghi-Asl[3], Saghi Sepehri[4] and Ramin Miri[2,3*]

Abstract

Background and purpose of the study: Acenaphtho derivatives have been reported as antitumor agents. Due to this fact and also with the aim of developing the chemistry of potentially bioactive heterocyclic compounds via efficient reactions, a facile procedure for the synthesis of 9-(alkylthio)-acenaphtho[1,2-e]-1,2,4-triazines via two step condensation of thiosemicarbazide and acenaphtylene-9,10-quinone to form acenaphtho[1,2-e]-1,2,4-triazine-9(8H)-thiones and subsequent reaction with benzyl chloride derivatives is reported.

Methods: 9-(alkylthio) acenaphtho[1,2-e]-1,2,4-triazines were synthesized via the reaction of acenaphtho-9,10-quinone with thiosemicarbazide, and then with the benzyl chloride derivatives. Cytotoxicity of some prepared compounds was assessed through MTT assay on three different human cancerous cell lines (HL-60, MCF7, and MOLT-4 cells). Molecular docking studies were performed via AutoDock4.2 software in order to confirm an apoptosis-inducing activity of acenaphtho scaffolds via the Bcl-2 protein.

Results: Excellent yields of the products, short reaction times and simple work-up are attractive features of this synthetic protocol. The evaluated compounds exhibited moderate to good cytotoxic activities. Docking results on the active site of B-cell lymphoma 2 (Bcl-2) supported the experimental biological data and agreed well with previous *in silico* data for commonly used anti-cancer drugs. Moreover; results were analyzed considering binding efficiency indices.

Conclusions: The outcomes of the present study may be helpful in future targeting of Bcl-2 with the aim of developing apoptosis-inducing agents.

Keywords: Synthesis, Acenaphtho-9,10-quinone, Cytotoxic activity, Docking

Introduction

Economic generation of bioactive compounds has been a major concern in modern organic chemistry [1]. In this regard, development of novel compounds and especially diverse small molecule scaffolds caused higher attention of medicinal and biological chemists [2-4]. This can be attributed to the growing requirement in assembling libraries of structurally complex substances to be evaluated as hit/lead compounds in drug discovery projects.

Polycyclic aromatic hydrocarbon (PAH) heterocycles are highly important structural units in a variety of pharmacologically active substances [5-9]. At first glance, rigid polycyclic structures seem to have role in the development of antitumor agents owing to their ability in insertion between stacked base pairs of oligonucleotides and action as intercalator [10-12]. Particularly important is that when these planar polycyclic heterocycles bear appropriate side chains, further interactions with other important macromolecules might be envisaged [11,13].

* Correspondence: mirir@sums.ac.ir
[2]Medicinal and Natural Products Chemistry Research Center, Shiraz, University of Medical Sciences, PO Box 3288–71345, Shiraz, Iran
[3]Departments of Medicinal Chemistry, School of Pharmacy, Shiraz University of Medical Sciences, Shiraz, Iran
Full list of author information is available at the end of the article

In this view, privileged heterocyclic structures have been constructed around the acenaphtho core [14,15]. Some of the acenaphtho derivatives containing thiazole backbone have been reported as antitumor agents [16]. Recently in an attempt to develop protein-targeted instead of DNA-targeted antitumor agents, some derivatives of 8H-acenaphtho[1,2-b]pyrrole have been constructed [17].

The authors demonstrated that 8-oxo-3-thiomorpholin-4-yl-8H-acenaphtho[1,2-b]pyrrole-9-carbonitrile could serve as an apoptosis-inducing agent via interacting Bcl-2 protein [17]. It is well known that the Bcl-2 family of proteins is comprised of pro-apoptotic and anti-apoptotic proteins and all members of this family are not anti-apoptotic. Anti-apoptotic Bcl-2 family proteins, including Bcl-2, Bcl-XL, Bcl-w, Mcl-1 and A1, prevent cell death by binding and sequestering pro-apoptotic proteins so, inhibition of these anti-apoptotic proteins might be lethal to cancer cells.

Indeed, Bcl-2 proteins have been regarded as important targets for anti-neoplastic drug development and Bcl-2 gen has been identified as over expressed in various cancers. Bcl-2 is an anti-apoptotic protein possessing an important role in various types of cancers. Bcl-2 is the member of the Bcl-2 family of apoptosis regulator proteins which is encoded by the BCL2 gene [18,19].

Various reactions of acenaphthaquinone with nucleophiles, organic and inorganic reagents have been reviewed elsewhere [20,21]. In the framework of our program to develop the chemistry of potentially bioactive heterocyclic compounds [22] and in connection with our ongoing interests in this field [23-25], we represent here a facile procedure for the synthesis of 9-(alkylthio)-acenaphtho [1,2-e]-1,2,4-triazines via two step condensation of thiosemicarbazide and acenaphtylene-9,10-quinone to form acenaphtho[1,2-e]-1,2,4-triazine-9(8H)-thiones and subsequent reaction with benzyl chloride derivatives. Prepared compounds were subjected to cytotoxic assay in three different cancerous cell lines. Moreover; molecular docking was used to gain further insight into the binding mode and binding affinity of acenaphtho derivatives in the active site of Bcl-2.

Material and methods

All of the reagents were purchased from commercial sources and were freshly used after being purified by standard procedures. Melting points were determined on the Electro-thermal Melting Point apparatus and were uncorrected. Infrared spectra were recorded on the Shimadzu-420 infrared spectrophotometer. ^{1}H-NMR and ^{13}C-NMR spectra were recorded in DMSO-d$_6$ or CDCl$_3$ on Brucker 300 MHz spectrometer (Chemical shifts are given in parts per million or ppm). Mass spectra were recorded on a MS model 5973 Network apparatus at

ionization potential of 70 eV. Elemental analyses (C, H, N) were performed by the Microanalytical Unit.

General procedure for preparation of acenaphtho [1,2-e]-1,2,4-triazine-9(8H)-thione (3)

To the acenaphtylene-9,10-quinone (5 mmol) and thiosemicarbazide (5 mmol) in chloroform (30 mL), small amount of acetic acid was added as an catalyst. The reaction mixture was stirred under reflux condition. The progress of the reaction was monitored with TLC and at the completion of the reaction, The precipitated product was filtered off, washed with mixture of H$_2$O/EtOH, dried and recrystallized from ethanol to give yellow crystalline acenaphtho[1,2-e]-1,2,4-triazine-9(8H)-thione (Scheme 1).

General procedure for preparation of 9-(alkylthio)-acenaphtho [1,2-e]-1,2,4-triazines (5a-g)

To a well-stirred solution of acenaphtho[1,2-e]-1,2,4-triazine-9(8H)-thione (3) in 10 ml Chloroform was added triethylamine (3 mmol).

The solution was stirred and then the benzyl chloride derivatives, methyl iodide or ethyl iodide were added and the mixture was heated and stirred under reflux condition. After completion of the reactions, the precipitated residue was filtered, recrystallized in ethanol, filtered, washed with water (2 × 5 mL) and then completely dried in electrical oven (Scheme 1). All prepared compounds were characterized using FT-IR, ^{1}H NMR, ^{13}C NMR and mass spectroscopy (Additional file 1: Table S1).

Acenaphtho[1,2-e]-1,2,4-triazine-9(8H)-thione (3)

Yield 88%, m.p. 148-150°C. ^{1}HNMR (300 MHz, DMSO-d$_6$) δ: 7.81 (d, 2H, J = 7.5Hz, CH-aromatic), 7.65 (dd, 2H, J = 7.6, 5.9 Hz, CH-aromatic), 7.46 (d, 2H, J = 8Hz CH-aromatic), 3.21 (s, 1H, SH); IR (KBr, cm^{-1}): 3245, 3151, 2922, 1689, 1607, 777; ^{13}C-NMR (75 MHz, DMSO-d$_6$) δ: 163, 150, 131, 128, 126, 124, 123; MS: m/z (%) 255 (M$^+$, 51), 213 (100), 180 (75), 152 (49), 139 (44); Anal. Calcd for C$_{13}$H$_7$N$_3$S: C, 65.80; H, 2.97; N, 17.71. Found: C, 65.62; H, 2.98; N, 17.58.

9-(benzylthio)-acenaphtho[1,2-e]-1,2,4-triazine (5a)

Yield 94%, m.p. 151-153°C. ^{1}HNMR (300 MHz, DMSO-d$_6$) δ: 7.78 (d, 2H, J = 7.6Hz, CH-aromatic), 7.61 (dd, 2H, J = 7.6, 6.6 Hz, CH-aromatic), 7.46 (d, 2H, J = 8.5Hz, CH-aromatic), 7.05-7.19 (m, 5H, CH-phenyl), 3.26 (s, 2H, CH$_2$-benzylic); IR (KBr, cm^{-1}): 3153, 3050, 1694, 1606; ^{13}C-NMR (75 MHz, DMSO-d6) δ: 170.9, 139.7, 142.4, 138.9, 133.5, 128.5, 128.3, 128, 127.8, 127.7, 127.3, 127.2, 126.6, 124.5, 42.2; MS: m/z (%) 327 (M$^+$, 100), 294 (63), 208 (71), 164 (52), 91 (75); Anal. Calcd for C$_{20}$H$_{13}$N$_3$S: C, 73.37; H, 4.00; N, 12.83. Found: C, 73.62; H, 3.88; N, 12.58.

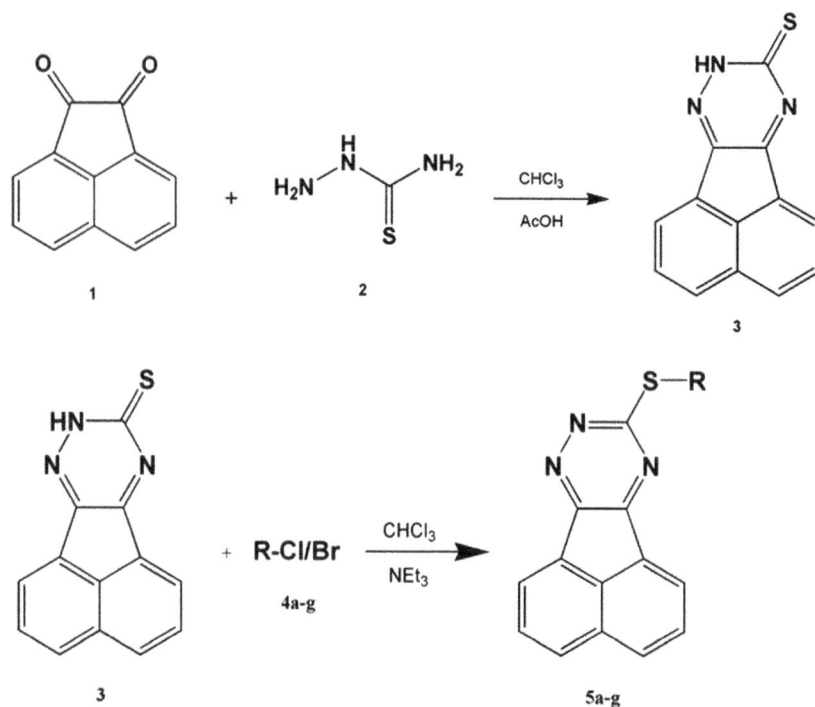

Scheme 1 Synthetic rout to acenaphtho[1,2-e]-1,2,4-triazine-9(8H)-thione and 9-(alkylthio)-acenaphtho[1,2-e]-1,2,4-triazines.

9-(4-nitro-benzylthio)-acenaphtho[1,2-e]-1,2,4-triazine (5b)
Yield 79%, m.p. 156-158°C. ^{1}HNMR (300 MHz, DMSO-d$_6$) δ: 8.08 (d, 2H, J = 7.5Hz, CH-phenyl), 7.83 (d, 2H, J = 7.6Hz, CH-aromatic), 7.75 (dd, 2H, J = 7.3, 6.6 Hz, CH-aromatic), 7.46 (d, 2H, J = 7.6Hz, CH-phenyl), 7.48 (d, 2H, CH-phenyl), 3.32 (s, 2H, CH$_2$-benzylic); IR (KBr, cm^{-1}): 3121, 3035, 1670, 1585, 1532, 1486, 937; ^{13}C-NMR (75 MHz, DMSO-d6) δ: 172.4, 149.8, 145.8, 142.4, 133.5, 131.7, 130.3, 127.6, 127.8, 127.3, 128.9, 128.5, 127.5, 124.1, 44.5; MS: m/z (%) 372 (M$^+$, 12), 255 (48), 213 (100), 180 (87), 152 (62); Anal. Calcd for C$_{20}$H$_{12}$N$_4$O$_2$S: C, 64.50; H, 3.25; N, 15.04. Found: C, 64.62; H, 3.18; N, 15.28.

9-(2,4-dichloro-benzylthio)-acenaphtho[1,2-e]-1,2,4-triazine (5c)
Yield 83%, m.p. 187-188°C. ^{1}HNMR (300 MHz, DMSO-d$_6$) δ: 7.79 (d, 2H, J = 7.5Hz, CH-aromatic), 7.60 (dd, 2H, J = 7.5, 6.1 Hz, CH-aromatic), 7.46 (d, 2H, J = 8.3Hz CH-aromatic), 7.19 (s, 1H, CH-phenyl), 7.09 (d, 1H, J = 7.3Hz, CH-phenyl), 6.98 (d, 1H, J = 7.3Hz, CH-phenyl), 3.33 (s, 2H, CH$_2$-benzylic); IR (KBr, cm^{-1}): 3175, 3095, 1656, 1578, 951, 875, 839; ^{13}C-NMR (75 MHz, DMSO-d6) δ: 171.8, 145.4, 134.5, 134.1, 133.5, 131.4, 130.8, 130.4, 129.2, 128.6, 128.1, 127.9, 127.6, 127.3, 127.1, 125.6, 40.4; MS: m/z (%) 395 (M$^+$, 29), 360 (100), 208 (94), 164 (58); Anal. Calcd for C$_{20}$H$_{11}$Cl$_2$N$_3$S: C, 60.62; H, 2.80; N, 10.60. Found: C, 60.42; H, 2.91; N, 10.73.

9-(3,4-dichloro -benzylthio)-acenaphtho[1,2-e]-1,2,4-triazine (5d)
Yield 60%, m.p. 156-159°C. ^{1}HNMR (300 MHz, DMSO-d$_6$) δ: 7.80 (d, 2H, J = 7.5Hz, CH-aromatic), 7.52 (dd, 2H, J = 7.4, 6.2 Hz, CH-aromatic), 7.41 (d, 2H, J = 8.3Hz CH-aromatic), 7.18 (d, 1H, J = 7.3Hz, CH-phenyl), 7.08 (s, 1H, CH-phenyl), 6.93 (d, 1H, J = 7.4Hz, CH-phenyl), 3.29 (s, 2H, CH$_2$-benzylic); IR (KBr, cm^{-1}): 3106, 3019, 1686, 1557, 984, 854; ^{13}C-NMR (75 MHz, DMSO-d6) δ: 170.5, 143.4, 139.2, 133.8, 133.4, 131.8, 130.9, 129.5, 129, 128.6, 128.3, 128.1, 127.6, 127.1, 126.9, 126.5, 38.9; MS: m/z (%) 395 (M$^+$, 46), 362 (13), 255 (53), 213 (100), 180 (85), 152 (54), 86 (83); Anal. Calcd for C$_{20}$H$_{11}$Cl$_2$N$_3$S: C, 60.62; H, 2.80; N, 10.60. Found: C, 60.53; H, 2.99; N, 10.44.

9-(4-chloro-benzylthio)-acenaphtho[1,2-e]-1,2,4-triazine (5e)
Yield 84%, m.p. 153-156°C. ^{1}HNMR (300 MHz, DMSO-d$_6$) δ: 7.89 (d, 2H, J = 7.7Hz, CH-aromatic), 7.58 (dd, 2H, J = 7.5, 6.5 Hz, CH-aromatic), 7.42 (d, 2H, J = 8.6Hz CH-aromatic), 7.13 (d, 2H, J = 7.5Hz, CH-phenyl); 6.99 (d, 2H, J = 7.4Hz, CH-phenyl), 3.36 (s, 2H, CH$_2$-benzylic); IR (KBr, cm^{-1}): 3126, 3058, 1629, 1612, 1597, 1005, 917; ^{13}C-NMR (75 MHz, DMSO-d6) δ: 169.9, 142.4, 138.7, 137.8, 132.7, 133.5, 129.2, 128.9, 128.3, 128, 127.7, 127.3, 126.1, 125.5, 38.5; MS: m/z (%) 361 (M$^+$, 100), 328 (42), 208 (83), 180 (38), 164 (58), 125 (61); Anal. Calcd for C$_{20}$H$_{12}$ClN$_3$S: C, 66.39; H, 3.34; N, 11.61. Found: C, 66.62; H, 3.38; N, 11.40.

9-(methylthio)-acenaphtho[1,2-e]-1,2,4-triazine (5f)

Yield 31%, ^{1}HNMR (500 MHz, CDCl$_3$): 8.44-8.46 (m, 2H, CH-aromatic), 8.24 (m, 1H, CH-aromatic), 8.14 (d, 1H, J = 8.25 Hz, CH-aromatic), 7.86-7.90 (m, 2H, CH-aromatic), 2.84 (s, 3H, -CH$_3$); IR (KBr, cm $^{-1}$): 3150, 2923, 1615, 1416 and 1382; Anal. Calcd for C$_{14}$H$_9$N$_3$S: C, 66.91; H, 3.61; N, 16.72. Found: C, 66.82; H, 3.68; N, 16.59.

9-(ethylthio)-acenaphtho[1,2-e]-1,2,4-triazine (5g)

Yield 30%, ^{1}HNMR (500 MHz, DMSO-d$_6$): 8.38-8.44 (m, 3H, CH-aromatic), 8.29 (d, 1H, J = 8.1 Hz, CH-aromatic), 7.91-7.96 (m, 2H, CH-aromatic), 3.33 (q, 2H, CH$_2$-CH$_3$), 1.44-1.47 (t, 3H, J = 7.2 Hz, CH$_2$-CH$_3$); IR (KBr, cm $^{-1}$): 3148, 2944, 1617, 1420 and 1381; Anal. Calcd for C$_{15}$H$_{11}$N$_3$S: C, 67.90; H, 4.18; N, 15.84. Found: C, 68.06; H, 4.28; N, 15.73.

Cytotoxicity assay

RPMI 1640, fetal bovine serum (FBS), trypsin and phosphate buffered saline (PBS) were purchased from Biosera (Ringmer, UK). 3-(4,5-dimethylthiazol-2-yl)-2,5-diphenyl-tetrazolium bromide (MTT) was obtained from Sigma (Saint Louis, MO, USA) and penicillin/streptomycin was purchased from Invitrogen (San Diego, CA, USA). Doxorubicin and dimethyl sulphoxide were obtained from EBEWE Pharma (Unterach, Austria) and Merck (Darmstadt, Germany), respectively.

HL-60 (human promyelocytic leukemia), MCF-7 (human breast adenocarcinoma) and MOLT-4 (human acute lymphoblastic leukemia) cells were obtained from the National Cell Bank of Iran, Pasteur Institute, Tehran, Iran. All cell lines were maintained in RPMI 1640 supplemented with 10% FBS, and 100 units/mL penicillin-G and 100 µg/mL streptomycin. Cells were grown in monolayer cultures.

Cell viability following exposure to synthetic compounds was evaluated by using the MTT reduction assay. HL-60, MCF7, and MOLT-4 cells were plated in 96-well microplates at a density of 5×10^4 cells/ mL (100 µl per well). Positive control wells contained cisplatin and doxorubicin and blank wells contained only growth medium for background correction. After overnight incubation at 37°C, half of the growth medium was removed and 50 µL of medium supplemented with different concentrations of synthetic compounds dissolved in DMSO were added in quadruplicate. Maximum concentration of DMSO in the wells was 0.5% (The solution of 0.5% DMSO was also tested as a cytotoxicity control). Cells were further incubated for 72 h. At the end of the incubation time, the medium was removed and MTT was added to each well at a final concentration of 0.5 mg/mL and plates were incubated for another 4 h at 37°C. Then formazan crystals were solubilized in 200 µl DMSO. The optical density was measured at 570 nm with background correction at 655 nm using a Bio-Rad microplate reader (Model 680). The percentage of viability compared to control wells was calculated for each concentration of the compound and IC50 values were calculated with the software CurveExpert version 1.34 for Windows. Each experiment was repeated 3–4 times. Data are represented as mean ± S.E.M.

Molecular docking study

The ligand-flexible docking studies were performed using the widely distributed molecular docking software, AutoDock 4.2 [26]. Lamarckian Genetic Algorithm of the AutoDock 4.2 program was used to perform the flexible-ligand docking studies [27]. All the x-ray crystallographic *holo* structures of Bcl-2 were retrieved from the Brookhaven protein data bank (http://www.rcsb.org/). The protein structure was subjected to optimization step in order to minimize the crystallographic induced bond clashes using steepest descent method. All the preprocessing steps for receptor and ligand files were done by Auto-Dock Tools 1.5.4 (ADT) [28]. For the preparation of protein, Kollman united atom charges and polar hydrogen's were added to the receptor and crystallographic waters were removed. For docked ligands, Gasteiger charge was assigned, non-polar hydrogens were merged into the related carbon atoms of the receptor and torsions degrees of freedom were also allocated by ADT program.

Lamarckian genetic algorithm (LGA) was used to simulate the binding affinity and binding mode of acenaphtho derivatives in the active site of Bcl-2. 100 independent genetic algorithm (GA) runs were considered for each ligand under study. For Lamarckian GA; 27000 maximum generations; a gene mutation rate of 0.02; and

Table 1 Cell growth inhibitory activity of synthetic acenaphtho derivatives assessed by the MTT reduction assay

Comp. no.	IC$_{50}$^{a} (µM)		
	HL-60 cells	MCF-7 cells	MOLT-4 cells
5a	48.4 ± 8.7	NA^b	30.1 ± 5.6
5b	36.0 ± 5.4	NA	28.0 ± 4.6
5c	51.2 ± 7.6	NA	30.3 ± 8.2
5d	NA	NA	NA
5e	30.1 ± 3.6	NA	33.6 ± 2.9
5f	ND^c	61.9 ± 20.6	65.5 ± 20.4
5g	ND	NA	NA
Cisplatin	3.0 ± 0.1	23.7 ± 6.8	3.0 ± 0.2
Doxorubicin	0.014 ± 0.002	0.221 ± 0.095	0.017 ± 0.002

^{a}Values represent mean ± S.E.M..
^{b}NA: not active.
^{c}ND: not determined.

Table 2 Top ranked AutoDock scores based on the binding free energies (ΔG) of acenaphtho structures docked into the Bcl-2 active site (Isoform 1: 1G5M) along with interacted amino acids of Bcl-2

Comp. no.	ΔG_b (kcal/mol)	H-bonds		Amino acids in non-bonded contacts
		Amino acid	Distance (Å)	
5a	−7.03	Arg12	2.22	Glu13, Met16, Lys17, His20, Ala32, Asp35, Val36, Glu38, Asn39, Thr41
		Glu48	1.95	
5b	−9.29	Ser49	2.50	Asp10, Gly46, Glu50
		Lys17	1.73	
5c	−8.09	Arg12	1.96	Glu13, Met16, Ala32, Val36, Glu38, Asn39, Thr41
5d	−8.22	Arg12	2.20	Glu13, Met16, Ala32, Asp35, Val36, Glu38, Asn39, Thr41
5e	−7.73	Arg12	2.16	Glu13, Met16, Ala32, Asp35, Val36, Glu38, Asn39, Thr41

a crossover rate of 0.8 were applied. The grid maps of the protein were calculated using AutoGrid (part of the AutoDock package). The size of grid was set in a way to include not only the active site but also considerable portions of the surrounding surface. For this purpose, a grid of 60 × 60 × 60 points in x, y, and z directions was built centered on the center of mass of the catalytic site of Bcl-2 with a spacing of 0.375 Å. Cluster analysis was performed on the docked results using an Root mean square deviation (RMSD) tolerance of 2 Å.

Ligand-receptor interactions were all detected on the basis of docking results using LIGPLOT [29]. Molecular images were produced using VMD program [30].

Results and discussion
Chemistry
Some new acenaphtho derivatives were obtained by condensation of acenaphtylene-9,10-quinone and thiosemicarbazide followed by reaction with different benzyl chloride derivatives under mild conditions in chloroform solution (Scheme 1). The isolated compounds were then characterized by elemental analyses, FT-IR, MS and NMR spectroscopy. The applied synthetic method afforded all the 9-(alkylthio)-acenaphtho[1,2-e]-1,2,4-triazines in high yields and short reaction times except for 9-(methylthio) and 9-(ethylthio) derivatives that were produced in lower yields (Additional file 1: Table S1).

Cytotoxicity assay
The *in vitro* cytotoxic activities for prepared acenaphtho derivatives are shown in Table 1.

All the compounds under study exhibited medium cytotoxic activity on the evaluated cancerous cell lines except for 9-(methylthio) (5f) and 9-(ethylthio) (5 g) derivatives. Compound 5 g was inactive in MCF-7 and MOLT-4 cells. Compound 5b showed higher cytotoxicity in MOLT-4 cells. In HL-60 cells, compound 5e exhibited superior cytotoxic activity. The order of cytotoxic effects in HL-60 and MOLT-4 cell lines could be shown as 5e > 5b > 5a > 5c > 5d and 5b > 5a > 5c > 5e > 5f > 5d = 5 g. Variations of cytotoxic results were less pronounced for MOLT-4 cell lines. Moreover, all of the tested compounds were inactive on MCF-7 cells except for 5f which exhibited an IC$_{50}$ value of 61.9 μM.

With the exception of compound **5e**, a common trend, might be deduced that the presence of electron withdrawing/hydrogen acceptor nitro group on the phenyl ring of 9-(alkylthio)-acenaphtho[1,2-e]-1,2,4-triazines afforded higher cytotoxic effects while halogenated compounds showed lower *in vitro* potencies. It was also revealed that acenaphtho derivatives bearing aralkyl substituents on their sulfur atom (5a-e) might exhibit better cytotoxicity profiles than acenaphtho derivatives bearing alkyl substituents (5f and 5 g). Further structure activity relationship developments is under investigation via preparing more diverse sets of these derivatives.

Table 3 Top ranked AutoDock scores based on the binding free energies (ΔG) of acenaphtho structures docked into the Bcl-2 active site (Isoform 2: 1GJH) along with interacted amino acids of Bcl-2

Comp. no.	ΔG_b (kcal/mol)	H-bonds		Amino acids in non-bonded contacts
		Amino acid	Distance (Å)	
5a	−6.78	Ser49	2.18	Thr7, Pro44, Gly46, Glu48, Glu50
5b	−9.13	Asp10	1.87	Thr7, Gly8, Tyr9, Glu13, Thr41, Glu42, Ala43, Pro44, Gly46, Ser49
5c	−8.11	Ala32	2.36	Glu13, Met16, His20, Trp30, Asp31, Gly33, Val36
5d	−7.74	-		Glu13, Met16, His20, Glu29, Trp30, Ala32
5e	−7.84	-		Glu13, Met16, His20, Glu29, Trp30, Ala32

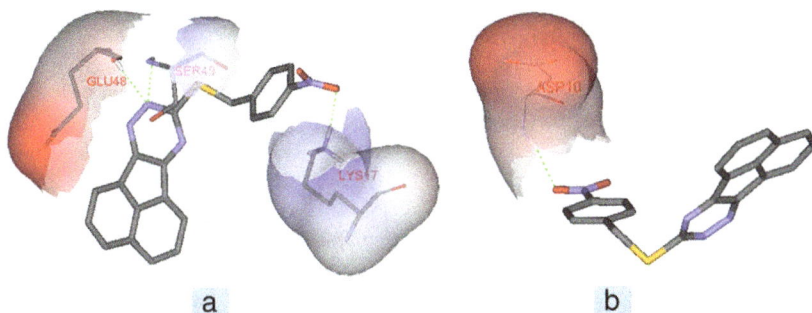

Figure 1 H-bond interactions of compound 5b in the active site of Bcl-2 isoforms a) PDB ID: 1G5M and b) PDB ID: 1GJH.

Molecular modeling studies

We decided to gain some information on binding modes of tested compounds on the Bcl-2 active site via molecular docking. Previous reports proposed that despite the similarity in the structures of two Bcl-2 isoforms, they behave differently in binding to the pro-apoptotic members of the Bcl-2 family [31]. For this purpose we decided to conduct our modeling studies on the structures of the two isoforms of Bcl-2 protein (isoforms 1: 1G5M and isoform 2: 1GJH).

Due to the lower cytotoxic activities of 9-(methylthio) and 9-(ethylthio) derivatives and also considering our main focus on 9-(Aralkylthio)-acenaphtho[1,2-e]-1,2,4-triazines rather than 9-(alkylthio)-acenaphtho[1,2-e]-1,2,4-triazines, all modeling studies were performed on 9-(benzylthio) derivatives.

Validation of molecular docking

A performance of a typical docking protocol can be checked via testing its ability in predicting predominant binding mode of a cognate (co-crystallographic) ligand. This procedure is performed via extracting the structure of a cognate ligand and re-docking it into its receptor (self-docking). RMSD of the Cartesian coordinates of the atoms of the ligand in the docked and crystallographic conformations will be the criterion of the docking validation (RMSD ≤ 2 Å).

Various PDB derived Bcl-2 structures were subjected to docking validation procedure. PDB structures were chosen on the basis of crystallographic resolutions. Regarding RMSD values and also conformation population in the top-ranked cluster of AutoDock output file, 1G5M and 1GJH were selected as the most appropriate crystallographic structure for further modeling studies.

Docking simulation of acenaphtho derivatives

Considering the well obtained *in vitro* results, it was thought worthy to perform molecular docking studies, hence considering both *in silico* and *in vitro* results.

Owing to the potential apoptosis-inducing activity of acenaphtho scaffolds via the Bcl-2 protein [17], we decided to model the binding interactions of assayed 9-(alkylthio)-acenaphtho[1,2-e]-1,2,4-triazines in the active site of Bcl-2 via docking simulation. For this purpose, 9-(alkylthio)-acenaphtho[1,2-e]-1,2,4-triazines were all docked into the active site of selected receptors *i.e.* various isoforms of Bcl-2 (1G5M and 1GJH) which differed in two amino acids [31].

Docking results with isoforms 1 (PDB code: 1G5M) and 2 (PDB code: 1GJH) are summarized in Tables 2 and 3, respectively. Top ranked binding energies (kcal/mol) in AutoDock dlg output files were considered as the best docking result in each case. It should be noted that all top ranked clusters were supported by high conformation populations. This observation could be expected since literature evidence implied that docking studies with compounds bearing less active torsions can significantly promote the docking success rates due to the limited conformational degrees of freedom [32].

In silico results revealed that synthesized molecules showed relatively good binding energies toward Bcl-2 active site ranging from –7.03 to –9.29 kcal/mol in isoform1 (1G5M) and –6.78 to –9.13 kcal/mol in isoform 2 (1GJH). Estimated binding energies were in the order of 5b > 5d > 5c > 5e > 5a in the active site of isoform 1 and 5b > 5c > 5d > 5e > 5a in the active site of isoform 2. The trends may also highlight slight conformational differences for two Bcl-2 isoforms [31].

Molecular docking study revealed that 9-(alkylthio)-acenaphtho[1,2-e]-1,2,4-triazine derivatives (5a-e) may inhibit Bcl-2 protein via H-bond and hydrophobic interactions (Tables 2 and 3). Compound 5b exhibited the best docking score (Tables 2 and 3) while being most potent in human MOLT-4 cells (Table 1). It seemed that the presence of *para*-nitro substituent on phenyl ring of 5b might be responsible for additional H-bonds with the active site of the receptor. This H-bond acceptor site would potentially support one key H-bond interactions with NH of Lys17 in isoform 1 and NH of Asp10 in isoform 2 through oxygen atom of a nitro substituent (Figure 1). The profile of interaction in 5b (Figure 1) further announced us that *para* nitro substituent in *9-(4-nitro-alkylthio)-acenaphtho[1,2-e]-1,2,4-triazine* (5b) might have some directional effect on the active site oriented conformation of the ligand. This rationale could be shown in Figure 2 in which different orientation of acenaphtho cycle in 5b compared to other compounds is obviously detectable. This new orientation would relocate a triazine ring in a position to make H-bond

interactions with Ser49 and Glu48 via polar hydrogen of N15 atom (Figures 1 and 3). From another aspect of view, docking simulation could be applied to find the binding mode and mechanism of less active derivatives.

To add more, it seemed that H-bond connections contributed more significantly in complex stabilization in the case of 5b and Bcl-2 isoform 1 (1G5M) rather than isoform 2 (1GJH). Compounds 5a, 5c, 5d and 5e all participated in key H-bonds with nitrogen atoms of a triazine ring (Figure 2). We found that Arg12 interacted via its guanine side chain (NH1; Figure 2) with nitrogen

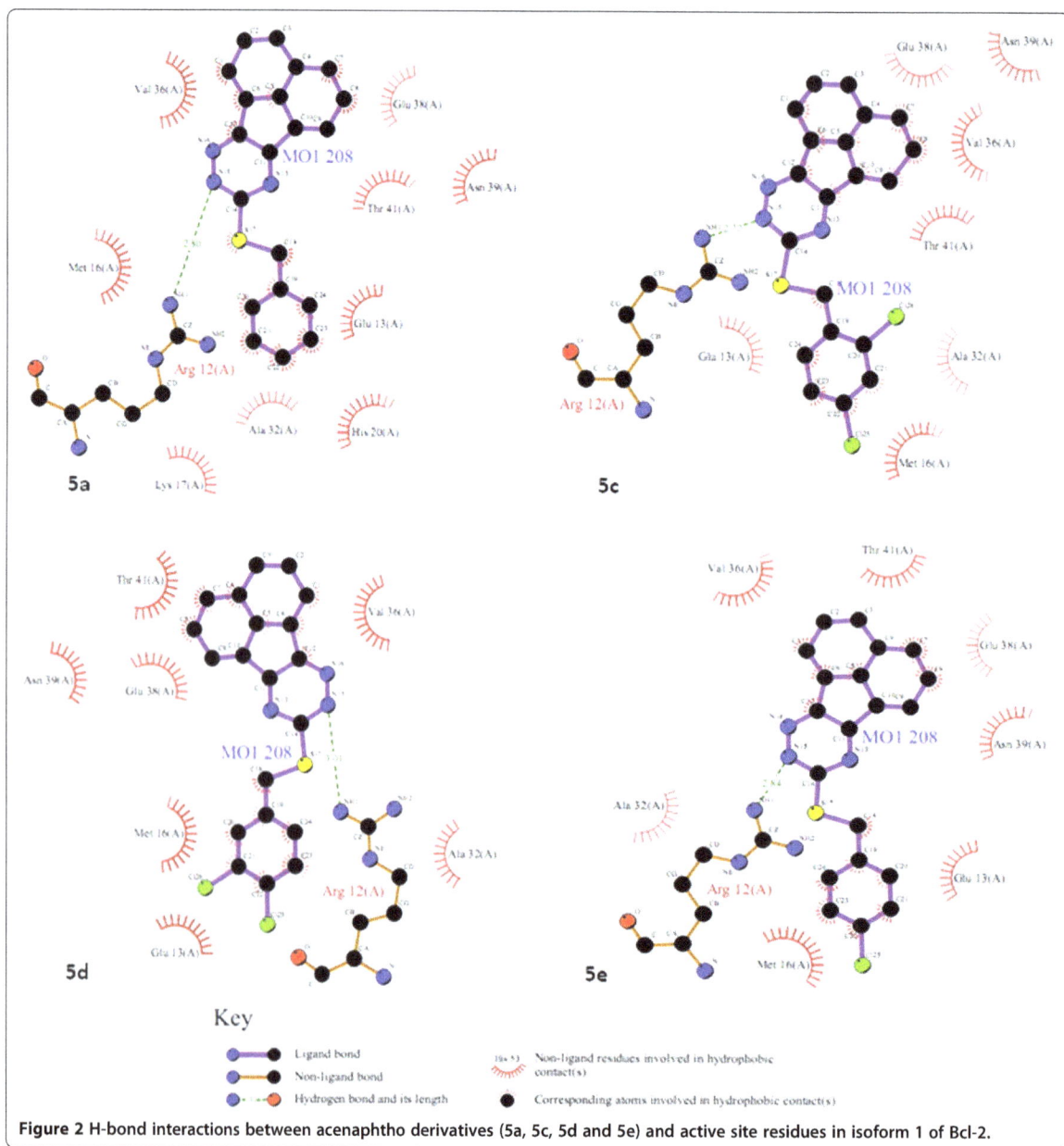

Figure 2 H-bond interactions between acenaphtho derivatives (5a, 5c, 5d and 5e) and active site residues in isoform 1 of Bcl-2.

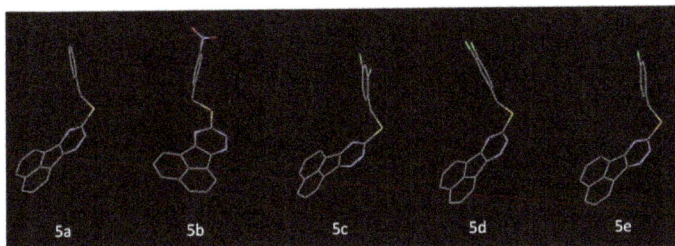

Figure 3 Different active site oriented conformations for docked acenaphtho derivatives (5a, 5b, 5c, 5d and 5e) in the active site of Bcl-2 isoform 1.

atom of a triazine ring in acenaphtho derivatives (N15; Figure 2).

Docking of commonly used neoplastic drugs *i.e.* Geftinib, Cisplatin, 5-FU, Gemcitabine and Vinorelbine into the active site of Bcl-2 (isoform 1; 15GM) has been reported elsewhere [6]. It was revealed that Asp10, Glu13, Lys17, Glu42 and Ser49 contributed to H-bond formation with the docked drugs [6]. Same residues were found to be key H-bond/non-bonded participants for inhibitor recognition in our study. Docking results showed that Glu13 contributed to non-bonded contacts with 5a, 5b, 5c and 5d (Table 1) while Asp10 participated in non-bonded contacts with 5b. Moreover; H-bond network in the case of Cisplatin (Asp10, Lys17 and Ser49) was very similar to that of 5b (Lys17, Glu48 and Ser49). The residue atoms involved in the binding pattern were the same for cisplatin and 5b in the case of Lys17 (quaternary NH of side chain; Figure 1) while for Ser49, cisplatin interacted with hydroxyl group of the Ser49 side chain but compound 5b made hydrogen bond via Ser49 backbone NH (Figure 1). Lys17 has also been reported to be involved in efficient H-bonds with Geftinib, Gemcitabine and Vinorelbine while stabilizing H-bonds were detected in the case of Glu13 for Gemcitabine and Vinorelbine [6].

Literature data revealed the effect of position of substituent(s) on phenyl moiety in comparison to our results [33]. It has been discussed that considering substituent

groups being attached to the *para* or *meta*-position, the hydrophobic pocket of Bcl-2 exhibited varied tolerability. This further identified the size of the hydrophobic pocket of Bcl-2 to be limited. *Meta* or *para*-halogen atoms on phenyl ring induce different conformations leading to decreased interactions with hydrophobic pocket of Bcl-2 (compounds 5d and 5f) (Figure 4).

Molecular docking on human anti-apoptotic Bcl-2 further supported the biological data. Regarding the obtained results, compound 5b could serve as an appropriate starting point for designing new chemical entities as potent Bcl-2 inhibitors.

Binding efficiency indices

Another criterion which has recently absorbed much attention in ligand-receptor interaction studies is the ligand efficiency (LE) parameter. Nowadays LE indices are regarded as undeniable tools in modern drug discovery projects [34]. The model of analyzing ligand binding in terms of the free energy per heavy atom (heavy atom count; HAC) was first introduced by Andrews [35]. Concept of the binding energy per atom or binding efficiency of a ligand could be a useful parameter in the selection of lead compounds, considering the real potency of a compound and hence might consider optimized fragments [36]. Generally speaking, molecules achieving a desirable potency with fewer HACs are by definition

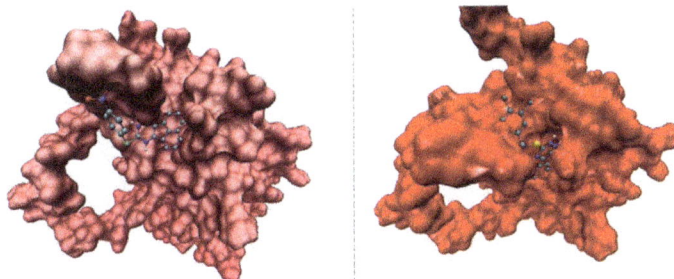

Figure 4 Compounds 5b (left) and 5d (right) in the active site of Bcl-2.

Table 4 Experimental/theoretical binding/ligand efficiency indices for 9-(benzylthio)-acenaphtho[1,2-e]-1,2,4-triazine derivatives (Bcl-2, isoforms 1 & 2, PDB IDs: 1G5M & 1GJH)

HL-60 cells

Molecule no.	Related PDB code	IC50 (µM)	pIC50	Experimental LE[a] (kcal.mol⁻¹.HAC⁻¹)	Estimated LE[b] (kcal.mol⁻¹.HAC⁻¹)	Experimental BEI[c]	Estimated BEI (kcal.mol⁻¹.kDa⁻¹)
5a	1G5M	48.4	4.32	0.179	0.208	13.20	15.77
5b	1G5M	36.0	4.44	0.114	0.134	11.95	14.36
5c	1G5M	51.2	4.29	0.165	0.228	10.86	15.01
5d	1G5M	-	-	-	0.218	-	15.26
5e	1G5M	30.1	4.52	0.170	0.219	12.52	15.69
5a	1GJH	48.4	4.31	0.179	0.214	13.20	15.24
5b	1GJH	36.0	4.44	0.114	0.137	11.95	14.05
5c	1GJH	51.2	4.29	0.165	0.228	10.86	15.04
5d	1GJH	-	-	-	0.232	-	14.36
5e	1GJH	30.1	4.52	0.170	0.237	12.52	15.18

MOLT-4 cells

Molecule no.	Related PDB code	IC50 (µM)	pIC50	Experimental LE	Estimated LE (kcal.mol⁻¹.HAC⁻¹)	Experimental BEI	Estimated BEI (kcal.mol⁻¹.kDa⁻¹)
5a	1G5M	30.1	4.52	0.188	0.208	13.83	15.77
5b	1G5M	28.0	4.55	0.190	0.134	12.24	14.36
5c	1G5M	30.3	4.52	0.188	0.228	11.44	15.01
5d	1G5M	-	-	-	0.218	-	15.26
5e	1G5M	33.6	4.47	0.186	0.219	12.39	15.69
5a	1GJH	30.1	4.52	0.188	0.214	13.83	15.24
5b	1GJH	28.0	4.55	0.190	0.137	12.24	14.05
5c	1GJH	30.3	4.52	0.188	0.228	11.44	15.04
5d	1GJH	-	-	-	0.232	-	14.36
5e	1GJH	33.6	4.47	0.186	0.237	12.39	15.18

[a] LE values are defined in the range of 0–1 [34].
[b] Estimated LEs were calculated according to equation (2).
[c] Reference value for BEI is 27 [35].

more efficient. LE index can be simply calculated using the equations (1) or (2):

$$LE = -\frac{\Delta G_b}{HAC} \tag{1}$$

$$LE = -\frac{pK_i; pK_d; or\ pIC50}{HAC} \tag{2}$$

Regarding the ligand efficiencies, it was postulated that molecular weights are prior to the HACs in considering the contribution of heteroatoms from different rows of the periodic table [37]. Thus a modified efficiency value was suggested as binding efficiency index (BEI). The importance of BEI can be emphasized regarding an increase in molecular weight at the clinical candidate step, which is regarded as an undeniable paradox with a common trend towards lower MWs and better pharmacokinetic profiles in marketable drugs [38]. BEI could be easily estimated from equation (3):

$$BEI = -\frac{pK_i; \ or\ pIC50}{MW\ (kDa)} \tag{3}$$

Accordingly, assayed acenaphtho derivatives were re-evaluated on the basis of their experimental and theoretical BEI/LE values (Table 4).

Regarding the summarized data in Table 4, following rationales might be pointed out:

- In our calculations, estimated LEs in terms of pKi values (equation 2) produced results more compatible to the experimental LEs (cellular assays) when compared to the LEs in terms of ΔG_b values (equation 1; the related data are not shown in the Table).
- Compound 5b is the top ranked bioactive molecule in docking results and also MOLT-4 based cellular assay. But this compound achieved relatively lower scores in terms of experimental/theoretical efficiency indices. The observed paradox demonstrated that larger bioactive compounds may require special attention in their design toward efficiency indices [25].
- Efficient bioactive molecules may be better categorized considering estimated BEIs rather than LEs. In some cases, especially for molecules bearing larger atoms, incorporating molecular weights rather than number of heavy atoms in the calculation of efficiency indices produced less biased results.
- The application of theoretical ligand/binding efficiency indices in the cell –based cytotoxicity protocols should be considered with care due to the multi-target nature of the cytotoxic agents. For example, compound 5d which is the structural isomer of compound 5c, was inactive in MTT assays.

Conclusion

Various studies have demonstrated that chemical structures bearing sulfur atom(s) may possibly induce apoptosis [39,40]. On the basis of results from this study, corresponding 9-(benzylthio) acenaphtho[1,2-e]-1,2,4-triazines might be regarded as valuable cytotoxic polycyclic heterocycles and potential candidates for additional molecular modifications with the aim of developing potent cytotoxic agents. Experimental and modeling studies confirmed the previous reports on acenaphtho derivatives and moreover; the docking results agreed well with the observed *in silico* data for commonly used anticancer drugs. Despite the closeness of docking scores, relatively different binding profiles for acenaphtho derivatives might confirm the previous results on conformational difference between two Bcl-2 isoforms. Concept of binding efficiency as a common and well–approached tool in modern drug discovery strategies was reviewed in our study. Confirming previous reports, it was demonstrated that bioactive molecular design on the basis of potency alone or binding efficiency values might be considered as different strategies leading to dissimilar results in lead/drug development campaigns. However several literature reports demonstrated that lead/drug discovery projects on the basis of binding efficiency indices would afford bioactive compounds with better pharmacokinetic outcomes. Extended cytotoxicity assays on diverse sets of acenaphtho-based scaffolds with the aim of establishing more rational structure activity relationships are under investigation.

Additional file

Additional file 1: Table S1. Physical and analytical data of 9-(alkylthio)-acenaphtho[1,2-e]-1,2,4-triazines 5a-h.

Competing interests
The authors declare that they have no competing interests.

Authors' contributions
MKM: Synthesis of some target compounds. OF: Supervision of biological tests. MKH: Design of target compounds and collaboration in manuscript preparation. NR-A: Performed the molecular docking study and collaboration in manuscript preparation. SS: Performed the molecular docking study. RM: supervision of the design, synthetic and pharmacological parts. All authors read and approved the final manuscript.

Acknowledgement
Financial supports of this project by Vice-chancellor Research of Shiraz University of Medical Sciences are acknowledged.

Author details
[1]Faculty of sciences, Ahvaz Branch, Islamic Azad University, Ahvaz, Iran. [2]Medicinal and Natural Products Chemistry Research Center, Shiraz, University of Medical Sciences, PO Box 3288–71345, Shiraz, Iran. [3]Departments of Medicinal Chemistry, School of Pharmacy, Shiraz University of Medical Sciences, Shiraz, Iran. [4]Departments of Medicinal Chemistry, Faculty of Pharmacy, Isfahan University of Medical Sciences, Isfahan, Iran.

References

1. Weber L, Illgen K, Almstetter M: Discovery of new multi component reactions with combinatorial methods. *Synlett* 1999, 3:366–374.

2. Tietze LF, Modi A: Multicomponent domino reactions for the synthesis of biologically active natural products and drugs. *Med Res Rev* 2000, 20:304–322.

3. Ganem B: Strategies for innovation in multicomponent reaction design. *Acc Chem Res* 2009, 42:463–472.

4. Marcaurelle LA, Johannes CW: Application of natural product-inspired diversity-oriented synthesis to drug discovery. *Prog Drug Res* 2008, 66:187–216.

5. Ulaczyk-Lesanko A, Hall DG: Wanted: New multicomponent reactions for generating libraries of polycyclic natural products. *Curr Opin Chem Biol* 2005, 9:266–276.

6. Ahmed A, Daneshtalab M: Polycyclic quinolones (part 1)-thieno[2,3-b] benzo[h]-quinoline derivatives: design, synthesis, preliminary in vitro and in silico studies. *Heterocycles* 2012, 85:103–122.

7. Kock I, Heber D, Weide M, Wolschendorf U, Clement B: Synthesis and biological evaluation of 11-substituted 6-aminobenzo [c] phenanthridine derivatives, a new class of antitumor agents. *J Med Chem* 2005, 48:2772–2777.

8. Khan IA, Kulkarni MV, Gopal M, Shahabuddin MS, Sun CM: Synthesis and biological evaluation of novel angularly fused polycyclic coumarins. *Bioorg Med Chem Lett* 2005, 15:3584–3587.

9. Noushini S, Emami S, Safavi M, Ardestani SK, Gohari AR, Shafiee A, Foroumadi A: Synthesis and cytotoxic properties of novel (E)-3-benzylidene-7-methoxychroman-4-one derivatives. *DARU J Pharm Sci* 2013, 21:31.

10. Rescifina A, Zagni C, Romeo G, Sortino S: Synthesis and biological activity of novel bifunctional isoxazolidinyl polycyclic aromatic hydrocarbons. *Bioorg Med Chem* 2012, 20:4978–4984.

11. Banik BK, Becker FF: Polycyclic aromatic compounds as anticancer agents: structure-activity relationships of chrysene and pyrene derivatives. *Bioorg Med Chem* 2001, 9:593–605.

12. Madakar Sobhani A, Rasoul Amini S, Tyndall JDA, Azizi E, Daneshtalab M, Khalaj A: A theory of mode of action of azolylalkylquinolines as DNA binding agents using automated flexible ligand docking. *J Mol Graph Model* 2006, 25:459–469.

13. Lee CH, Jiang M, Cowart M, Gfesser G, Perner R, Kim KH, Gu YG, Williams M, Jarvis MF, Kowaluk EA: Discovery of 4-amino-5-(3-bromophenyl)-7-(6-morpholino-pyridin-3-yl) pyrido [2, 3-d] pyrimidine, an orally active, non-nucleoside adenosine kinase inhibitor. *J Med Chem* 2001, 44:2133–2138.

14. Jellimann C, Mathe-Allainmat M, Andrieux J, Kloubert S, Boutin JA, Nicolas JP, Bennejean C, Delagrange P, Langlois M: Synthesis of phenalene and acenaphthene derivatives as new conformationally restricted ligands for melatonin receptors. *J Med Chem* 2000, 43:4051–4062.

15. Kozlov NS, Shmanai GS, Tai DN: Synthesis and spectral characteristics of acenaphtho derivatives of benzo [f] quinoline. *Chem Heterocyc Compd* 1986, 22:894–898.

16. Xie YM, Deng Y, Dai XY, Liu J, Ouyang L, Wei YQ, Zhao YL: Synthesis and biological evaluation of novel acenaphtho derivatives as potential antitumor agents. *Molecules* 2011, 16:2519–2526.

17. Zhang Z, Jin L, Qian X, Wei M, Wang Y, Wang J, Yang Y, Xu Q, Xu Y, Liu F: Novel Bcl-2 inhibitors: discovery and mechanism study of small organic apoptosis-inducing agents. *Chembiochem* 2007, 8:113–121.

18. Tsujimoto Y, Finger LR, Yunis J, Nowell PC, Croce CM: Cloning of the chromosome breakpoint of neoplastic B cells with the t (14; 18) chromosome translocation. *Science* 1984, 226:1097–1099.

19. Cleary ML, Smith SD, Sklar J: Cloning and structural analysis of cDNAs for bcl-2 and a hybrid bcl-2/immunoglobulin transcript resulting from the t(14;18) translocation. *Cell* 1986, 47:19–28.

20. El Ashry ESH, Abdel HH, Shoukry M: Synthesis and reaction of acenaphthoquinones. part-1. A review. *Ind J Heterocycl Chem* 1998, 7:313–320.

21. El Ashry ESH, Hamid HA, Kassem AA, Shoukry M: Synthesis and reactions of acenaphthoquinones-part-2. The reactions of acenaphthoquinones. *Mol* 2002, 7:155–188.

22. Vosooghi M, Yahyavi H, Divsalar K, Shamsa H, Kheirollahi A, Safavi M, Ardestani SK, Sadeghi-Neshat S, Mohammadhosseini N, Edraki N,

23. Khoshneviszadeh M, Shafiee A, Foroumadi A: Synthesis and in vitrocytotoxic activity evaluation of (E)-16-(substituted benzylidene) derivatives of dehydroepiandrosterone. *DARU J Pharm Sci* 2013, 21:34.

23. Miri R, Firuzi O, Peymani P, Zamani M, Mehdipour AR, Heydari Z, Masteri Farahani M, Shafiee A: Synthesis, cytotoxicity, and QSAR study of new aza-cyclopenta [b] fluorene1, 9-dione derivatives. *Chem Biol Drug Des* 2012, 79:68–75.

24. Azizian J, Mohammadi MK, Firuzi O, Mirza B, Miri R: Microwave-assisted solvent-free synthesis of bis(dihydropyrimidinone)benzenes and evaluation of their cytotoxic activity. *Chem Biol Drug Des* 2010, 75:375–380.

25. Azizian J, Mohammadi MK, Firuzi O, Razzaghi-asl N, Miri R: Synthesis, biological activity and docking study of some new isatin Schiff base derivatives. *Med Chem Res* 2012, 21:3730–3740.

26. Morris GM, Huey R, Lindstrom W, Sanner MF, Belew RK, Goodsell DS, Olson AJ: AutoDock4 and AutoDockTools4: automated docking with selective receptor flexibility. *J Comput Chem* 2009, 30:2785–2791.

27. Morris GM, Goodsell DS, Halliday RS, Huey R, Hart WE, Belew RK, Olson AJ: Automated docking using a Lamarckian genetic algorithm and an empirical binding free energy function. *J Comput Chem* 1998, 19:1639–1662.

28. Morris GM, Huey R, Olson AJ: Using AutoDock for ligand-receptor docking. *Curr Protoc Bioinformatics* 2008, 11:34–37.

29. Wallace AC, Laskowski RA, Thornton JM: LIGPLOT: a program to generate schematic diagrams of protein-ligand interactions. *Protein Eng* 1995, 8:127–134.

30. Humphrey W, Dalke A, Schulten K: VMD: visual molecular dynamics. *J Mol Graphics* 1996, 14:33–38.

31. Petros AM, Medek A, Nettesheim DG, Kim DH, Yoon HS, Swift K, Matayoshi ED, Oltersdorf T, Fesik SW: Solution structure of the antiapoptotic protein bcl-2. *Proc Natl Acad Sci* 2001, 98:3012–3017.

32. Erickson JA, Jalaie M, Robertson DH, Lewis RA, Vieth M: Lessons in molecular recognition: the effects of ligand and protein flexibility on molecular docking accuracy. *J Med Chem* 2004, 47:45–55.

33. Zhang Z, Yang H, Wu G, Li Z, Song T: Probing the difference between BH3 groove of Mcl-1 and Bcl-2 protein: implications for dual inhibitors design. *Eur J Med Chem* 2011, 46:3909–3916.

34. Tanaka D, Tsuda Y, Shiyama T, Nishimura T, Chiyo N, Tominaga Y, Sawada N, Mimoto T, Kusunose N: A practical use of ligand efficiency indices out of the fragment-based approach: Ligand efficiency-guided lead identification of soluble epoxide hydrolase inhibitors. *J Med Chem* 2011, 54:851–857.

35. Andrews PR, Craik DJ, Martin JL: Functional group contributions to drug-receptor interactions. *J Med Chem* 1984, 27:1648–1657.

36. Hopkins AL, Groom CR, Alex A: Ligand efficiency: a useful metric for lead selection. *Drug Discov Today* 2004, 9:430.

37. Abad-Zapatero C, Metz JT: Ligand efficiency indices as guideposts for drug discovery. *Drug Discov Today* 2005, 10:464–469.

38. Wenlock MC, Austin RP, Barton P, Davis AM, Leeson PD: A comparison of physiochemical property profiles of development and marketed oral drugs. *J Med Chem* 2003, 46:1250–1256.

39. Becattini B, Sareth S, Zhai D, Crowell KJ, Leone M, Reed JC, Pellecchia M: Targeting apoptosis via chemical design: inhibition of bid-induced cell death by small organic molecules. *Chem Biol* 2004, 11:1107–1117.

40. Rahman MA, Dhar DK, Masunaga R, Yamanoi A, Kohno H, Nagasue N: Sulindac and exisulind exhibit a significant antiproliferative effect and induce apoptosis in human hepatocellular carcinoma cell lines. *Cancer Res* 2000, 60:2085–2089.

A case report of hearing loss post use of hydroxychloroquine in a HIV-infected patient

Hossein Khalili[1*], Farzaneh Dastan[1] and Seyed Ali Dehghan Manshadi[2]

Abstract

Objective: A case with reversible symmetrical sensorineural hearing loss following hydroxychloroquine therapy is described.

Case summary: A 57-year-old, human immunodeficiency virus (HIV) positive man was referred to the HIV clinic of Imam Khomeini Hospital, Tehran with chief complaint of bilateral slowly progressive hearing loss starting from two months ago. The man had history of rheumatoid arthritis diagnosed from 3 months ago and was administered hydroxychloroquine 200 mg and prednisolone 5 mg twice daily. Audiometry test showed moderate to severe neuronal hearing loss and reduced speech recognition in both ears of the patient. With suspicion of hydroxychloroquine-induced hearing loss, this drug was discontinued. After 2 months of hydroxychloroquine discontinuation, his audiometry findings were improved.

Discussion: A few cases of hydroxychloroquine-induced hearing loss have been reported. All of the cases were non-HIV positive individuals. Irreversible hearing loss was developed following long-term therapy with hydroxychloroquine. The present case was a HIV-positive man who developed hearing loss following short course (one month) hydroxychloroquine therapy and his problem was resolved following discontinuation of hydroxychloroquine and continuation of prednisolone.

Conclusions: Hydroxychloroquine-induced hearing loss may reversibly occur following short term therapy in HIV patients.

Keywords: Acquired immunodeficiency syndrome, Case report, Hearing loss, Human immunodeficiency virus, Hydroxychloroquine

Introduction

Hydroxychloroquine (HQ), a quinoline compound, rarely causes ototoxicity. Its ototoxicity is associated with varying degree of destruction of the cochlear sensory hair cells, a decrease in neuronal population, alteration in supporting structures and atrophy and vacuolization of the stria vascularis as a possible consequence of ischemia [1,2]. Clinically significant HQ-related adverse reactions including retinopathy and other visual disorders are usually detected during long-term therapy [3]. Deafness following prolonged therapy with HQ has been also reported [4]. In the previous report, ototoxicity of HQ was irreversible and manifested by auditory dysfunction without vestibular changes [5]. In the present case, HQ-induced bilateral reversible hearing loss is described in a HIV positive man suffering from rheumatoid arthritis (RA).

Case report

A 57-year-old HIV positive man was referred to the HIV clinic of Imam Khomeini Hospital, Tehran, Iran, with chief complaint of bilateral slowly progressive hearing loss starting from two months ago. He had no previous cochleo-vestibular symptoms and the hearing loss was described without tinnitus, vertigo or balance changes. He had no history of head trauma prior to the beginning of the hearing loss. He was a known case of HIV infection following blood transfusion from 2 years ago. In his medical history, RA was diagnosed from 3 months ago when he was receiving HQ 200 mg and prednisolone 5 mg twice daily. He did not consume any antiretroviral supplements or herbal products.

* Correspondence: khalilih@tums.ac.ir
[1]Department of Clinical Pharmacy, Faculty of Pharmacy, Tehran University of Medical Sciences, Tehran 1417614411, Iran
Full list of author information is available at the end of the article

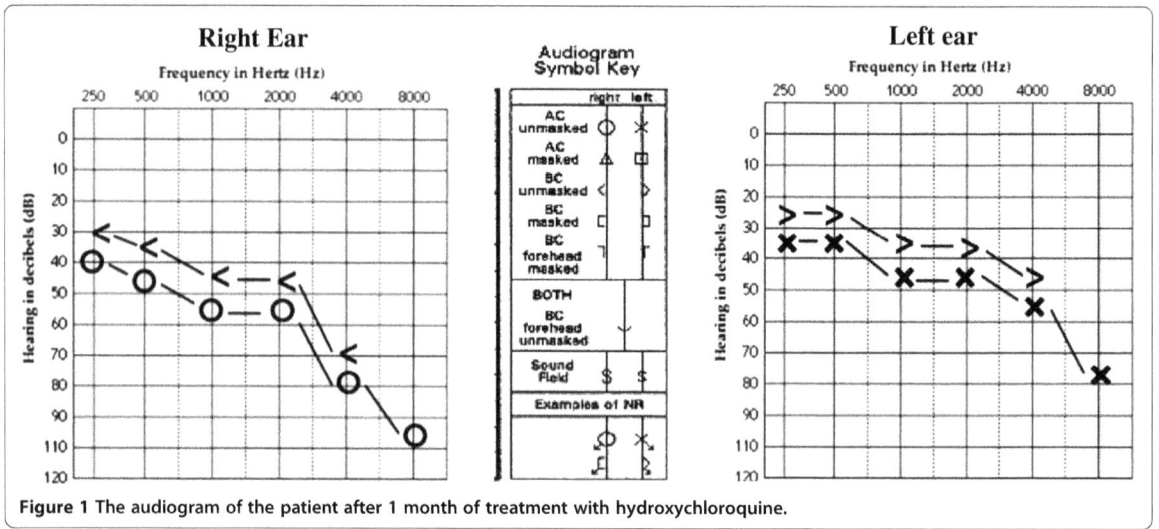

Figure 1 The audiogram of the patient after 1 month of treatment with hydroxychloroquine.

His laboratory findings showed CD4 count of 107/L and CD4/CD8 ratio of 0.13. All the other routine laboratory parameters were within the normal range. Based on the patient clinical status and his CD4 count, antiretroviral regimen including lamivudine, zidovudine and efavirenz was started. Also sulfamethoxazole/trimethoprim and isoniazid was considered for prophylaxis of pneumocystis and tuberculosis respectively in this patient.

Otolaryngological consultation reported normal otoscopic and neurologic examinations for the patient. Pure-tone (air and bone conduction) and speech audiometry showed moderate to severe neuronal hearing loss and reduced speech recognition in his both ears (45 and 40 dB in the right and left ears respectively) (Figure 1). Absence of middle ear pathologic conditions was confirmed by

pneumatic otoscopy and tympanometry. Furthermore, acoustic reflexes were latent in the patient.

With suspicious of HQ-induced hearing loss, the drug was discontinued and prednisolone was continued to control his RA symptoms. Two months later, his audiometric findings improved. Pure-tone and speech audiometry revealed mild to moderate hearing loss and slight to mild disability in speech recognition in the right and left ears, respectively (Figure 2). His acoustic reflexes were still latent.

Discussion

Idiopathic sudden sensorineural hearing loss usually occurs 5–20 per 100,000 populations mostly due to viral infections, vascular occlusion with microcirculatory

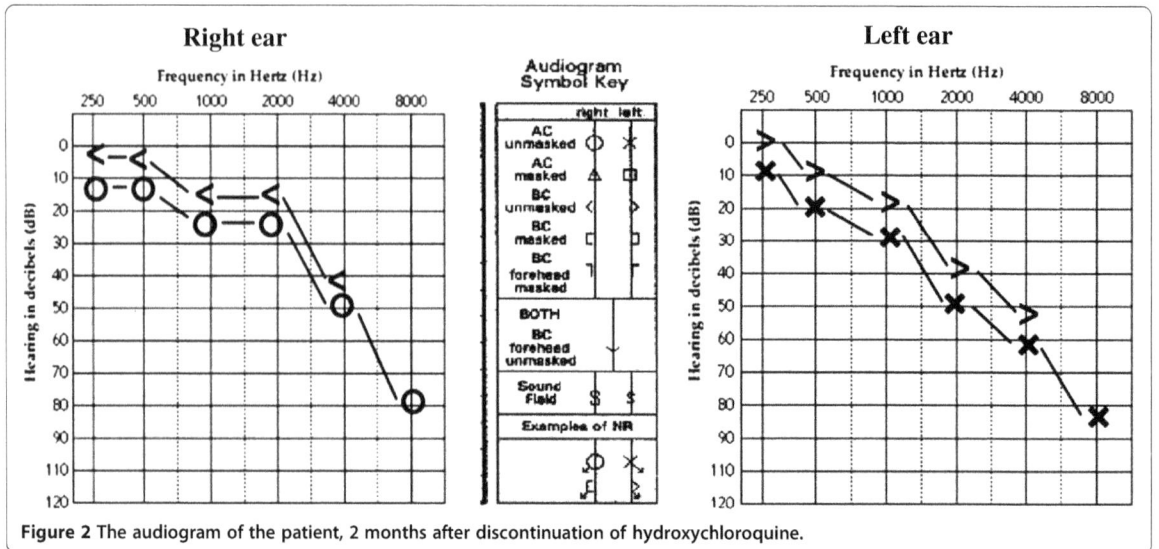

Figure 2 The audiogram of the patient, 2 months after discontinuation of hydroxychloroquine.

disturbances, immunologic diseases, or intralabyrinthine membrane breaks [6]. Some drugs may cause vestibulocochlear toxicity. Chloroquine another quinoline compound aggregates in melanocytes and results in variable injuries to the cochlear sensory hair cells, decrease in neuronal population, loss of supporting hair cells, and atrophy of stria vascularis. These changes might be caused by an ischemic process [1,7]. There are some reports about chloroquine-induced ototoxicity [7-9]. Severe chloroquine-induced cochleovestibular toxicity was reported in a pregnant woman [8]. Absence of inner and outer hair cells of the cochlea was also detected in a child whose mother took chloroquine during her pregnancy [9]. Scherbel *et al.* reported tinnitus, a sense of imbalance and nerve deafness after prolonged chloroquine administration [7].

Only a few cases of HQ-induced hearing loss have been reported. First case was a 44-year-old woman and the second case was a 44-year-old man with lupus erythematous. Both of these patients developed irreversible hearing loss following several years of HQ treatment [5]. The third patient was a 34-year-old woman with diagnosis of RA, who developed reversible, bilateral hearing loss following five months of HQ therapy [10]. Another report was unilateral sensorineural hearing loss in a 7-year-old girl with idiopathic pulmonary hamosiderosis. Her problem was diagnosed after 2 years of HQ administration [11].

All of the previous cases were non-HIV positive individuals. In these patients HQ-induced ototoxicity developed following long term HQ administration. In most of them, hearing loss was irreversible. Our case was a HIV-positive man who developed hearing loss following short course (one month) HQ therapy and his problem was resolved following HQ discontinuation.

HQ is structurally related to chloroquine and shows similar ototoxicity pattern. Chloroquine-induced hearing loss is reversible if prompt chloroquine cessation and steroid administration is done [12]. Our patient was receiving prednisolone concomitant with HQ and it is justifiable to suppose that the reversibility of his hearing loss was due to concomitant administration of this anti-inflammatory agent.

Our case is the first report of reversible symmetrical hearing loss following HQ therapy in a HIV-infected patient. The patient received daily HQ with dose of 200 mg twice daily for 3 months. No other causes of hearing loss were detected in this patient. Hearing loss in HIV infected persons may result from opportunistic infections such as cryptococcal meningitis or neurosyphilis [13] and ototoxic medications [14]. Although hearing loss was reported following antiretroviral therapy [15], in our patient these drugs were started two months after the beginning of his hearing loss. There is no any difference in audiometric findings in patients with RA compared with non-RA subjects [16].

According to the Naranjo probability scale [17], hearing loss in the present patient was probably related to HQ administration. According to definition of adverse reaction severity [18], that reaction was categorized as grade 3.

Corticosteroids are only confirmed effective treatment of sudden sensorineural hearing loss. It is important to notice that prednisone should be started as soon as possible after the onset of hearing loss [19].

In conclusion HQ-induced hearing loss may appear following short-term administration especially in patients with underlying viral infections and may be reversible by corticosteroid therapy.

Consent

Written informed consent was obtained from the patient for the publication of this report and any accompanying images.

Competing interests

The authors declare that they have no competing interests.

Authors' contribution

HK: Followed the case and edited the manuscript. FD: The case was detected and followed by FD in HIV clinic of the hospital. She also drafted the manuscript. AD: Did clinical assessment of the patient. All authors read and approved the final manuscript.

Author details

[1]Department of Clinical Pharmacy, Faculty of Pharmacy, Tehran University of Medical Sciences, Tehran 1417614411, Iran. [2]Department of Infectious Diseases, Faculty of Medicine, Tehran University of Medical Sciences, Tehran, Iran.

References

1. Hadi U, Nuwayhtd N, Hasbini AS: Chloroquine ototoxicity: an idiosyncratic phenomenon. *Otolaryngol Head Neck Surg* 1996, **114**:491–493.
2. Bernard P: Alteration of auditory evoked potentials during the course of chloroquine treatment. *Acta Otolaryngol* 1985, **99**:387–392.
3. Yam JCS, Kwok AKH: Ocular toxicity of hydroxychloroquine. *Hong Kong Med J* 2006, **12**:294–304.
4. Rodrigo B, Mittermayer S: Chloroquine ototoxicity. *Clin Rheumatol* 2007, **26**:1809–1810.
5. Johansen PB, Gran JT: Ototoxicity due to hydroxychloroquine: report of two cases. *Clin Exp Rheumatol* 1998, **16**:472–474.
6. Byl FM: Sudden hearing loss: eight years' experience and suggested prognostic table. *Laryngoscope* 1984, **94**:647–661.
7. Scherbel AL, Harrison JW, Atojian M: Further observations on use of a 4-amino-quinolone compounds in patients with rheumatoid arthritis or related diseases. *Clinical Quarterly* 1958, **25**:95–111.
8. Hart EW, Naunton RE: The ototoxicity of chloroquine phosphate. *Arch Otolaryngol* 1964, **80**:407–412.
9. Matz GJ, Naunton RF: Ototoxicity of chloroquine. *Arch Otolaryngol* 1968, **88**:370–372.
10. Seckin U, Ozoran K, Ikinciogullari A, et al: Hydroxychloroquine ototoxicity in a patient with rheumatoid arthritis. *Rheumatol Int* 2000, **19**:203–204.
11. Coutinho MB, Duarte I: Hydroxychloroquine ototoxicity in a child with idiopathic pulmonary haemosiderosis. *Int J Pediatr Otorhinolaryngol* 2002, **62**:53–57.
12. Scott PMJ, Griffiths MV: A clinical review of ototoxicity. *Clin Otolaryngol* 1994, **19**:38.

13. Smith M, Canalis R: Otologic manifestations of AIDS: the otosyphilis connection. *Laryngoscope* 1989, **99**:365–372.

14. Nadol JB: Hearing loss. *N Engl J Med* 1993, **329**:1092–1102.

15. Christina M, Marra MD, Hope A, *et al*: Hearing loss and antiretroviral therapy in patients infected with HIV-1. *Arch Neurol* 1997, **54**:407–410.

16. Halligan CS, Bauch CD, Brey RH: Hearing loss in rheumatoid arthritis. *Laryngoscope* 2006, **116**:2044–2049.

17. Naranjo CA, Busto U, Sellers EM, *et al*: A method for estimating the probability of adverse drug reactions. *Clin Pharmacol Ther* 1981, **30**:239–245. 10.1038/clpt.1981.154.

18. Hartwig SC, Siegel J, Schneider PJ: Preventability and severity assessment in reporting adverse drug reactions. *Am J Hosp Pharm* 1992, **49**:2229–2232.

19. Spear SA, *et al*: Intratympanic steroids for sudden sensorineural hearing loss, a systematic review. *Otolaryngol Head Neck Surg* 2011, **145**(4):534–543.

Synthesis, analgesic and anti-inflammatory activities of new methyl-imidazolyl-1,3,4-oxadiazoles and 1,2,4-triazoles

Ali Almasirad[1*], Zahra Mousavi[2], Mohammad Tajik[3], Mohammad Javad Assarzadeh[1] and Abbas Shafiee[3]

Abstract

Background: Long-term clinical employment of nonsteroidal anti-inflammatory drugs (NSAIDs) is associated with significant side effects including gastrointestinal (GI) lesions and kidney toxicity. In this paper we designed and synthesized new imidazolyl-1,3,4-oxadiazoles and 1,2,4-triazoles by molecular hybridization of previously described anti-inflammatory compounds in the hope of obtaining new safer analgesic and anti-inflammatory agents.

Methods: The target structures were synthesized by preparation of 5-methyl-1H-imidazole-4-carboxylic acid ethyl ester 5. The reaction of hydrazine hydrate with this ester afforded the 5-methyl-1H-imidazole-4-carboxylic acid hydrazide 6 which was converted to target compounds 7-15 according to the known procedures. *In silico* toxicity risk assessment and drug likeness predictions were done, in order to consider the privileges of the synthesized structures as drug candidates.

Results and discussion: The analgesic and anti-inflammatory profile of the synthesized compounds were evaluated by writhing and carrageenan induced rat paw edema tests respectively. Compounds 8, 9 and 11-13 and 15 were active analgesic agents and compounds 8, 9 and 11-13 showed significant anti-inflammatory response in comparison with control. Compounds 11 and 13 were screened for their ulcerogenic activities and none of them showed significant ulcerogenic activity. The active Compounds 11 and 12 showed the highest drug likeness and drug score.

Conclusions: The analgesic and anti-inflammatory activities of title compounds were comparable to that of standard drug indomethacin with a safer profile of activity. The results revealed that both of oxadiazole and triazole scaffolds can be determined as pharmacophores. The *in silico* predictions and pharmacological evaluations showed that compounds 11 and 12 can be chosen as lead for further investigations.

Keywords: Analgesic, Anti-inflammatory, Non ulcerogenic, Imidazole, Oxadiazole, Triazole

Background

Cyclooxygenase (COX) and 5-Lipoxygenase (5-LO) are two key enzymes that play important roles in the metabolism of arachidonic acid (AA) to pro-inflammatory prostaglandins (PGs) and leukotrienes (LTs) respectively [1]. It has been pointed out that inhibiting COX enzyme could decrease cytoprotective PGs and increase the conversion of AA to LTs by 5-LO enzyme which are implicated in the ulceration induced by nonsteroidal anti-inflammatory drugs (NSAIDs) [2,3]. Conversion of

AA to Leukotrien B_4 (LTB_4) leads to hyperalgesic response and related with rheumatoid arthritis and inflammatory bowel disease. However, dual inhibition of COX and 5-LO would provide an anti-inflammatory agent with better efficacy and fewer side effects [4-6]. During recent years, various structural families such as di-tert-butylphenols, thiophene and pyrazoline derivatives and modified NSAIDs have been investigated as dual COX/5-LO inhibitors [7-9]. Amongst them several 1,3,4-oxadiazole, 1,3,4-triazole and hydrazone derivatives, compounds 1 and 2 were dual COX, 5-LO inhibitors and anti-inflammatory agents (Figure 1) [7-12]. As a part of our ongoing research program to find novel anti-inflammatory and analgesic compounds, herein,we describe

* Correspondence: almasirad.a@iaups.ac.ir
[1]Department of Medicinal Chemistry, Pharmaceutical Sciences Branch, Islamic Azad University, Tehran, Iran
Full list of author information is available at the end of the article

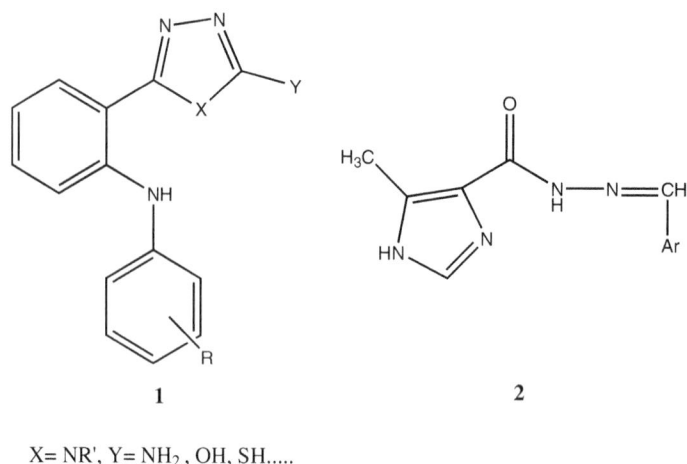

X= NR', Y= NH$_2$, OH, SH.....

Figure 1 Chemical structures of compounds 1 and 2 as dual COX/5-LO inhibitors and anti-inflammatory agents.

the synthesis of new imidazolyl-oxadiazole and triazole derivatives which were designed by molecular hybridization of previously described compounds, 1 and 2, in order to evaluate the plausible pharmacophoric contribution of the both imidazole and oxadiazole or triazole moieties in the pharmacological activities. *In silico* toxicity risk assessment and drug likeness predictions were done, in order to consider the privileges of the synthesized structures as drug candidates.

Methods

Chemistry

Chemicals were purchased from Merck Chemical Company (Tehran, Iran) and carrageenan was prepared from (Sigma-Aldrich, Dorset, UK). Melting points were taken on an electrothermal IA 9300 capillary melting-point apparatus (Ontario, Canada) and are uncorrected. ^{1}H-NMR spectra were obtained using a Bruker FT-400 spectrometer (Bruker, Rheinstetten, Germany). Tetramethyl silane was used as an internal standard. Mass spectra were obtained using a 5973 Network Mass Selective Detector at 70 eV (Agilent Technology). The FT-IR spectra were obtained using a Shimadzu FT-IR 8400S spectrographs (KBr disks).

5-Methyl-1H-Imidazole-4-carboxylic acid hydrazide (6)

To a stirring solution of ester 5 (10 g, 71.5 mmol) in 125 ml ethanol, at room temperature hydrazine hydrate (50 ml, 1000 mmol) was added and refluxed for 48 h. The resulting solution was concentrated, cooled and the precipitate was filtered, washed with dichloromethane and crystallized in ethanol to give 6.73 g (74%) of 6, mp 214-217°C. IR (KBr): υ cm^{-1} 3326, 3270 (NH$_2$, NH), 1656 (C = O). ^{1}H-NMR(DMSO-d6): δ(ppm) 11.95 (bs, 1H, NH), 8.61(bs, 1H, NH), 7.40(s, 1H, CH, imidazole),

4.09(bs, 2H, NH2), 2.51(s, 3H, CH3). MS: m/z (%) 140(M+, 100), 109(78), 54(20).

2-Amino-5-(5-methy-1H-imidazol-4-yl)-1,3,4-oxadiazole (7)

To a stirring suspension of hydrazide 6 (500 mg, 3.57 mmol) in dioxane (12 ml), sodium bicarbonate (300 mg) in water (1 ml) was added at room temperature. The mixture was stirred at room temperature for 5 min and cyanogen bromide (386 mg, 3.64 mmol) was added. After 24 h stirring at room temperature the solvent was evaporated and the resulting precipitate was purified by crystallization in methanol to give 400.7 mg(68%) of 7, mp 300-301°C. IR (KBr): υ cm^{-1} 3390, 3349 (NH$_2$, NH), 3135 (C-H). ^{1}H-NMR (DMSO-d$_6$): δ (ppm) 8.21 (bs, 1H, NH), 7.55(s, 1H, CH, imidazole), 6.85(bs, 2H, NH$_2$), 2.44(s, 3H, CH$_3$). MS: m/z (%) 165(M$^+$, 18), 69(58), 45(100).

5-(5-Methyl-1H-imidazol-4-yl)-1,3,4-oxadiazole-2(3H)-thione (8)

A mixtue of hyrazide 6 (500 mg, 3.57 mmol), potassium hydroxide (200 mg, 3.57 mmol), carbon disulfide (0.64 ml, 10.7 mmol) and ethanol (30 ml) was heated under reflux for 72 h. The solution was acidified with dilute hydrochloric acid. The resulting precipitate was removed by filtration and purified by crystallization in methanol to give 6.73 g (15%) of **8**, mp 261-262°C. IR (KBr): υ cm^{-1} 3477, 3281 (NH), 1626 (C = N), 1338 (C = S). ^{1}H-NMR (DMSO-d$_6$): δ (ppm) 13.97 (bs, 1H, NH), 8.20(bs, 1H, NH), 7.71 (s, 1H, CH, imidazole), 2.43(s, 3H, CH$_3$). MS: m/z (%) 182(M$^+$, 100), 122(87), 109(100).

5-(5-Methyl-1H-imidazol-4-yl)-1,3,4-oxadiazole-2(3H)-one (9)

To a solution of compound 6 (550 mg, 4 mmol) and triethyl amine (400 mg, 4 mmol) in DMF (50 ml), 1,1´-carbonyldiimidazole (0.84 g, 5.1 mmol) was added in one portion. The reaction mixture was refluxed for one week. The volatiles were removed in vacuo, and the residue was purified by TLC, eluting with ethyl acetate-petroleum ether (1:1) to provide 78.7 mg (11%) of **9**, mp 298-299°C. IR (KBr): υ cm^{-1} 3332(NH), 3206 (NH), 1714(C = O). ^{1}H-NMR (DMSO-d_6): δ (ppm) 9.1 (bs, 1H, NH), 8.1(bs, 1H,NH), 7.55(s, 1H, CH, imidazole), 2.43(s, 3H, CH$_3$). MS: m/z (%) 166(M$^+$, 10), 140(18), 109(100).

5-(5-Methyl-1H-imidazol-4-yl)-4H-1,2,4-triazole-3-thione (10)

A solution of hydrazide 6 (500 mg, 3.57 mmol), potassium thiocyanate (1 g, 10.71 mmol), concentrated hydrochloric acid (4 ml) and water 50 ml was stirred at room temperature for 24 h. To the resulting suspension, sodium hydroxide 4% (60 ml) was added and stirred for 24 h at 60-70°C.The resulting mixture was neutralized with hydrochloric acid and the resulting precipitate was filtered, washed with acetone and purified by two times crystallization in ethanol to give 219 mg (34%) of **10**, mp 225-227°C. IR (KBr): υ cm^{-1} 3400, 3134 (NH), 3114 (C-H), 1321 (C = S). ^{1}H-NMR (DMSO-d_6): δ (ppm) 13.87(bs, 1H, NH), 12.25(bs, 1H, NH), 9.1(bs, 1H, NH), 7.41(s, 1H, CH, imidazole), 2.31(s, 3H, CH$_3$). MS:m/z (%) 181(M$^+$, 13), 125(100), 107(90), 80(82), 67(58).

General procedures for the preparation of 4-substituted-5-(5-methyl-1H-imidazol-4-yl)-4H-1,2,4-triazole-3-thiones (11-15)

A mixture of compound 6 (500 mg, 3.57 mmol), corresponding isothiocyanate derivative (3.6 mmol) and absolute ethanol (5 ml) was stirred for 24 h. The resulting semicarbazide was filtered and washed with ether then added to 3% sodium hydroxide solution (50 ml) and refluxed for 24-48 h. The resulting solution was acidified with hydrochloric acid, the precipitate was filtered, dried and purified by crystallization.

4-Methyl-5-(5-methyl-1H-imidazol-4-yl)-4H-1,2,4-triazole-3-thione (11)

Yield 34%; mp 225-227°C (ethanol). IR (KBr): υ cm^{1-} 3376, 3149 (NH), 2526(weak, SH), 1337 (C = S). ^{1}H-NMR (DMSO-d_6): δ(ppm) 12.12(bs, 1H, NH), 8.25(bs, 1H, NH), 7.72(s, 1H, CH, imidazole), 3.74(s, 3H, CH3), 2.37 (s, 3H, CH$_3$). MS: m/z (%) 195(M$^+$, 100), 122(25), 108(30).

4-phenyl-5-(5-methyl-1H-imidazol-4-yl)-4H-1,2,4-triazole-3-thione (12)

Yield 13%; mp 275-277°C (THF/Water). IR (KBr): vcm^{1-} 3477(NH), 3410(NH), 3118(C-H, aromatic), 1326 (C = S). ^{1}H-NMR (DMSO-d_6): δ (ppm) 12.39 (bs, 1H, NH), 8.5 (bs, 1H, NH), 7.6-7.2(m, 6H, aromatic and CH, imidazole), 2.26 (s, 1H, CH$_3$). MS: m/z (%) 257(M$^+$, 100), 122(25), 108 (30).

5-(5-Methyl-1H-imidazol-4-yl)-4-(4-methylphenyl)-4H-1,2,4-triazole-3-thione (13)

Yield 24%; mp 268-270°C (Methanol). IR (KBr): υ cm^{-1} 3434(NH), 3210(NH), 3100(C-H,aromatic), 1340 (C = S). ^{1}H-NMR (DMSO-d_6): δ (ppm) 12.2(bs, 1H, NH), 8.5(bs, 1H, NH), 7.4(s, 1H, CH, imidazole), 7.3(d, J = 7.9Hz, 2H, aromatic), 7.1(d, J = 7.9 Hz, 2H, aromatic), 2.34(s, 1H, CH$_3$), 2.25(s, 3H, CH3). MS: m/z (%) 271(M$^+$, 20), 257 (100), 106(22), 77(30).

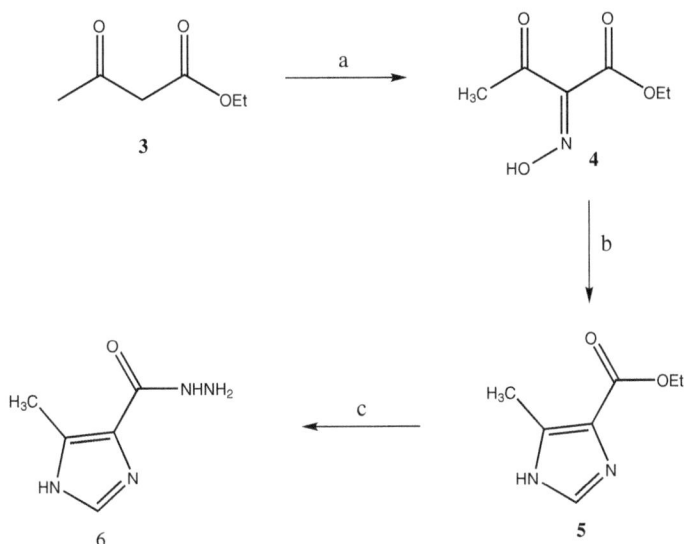

Scheme 1 Synthesis of hydrazide 6. (a) CH$_3$COOH, NaNO$_2$, 0°C; **(b)** HCHO, HCl, 0-5°C; NH$_3$, 70°C; **(c)** NH$_2$NH$_2$.H$_2$O, EtOH, reflux.

5-(5-Methyl-1H-imidazol-4-yl)-4-(4-methoxyphenyl)-4H-1,2,4-triazole-3-thione (14)

Yield 18%; mp 140-142°C (Ethylacetate/Acetone). IR (KBr): υ cm^{-1} 3430(NH), 3216(NH), 3144(C-H,aromatic), 1311(C = S). ^{1}H–NMR (DMSO-d_6): δ (ppm) 12.8(bs, 1H, NH), 8.5(bs, 1H, NH), 7.4(s, 1H, CH, imidazole), 7.2(d, J = 8.4Hz, 2H, aromatic), 6.9(d, J = 8.4Hz, 2H, aromatic), 3.76(s, 3H, OCH$_3$), 2.27(s, 3H, CH3). MS: m/z (%) 287(M$^+$, 100), 106(22), 77(30).

5-(5-Methyl-1H-imidazol-4-yl)-4-(4-fluorophenyl)-4H-1,2,4-triazole-3-thione (15)

Yield 20%; mp 150-152°C (Methanol). IR (KBr): υ cm^{-1} 3467 (NH), 3365 (NH), 3108(C-H, aromatic), 2520(weak, SH), 1321 (C = S). ^{1}H-NMR (DMSO-d_6): δ (ppm) 12.4 (bs, 1H, NH), 8.5 (bs, 1H, NH), 7.8-7.3 (m, 5H, aromatic and CH, imidazole), 2.25(s, 3H, CH$_3$). MS: m/z (%) 275 (M$^+$, 100), 106(22), 77(30).

Pharmacology

Male NMRI mice (20-25 g) and Wistar rats (100-150 g) were purchased from the animal breeding laboratories of Pasteur Institute (Karaj, Iran). Each group consisted of six animals. The animals were maintained in colony cages at 25 ± 2°C, relative humidity 45–55%, under a 12 h light-dark cycle; they were fed standard animal feed. All the animals were acclimatized for a week before use and all ethical manners for use of laboratory animals were considered carefully and the protocol was approved by Islamic Azad University of Pharmaceutical Sciences (IAUPS) ethical committee.

Analgesic activity evaluation

Acetic acid writhing test was performed on mice and indomethacin was used as standard drug [11]. Test compounds and the standard drug were administered intraperitoneally (ip) to the animals at the dose of 50 μmol/kg as

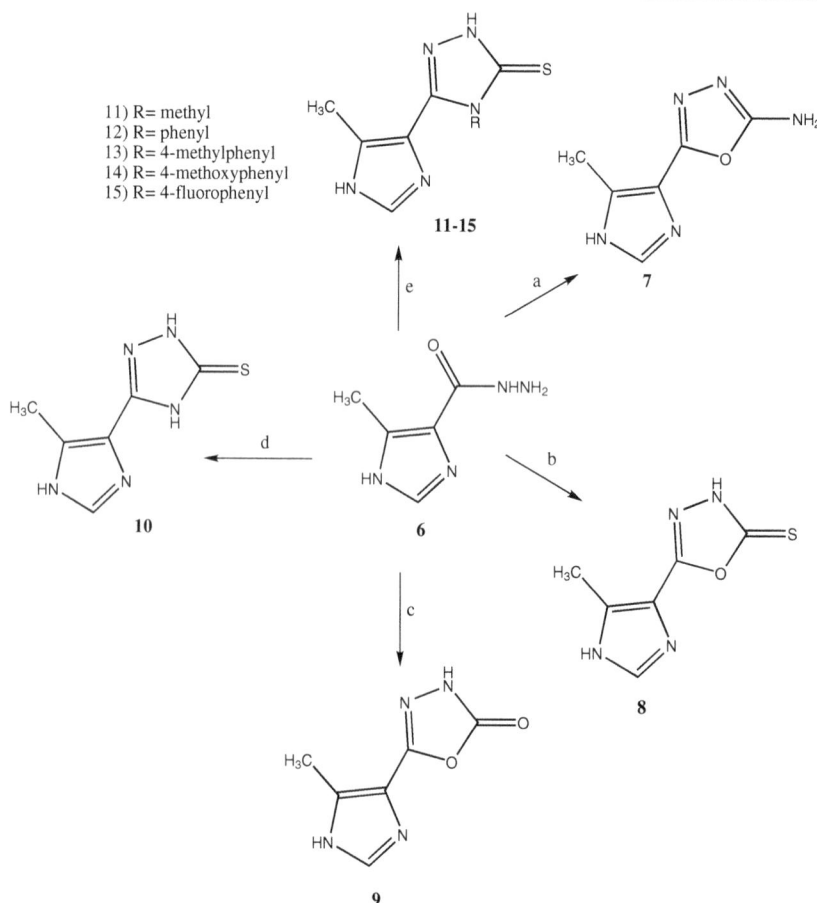

Scheme 2 Synthesis of target derivatives 7–15. (a) BrCN, Dioxane, rt; (b) CS$_2$, KOH, EtOH, reflux; (c) 1,1'-CDI, triethylamine, DMF, reflux; (d) (1) KSCN, HCl, H$_2$O, rt; (2) NaOH 3%, 60-70°C; (e) (1) Isothiocyanate derivatives, EtOH, rt; (2) NaOH, reflux.

suspension in saline and tween 80 (4% w/v). An acetic acid (0.6%, 0.1 ml/10 g) solution was administered ip 30 minutes after administration of compounds. The mean number of writhes for each experimental group and percentage decrease, compared with that of the control group were calculated during 30 minutes.

Anti-inflammatory activity against carrageenan induced rat paw edema

Effective compounds in analgesic test were screened for their anti-inflammatory activities using carrageenan induced paw edema on wistar male rats [13]. The standard and test groups received indomethacin as standard drug or target compounds, 50 μmol/kg body weight (ip) suspended in 4% tween in saline and the control animals received 4% tween in saline respectively. One hour after administration of drugs each rat received freshly prepared 0.1% w/v aqueous solution of carrageenan in the sub plantar region of right hind paw. The paw thickness was measured from the ventral to the dorsal surfaces using a dial caliper immediately prior to carrageenan injection and then at each hour, up to 5 h after the sub plantar injection. The edema was calculated as the thickness variation between the carrageenan and saline treated paw. Anti-inflammatory activity was expressed as the inhibition percent of the edema when compared with the control group.

Ulcerogenic activity

The ulcerogenic activity of newly synthesized compounds relative to known ulcerogenic drug, indomethacin was evaluated and scored by method of Cioli et al. [14]. Wistar rats (160-180 g) were fasted for 24 h before giving a single dose of each of vehicle, standard and test compounds (105 mg/kg in 0.5% v/v CMC suspension, peroral respectively and 17 h later, sacrificed under deep ether anesthesia and stomachs were removed and then examined by means of a magnifying glass to assess, the incidence of redness and spot ulcers. For each stomach, the mucosal damage was evaluated according to the following scoring system: 0.5: redness; 1.0: spot ulcers; 1.5: hemorrhagic streaks; 2.0: ulcers >3 but ≤5; 3.0: ulcers > 5. The mean score of each treated group minus the mean score of control group was regarded as gastric mucosal ulceration score.

In silico drug-score and toxicity assessments

Currently, there are several approaches to assess the drug-likeness of the drug candidates [15,16]. One such tool is the Osiris Property Explorer (OPE) a web based system which is able to calculate properties such as toxicity risk assessment and prediction of log p, solubility (log s), fragment-based drug-likeness and overall drug-score.

Results and discussion

Chemistry

The target compounds were prepared according to the Schemes 1 and 2. The ester 5 was synthesized as previously described method [17]. The key intermediate 6 was prepared from the reaction of hydrazine hydrate with ester 5. Reaction of hydrazide 6 with cyanogens bromide gave 2-amino-1,3,4-oxadiazole 7 [18]. The 1,3,4-oxadiazole-2-thone 8 and the 1,3,4-oxadiazole-2-one 9 were prepared by the reaction of hydrazide 6 with KOH and CS_2 or 1,1'-carbonyldiimidazole (1,1'-CDI) in the presence of triethylamine respectively [18,19]. The 1,2,4-triazole-3-thione 10 was synthesized via reaction of 6 with potassium thiocyanate and hydrochloric acid followed by cyclization of thiosemicarbazide intermediate with aqueous sodium hydroxide. Reaction of 6 with corresponding isothiocyanates yielded thiosemicarbazides as intermediate which were converted to 4-substituted-1,2,4-triazole-3-thiones 11-15 in aqueous sodium hydroxide [20-22]. The FCH group, Ukraine is the supplier of compound 11 and the synthesis of compound 12 has been previously reported [23].

Analgesic activity

The results of writing test revealed that several synthesized compounds 8, 9, 11-13 and 15 as well as indomethacin showed significant antinociceptive effect in comparison with control (P < 0.001) (Table 1). In compounds 7-9, existence of a more lipophilic group on the position 2 of the oxadiazole ring lead to a more potent

Table 1 Effects of new imidazolyl oxadiazole and triazole derivatives, and Indomethacin in the inhibition of abdominal constrictions induced by acetic acid (%0.6) in Mice

Compound	Constriction no. (mean ± SEM)[1]	Inhibition (%)[2]	Relative activity[3]
Vehicle control	59.67 ± 6.8	-	-
Indomethacin	13.50 ± 2.9	77.37	1[***]
7	44.33 ± 8.1	25.70	0.33
8	18.00 ± 3.7	69.83	0.90[***]
9	24.67 ± 5.5	58.65	0.76[***]
10	44.67 ± 2.8	25.14	0.32
11	23.83 ± 4.8	60.06	0.77[***]
12	24.33 ± 3.3	59.22	0.76[***]
13	17.67 ± 2.9	70.39	0.91[***]
14	ND[4]	-	-
15	15.50 ± 3.9	74.02	0.96[***]

[1]All compounds were administered i.p. at the dose of 50 μmol/kg, number of animals in each group n = 6.
[2]% of inhibition obtained by comparison with vehicle control group.
[3]Analgesic activity relative to Indomethacin,[***]P < 0.001 significant as compared to control.
[4]Not determined.

Table 2 Effects of new imidazolyl, oxadiazole and triazole derivatives 50(μmol/kg), and Indomethacin in the Carrageenan-induced rat paw edema

Compound	Time (h)[1]	Volume variation (μL)[2,3]	% inhibition[4]
Vehicle control	1	1.53 ± 0.12	-
	2	1.84 ± 0.17	-
	3	2.22 ± 0.24	-
	4	2.44 ± 0.26	-
	5	2.11 ± 0.21	-
Indomethacin	1	1.17 ± 0.01	23.53
	2	1.35 ± 0.01	26.63
	3	1.14 ± 0.02	48.6[**]
	4	1.03 ± 0.02	57.79[***]
	5	0.89 ± 0.01	57.82[***]
8	1	1.60 ± 0.15	-4.60
	2	1.82 ± 0.16	1.10
	3	1.68 ± 0.18	24.32
	4	1.53 ± 0.21	37.30[**]
	5	1.19 ± 0.18	43.60[**]
9	1	1.78 ± 0.14	-16.34
	2	1.90 ± 0.14	-3.26
	3	1.96 ± 0.16	11.71
	4	1.78 ± 0.14	27.05
	5	1.32 ± 0.07	37.44[*]
11	1	1.95 ± 0.04	-27.45
	2	2.11 ± 0.06	-14.67
	3	1.82 ± 0.16	18.02
	4	1.67 ± 0.20	31.56[*]
	5	1.38 ± 0.22	34.60[*]
12	1	1.27 ± 0.04	16.99
	2	1.44 ± 0.06	21.74
	3	1.49 ± 0.04	32.88[*]
	4	1.45 ± 0.07	40.57[*]
	5	1.22 ± 0.08	42.18[*]
13	1	1.19 ± 0.16	22.22
	2	1.70 ± 0.15	7.60
	3	1.55 ± 0.12	30.2[*]
	4	1.66 ± 0.11	31.97[*]
	5	1.41 ± 0.10	33.17[*]
14	1	1.39 ± 0.07	9.15
	2	1.64 ± 0.10	10.87
	3	1.90 ± 0.14	14.41
	4	1.91 ± 0.11	21.72
	5	1.69 ± 0.12	19.90
15	1	1.46 ± 0.08	4.57
	2	1.78 ± 0.08	3.26
	3	1.96 ± 0.10	11.71
	4	2.02 ± 0.26	17.21
	5	1.98 ± 019	6.16

[1]Time after carrageenan injection (0.1 mg/paw), number of animals in each group n = 6.
[2]All compounds were administered i.p, at the dose of 50 μmol/kg.
[3]Volume variation is the difference between the volumes of paw pre and post of Carrageenan injection.
[4]% of inhibition obtained by comparison with vehicle control group, *P < 0.05 , **p < 0.01, ***p < 0.001 significant from control.

compound 8. In addition, bioisosteric replacement of oxygen atom in compound 8 with NH to give compound 10, decreased the activity. Replacement of hydrogen atom in 4th position of triazole ring with alkyl or aryl groups, compounds 11-15 caused a noticeable analgesic activity. The most potent analgesic derivative was 15 and it can be concluded that existence of both electron withdrawing and donating substituents on the para position of the phenyl moiety (compounds 13 and 15) could enhance the analgesic activity of triazole derivatives.

Anti-inflammatory activity

In vivo anti-inflammatory evaluation of target compounds is summarized in Table 2. Compounds 8-9 and 11-13 were active anti-inflammatory agents (33-43% inhibition) after 5 h in comparison with control and their activity was comparable to indomethacin. As shown in Table 2, there wasn't any significant difference between the activity of compounds 9, 11 and 13 and the most active derivatives were 8 and 12. Similar to analgesic activity results, it can be deduced by comparison of these data that the best substituent on position 2 of oxadiazole ring is a sufur moiety. In contrast to analgesic activity, the introduction of electron donating or withdrawing moieties on the para position of phenyl ring has a deleterious effect on the anti-inflammatory activity.

Ulcerogenic activity

The compounds 11 and 13 as two active derivatives, in anti-Inflammatory and analgesic tests respectively, were evaluated for their acute ulcerogenic activity. A significant

Table 3 Acute ulcerogenic activity of compounds (11 and 13) in the method of Cioli

Compound	Dose (mg/kg)[1]	Ulcerogenic activity (Severity index ± SEM)	P value
11	105	0.50 ± 0.01	p > 0.05
13	105	0.58 ± 0.08	p > 0.05
Indomethacin	105	1.67 ± 0.333	P[*] < 0.001
Control	-	0.00 ± 0.00	-

[1]number of animals in each group n = 6, *p < 0.001 significant from control.

Table 4 Drug-likeness of target compounds predicted by Osiris Property Explorer tool in comparison with indomethacin and celecoxib

Compound	Toxicity risk[1]				cLogP	Solubility	MW	Drug- likeness	Drug-score
	M[2]	T[3]	I[4]	R[5]					
7	-	-	-	-	0.06	-2.57	165	-1.88	0.54
8	-	-	-	-	0.92	-2.2	182	0.87	0.81
9	-	-	-	-	0.25	-2.12	166	-1.75	0.55
10	-	-	-	-	0.75	-2.06	181	1.39	0.86
11	-	-	-	-	1.04	-1.7	195	2.39	0.94
12	-	-	-	-	2.29	-3.55	257	2.46	0.82
13	-	-	-	-	2.61	-3.89	271	0.76	0.68
14	+	±	-	-	2.19	-3.56	287	0.7	0.34
15	-	-	-	-	2.35	-3.86	275	0.7	0.69
Indomethacin	-	-	-	-	3.83	-5.4	357	7.59	0.57
Celecoxib	-	-	-	-	2.27	-5.4	365	-9.50	0.31

[1]Ranked according to: (-) no bad effect, (±) medium bad effect, (+) bad effect; [2] M, Mutagenic effect; [3] T, Tumorgenic effect; [4] I, Irritating effect; [5]R, Reproductive effect.

reduction in ulcerogenic activity with the stomach ulceration score between 0.50 ± 0.01 and 0.58 ± 0.08.

was observed in the tested compounds. In fact, not only the standard drug, indomethacin showed a high score of 1.67 ± 0.33, but also none of these two evaluated derivatives induced significant ulceration in comparison to control (Table 3).

In silico drug-likeness and toxicity results

In this work, open-source program OPE was used to evaluate the fragment-based drug-likeness of title compounds and comparing them with indomethacin and celecoxib. The overall drug-score which was mentioned earlier combines drug-likeness, clogp, clogs, molecular weight and toxicity risk factors in one single value, where the occurrence frequency of each fragment is determined within the collection of approved drugs and within the supposedly non-drug like chemicals of fluka company. A positive drug-likeness value (0.1-10) states that a molecule contains fragments which are present in commercial drugs. The OPE study revealed that except compound 14 which showed high risk of mutagenic and medium risk of tumorgenic effects, all compounds, indomethacin and celecoxib are supposed to be non-mutagenic, non-tumorgenic, non-irritant with no reproductive effects. The *in silico* drug-relevant properties obtained by OPE are given in Table 4. The potential drug-likeness values of all designed compounds were significantly higher than that of celecoxib but this value for compounds 7 and 9 is negative so their similarity to commercial chemicals is more than traded drugs. Generally, the drug-score values of compounds 7-15 (0.34-0.94) were more than that of celecoxib (0.31) and these scores for compounds 8, 10-13 and 15

(0.68-0.94) were more than indomethacin and for compounds 7 and 9 comparable with indomethacin.

Conclusion

A series of new methyl-imidazolyl-1,3,4-oxadiazoles and 1,2,4-triazoles were designed and synthesized. The *in vivo* analgesic, anti-inflammatory and ulcerogenic evaluations, revealed that most of them were active in both tests without any ulcerogenic potential in comparison to control. The results revealed that both of oxadiazole and triazole scaffolds can be determined as pharmacophores. However, compounds 11 and 12 showed the highest values of drug-likeness and drug-score and acceptable pharmacological activity in both tests, so they could be selected as lead compounds for further modifications.

Statistics

Statistics were performed with one-way analysis of variance (ANOVA), which was followed by Tukey multi-comparison test. All data are presented as mean $\pm$ SEM, $p < 0.05$ was considered to be significant.

Competing interests
The authors declare that they have no competing interests.

Authors' contributions
AA: Design of target compounds, supervision of the synthetic part and manuscript preparation. ZM: Supervision of pharmacological part. MT: Synthesis of target compounds. MJA: Performed the pharmacological tests. AS: Collaboration in identifying of the structures of target compounds. All authors read and approved the final manuscript.

Acknowledgement
This work was supported by a grant from the vice chancellor for research of pharmaceutical sciences branch, Islamic Azad University (IAUPS).

Author details
[1]Department of Medicinal Chemistry, Pharmaceutical Sciences Branch, Islamic Azad University, Tehran, Iran. [2]Department of Toxicology and Pharmacology, Pharmaceutical Sciences Branch, Islamic Azad University, Tehran, Iran. [3]Department of Medicinal Chemistry, Faculty of Pharmacy and Pharmaceutical Sciences Research Center, Tehran University of Medical Sciences, Tehran, Iran.

References

1. Gonzalez-Periz A, Claria J: New approaches to the modulation of the cyclooxygenase-2 and 5-lipoxygenase pathways. *Curr Top Med Chem* 2007, **7**(3):297–309.
2. Pontiki E, Hadjipavlou-Litina D, Litinas K, Nicolotti O, Carotti A: Design, synthesis and pharmacobiological evaluation of novel acrylic acid derivatives acting as lipoxygenase and cyclooxygenase-1 inhibitors with antioxidant and anti-inflammatory activities. *EurJ Med Chem* 2011, **46**(1):191–200.
3. Eleftheriou P, Geronikaki A, Hadjipavlou-Litina D, Vicini P, Filz O, Filimonov D, Poroikov V, Shailendra S, Chaudhaery E, Roy KK, Saxena AK: Fragment-based design, docking, synthesis, biological evaluation and structure–activity relationships of 2-benzo/benzisothiazolimino-5-aryliden-4-thiazolidinones as cycloxygenase/lipoxygenase inhibitors. *Eur J Med Chem* 2012, **47**:111–124.
4. Geronikaki AA, Lagunin AA, Hadjipavlou-Litina DI, Eleftheriou PT, Filimonov DA, Poroikov VV, Alam I, Saxena AA: Computer-aided discovery of anti-inflammatory thiazolidinones with dual cyclooxygenase/lipoxygenase inhibition. *J Med Chem* 2008, **51**(6):1601–1609.
5. Celotti F, Laufer S: Anti-inflammatory drugs: new multitarget compounds to face an old problem. The dual inhibition concept. *Pharm Res* 2001, **43**(5):429–436.
6. Araico A, Terencio MC, Alcaraz MJ, Dominguez JN, Leon C, Ferrandiz ML: Phenylsulfonyl urenyl chalcone derivatives as dual inhibitors of cyclo-oxygenase-2 and 5-lipoxygenase. *Life Sci* 2006, **78**:2911–2918.
7. Charlier C, Michaux: Dual inhibition of cyclooxygenase-2 (Cox-2) and lipoxygenase (5-Lox) as a new strategy to provide safer non-steroidal anti-inflammatory drugs. *Eur J Med Chem* 2003, **38**:645–659.
8. Moreau A, Chen QH, Roa PNP, Knaus EE: Design, synthesis and biological evaluation of (E)-3-(4-methanesulfonylphenyl)-2-(aryl)acrylic acids as dual inhibitors of cyclooxygenases and lipoxygenase. *Bioorg Med Chem* 2006, **14**:7716–7727.
9. Rao PNP, Chen QH, Knaus EE: Synthesis and biological evaluation of 1,3-diphenylprop-2-yn-1-ones as dual inhibitors of cyclooxygenase and lipoxygenase. *Bioorg Med Chem Lett* 2005, **15**:4842–4845.
10. Leval XD, Julemont F, Delarge J, Pirotte B, Dogne JM: New trends in dual 5-LOX/COX inhibition. *Curr Med Chem* 2002, **9**(9):941–962.
11. Figueiredo JM, Câmara CA, Amarante EG, Miranda ALP, Santos FM, Rodrigues CR, Fraga CAM, Barreiro EJ: Design and synthesis of novel potent antinociceptive agents: methyl-imidazolyl N-acylhydrazone derivatives. *Bioorg Med Chem* 2000, **8**(9):2243–2248.
12. Moradi A, Navidpour L, Amini M, Sadeghian H, Shadnia H, Firouzi O, Miri R, Ebrahimi ES, Abdollahi M, Zahmatkesh MH, Shafiee A: Design and Synthesis of 2-Phenoxynicotinic Acid Hydrazides as Anti-inflammatory and Analgesic Agents. *Arch Pharm Chem Life Sci* 2010, **9**:509–518.
13. Panchaxari DM, Pampana S, Pal T, Devabhaktuni B, Aravapalli AK: Design and characterization of diclofenac diethylamine transdermal patch using silicone and acrylic adhesives combination. *DARU J Pharmaceut Sci* 2013, **21**(1):6.
14. Cioli V, Silvestrini B, Dordoni F: Evaluation of potential of gastric ulceration after administration of certain drugs. *Exp Mol Pathol* 1967, **6**:68–75.
15. *Organic Chemistry Portal*; 2013. Available at http://www.organic-chemistry.org/prog/peo/. Accessed September 3.
16. Ayati A, Falahati M, Irannejad H, Emami S: Synthesis, in vitro antifungal evaluation and in silico study of 3-azolyl-4-chromanone phenylhydrazones. *DARU J Pharmaceut Sci* 2012, **20**:46.
17. Graboyes H, Kasper TJ, Vaidya PD: Process for preparing 5-methyl-4-imidazolecarboxylic acid esters. In *European Patent No. EP 0049638*. Munich, Germany: European Patent Organization; 1987.
18. Amir M, Shikha K: Synthesis and anti-inflammatory, analgesic, ulcerogenic and lipid peroxidation activities of some new 2-[(2,6-dichloroanilino) phenyl]acetic acid derivatives. *Eur J Med Chem* 2004, **39**(6):535–545.
19. Gilani SJ, Khan SA, Siddiqui N: Synthesis and pharmacological evaluation of condensed heterocyclic 6-substituted 1,2,4-triazolo-[3,4-b]-1,3,4-thia-diazole and 1,3,4-oxadiazole derivatives of isoniazid. *Bioorg Med Chem Lett* 2010, **20**(16):4762–4765.
20. Almasirad A, Vousooghi N, Tabatabai SA, Kebriaeezadeh A, Shafiee A: Synthesis, anticonvulsant and muscle relaxant activities of substituted 1,3,4-oxadiazole,1,3,4-thiadiazole and 1,2,4-triazole. *Acta Chim Slov* 2007, **54**(2):317–324.
21. Almasirad A, Shafiee A, Abdollahi M, Noeparast A, Shahrokhinejad N, Vousooghi N, Tabatabai SA, Khorasani R: Synthesis and analgesic activity of new 1, 3, 4-oxadiazoles and 1, 2, 4-triazoles. *Med Chem Res* 2011, **20**(4):435–442.
22. Cretu OD, Barbuceanu SF, Saramet G, Draghici C: Synthesis and characterization of some 1,2,4-triazole-3-thiones obtained from intramolecular cyclization of new 1-(4-(4-X-phenylsulfonyl)benzoyl)-4-(4-iodophenyl)-3-thiosemicarbazides. *J Serb Chem Soc* 2010, **75**(11):1463–1471.
23. Siwek A, Wujec M, Dobosz M, Wawrzycka-Gorczyca I: Study of direction of cyclization of 1-Azolil-4-Aryl/Alkyl-Thiosemicarbazides. *Het Chem* 2010, **21**(7):521–532.

Quantitative analysis of piroxicam using temperature-controlled ionic liquid dispersive liquid phase microextraction followed by stopped-flow injection spectrofluorimetry

Mohsen Zeeb[1*], Parisa Tayebi Jamil[1†], Ali Berenjian[1†], Mohammad Reza Ganjali[2†] and Mohamad Reza Talei Bavil Olyai[1†]

Abstract

Background: Piroxicam (PXM) belongs to the wide class of non-steroidal anti-inflammatory drugs (NSAIDs). PXM has been widely applied in the treatment of rheumatoid arthritis, gonarthrosis, osteoarthritis, backaches, neuralgia, mialgia. In the presented work, a green and benign sample pretreatment method called temperature-controlled ionic liquid dispersive liquid phase microextraction (TCIL-DLPME) was followed with stopped-flow injection spectrofluorimetry (SFIS) for quantitation of PXM in pharmaceutical formulations and biological samples.

Methods: Temperature-controlled ionic liquid dispersive liquid phase microextraction (TCIL-DLPME) was applied as an environmentally friendly sample enrichment method to extract and isolate PXM prior to quantitation. Dispersion of 1-hexyl-3-methylimidazolium hexafluorophosphate ([Hmim][PF$_6$]) ionic liquid (IL) through the sample aqueous solution was performed by applying a relatively high temperature. PXM was extracted into the extractor, and after phase separation, PXM in the final solution was determined by stopped-flow injection spectrofluorimetry (SFIS).

Results and Major Conclusion: Different factors affecting the designed method such as IL amount, diluting agent, pH and temperature were investigated in details and optimized. The method provided a linear dynamic range of 0.2-150 μg l^{-1}, a limit of detection (LOD) of 0.046 μg l^{-1} and a relative standard deviation (RSD) of 3.1%. Furthermore, in order to demonstrate the analytical applicability of the recommended method, it was applied for quantitation of PXM in real samples.

Keywords: 1-Hexyl-3-methylimidazolium hexafluorophosphate, Stopped-flow injection spectrofluorimetry, Pharmaceutical formulations, Biological samples

Background

Piroxicam (PXM, 4-hydroxy-2-methyl-N-(pyridine-2-yl)-2H-1, 2-benzo-thiazine-3-carboxamide-1,2-dioxide) belongs to the wide class of non-steroidal anti-inflammatory and analgesic drugs (NSAIDs) [1]. This drug has been widely used to treat podagrous and rheumatoid arthritis, gonarthrosis, osteoarthritis, backaches, neuralgia, mialgia, and other diseases accompanied by the pain syndrome or an inflammatory process [2,3]. To our knowledge, until now, some analytical techniques such as high performance liquid chromatography (HPLC) [4], capillary electrophoresis [5], liquid chromatography-mass spectrometry (LC/MS) [6], spectrometry [7], electrochemistry [8] have been reported for the quantitative analysis of PXM. The data obtained in these works reveal that the sensitivity and selectivity is not acceptable which is due to low amount of analyte in real sample and matrix impact. Thus, development and application of practical and benign sample pretreatment procedures prior to quantitation are important tasks of chemists. Combination of sample enrichment procedures with inexpensive, selective and sensitive determination tools such as spectrofluorimetry makes it possible to

* Correspondence: Zeeb.mohsen@gmail.com
†Equal contributors
¹Department of Applied Chemistry, Faculty of science, Islamic Azad University, South Tehran Branch, Tehran, Iran
Full list of author information is available at the end of the article

determine trace levels of analytes, provide better selectivity and extremely reduce the cost of analysis.

Previous studies reveal that ionic liquids (ILs) are suitable materials in sample enrichment procedures due to their special properties [9]. One of the practical advantages of ILs application in microextraction methods is the removal of toxic extraction materials. The most popular extraction techniques based on ILs are ionic liquid-based dispersive liquid-liquid microextraction (IL-DLLME) [10-13], cold-induced aggregation microextraction (CIAME) [14] and temperature-controlled ionic liquid dispersive liquid phase microextraction (TCIL-DLPME) [15].

In TCIL-DLPME procedure, dispersion of IL through the sample aqueous solution is occurred by applying a relatively high temperature. This phenomenon increases the chance of analyte extraction into extractor phase. By cooling the solution and centrifugation, it is possible to collect the IL-phase and transfer it to analytical tool for subsequent analysis. Based on the data obtained in our previous works, the out put of ionic liquid-sample enrichment methods meaningfully depends on variations in the values of ionic strength [16-19]. It is obvious that this factor can affect on the solubility of extractor. In order to obtained stable results, a common ion of extractor solvent (PF_6^-) was dissolved in the studied solution. Using this way, the volume of the extractor was not affected by changes occurred in the value of ionic strength.

In this study, spectrofluorimetric method was utilized for quantitation owning to some advantages including good selectivity and sensitivity, low cost of analysis and high response speed. To our knowledge, for the first time, TCIL-DLPME was combined with stopped-flow injection spectrofluorimetry (SFIS) for trace determination of PXM. The factors influencing the proposed method were studied in details and optimized. Finally, In order to demonstrate the analytical advantage of TCIL-DLPME -SFIS, It was utilized for quantitation of PXM in pharmaceutical and biological samples.

Material and methods
Instrumentation
Fluorescence signals were recorded using FP-6200 spectrofluorimeter (JASCO Corporation, Tokyo, Japan). Xenon discharge lamp, peristaltic sipper unit (model SHP-292), and micro-cell (path length of 3 mm and volume of 15 μL) were used as the accessories. The PC-based Windows® Spectra Manager™ software was applied for recording and processing of the analytical signals. A centrifuge was purchased from Hettich (Tuttlingen, Germany) and used for accelerating the phase separation. The pH-meter model 692 (Herisau, Switzerland) supplied with a glass-combined electrode was used for pH measuring.

Reagents and materials
Analytical-reagent grade of chemicals was used in all experiments. All aqueous solutions were prepared using ultra pure water. Piroxicam hydrochloride was obtained from Alhavi Pharmaceutical Company (Tehran, Iran). 1-Hexyl-3-methylimidazolium hexafluorophosphate [Hmim][PF_6], acetone, acetonitrile, methanol, ethanol, NH_3, HCl, NaOH and sodium hexafluorophosphate ($NaPF_6$) were purchased from Merck (Darmstadt, Germany). A stock solution of 200 mg ml^{-1} of $NaPF_6$ was obtained by dissolving required amount of $NaPF_6$ in water. Piroxicam has a low solubility in water (0.00004 M). Hence, a stock solution of piroxicam (1000 mg l^{-1}) was obtained by dissolving 10 mg of pure drug in 10 ml of 5 M NH_3. The obtained stock solution was stored at 5°C in the dark until use. Working solutions of lower concentrations were prepared daily from the above stock solution as required. Piroxicam capsules and tablets were obtained from a local pharmacy.

Microextraction procedure
In the presented microextraction procedure, aliquots of 10.0 ml sample solution (pH = 3) containing PXM in the concentration range of 0.2-150 μg l^{-1} were placed into a screw-glass test tube with conic bottom. Then, 55 mg of [Hmim][PF_6] IL and 0.9 ml of $NaPF_6$ (200 mg ml^{-1}) was added. After shaking, the conical tube was heated in a water bath with the temperature controlled at 40 °C for 5 min. Under this condition, the extractor was dissolved completely and the PXM was effectively extracted into the IL phase. After this step, the resulting solution was placed in ice-water bath and cooled for 7 min. After this process, a turbid condition was formed due to the decrease of the solubility of the extractor. The obtained solution was centrifuged for 5 min at 4000 rpm. The aqueous phase was removed using a proper syringe. For conditioning the extractor prior to quantitation by SFIS, the residue in the vessel was diluted to 250 μL by adding required amount of ethanol. Finally, the diluted IL-phase in the vessel was transferred to the spectrofluorimeter by the peristaltic sipper unit.

Stopped-flow injection spectrofluorimetry
In the presented work, fluorescence signals were recorded using stopped-flow injection technique. In order to apply stopped-flow injection mode, a peristaltic sipper unit supplied with a 15 μL quartz micro-cell was utilized to increase the speed of measurement and significantly reduce the required volume of the extractor. In order to control the enriched phase uptake, the rotation time of the peristaltic pump was changed. For transferring the extraction solvent to the spectrofluorimeter, the tube of the peristaltic pump unit was placed into the sample vessel, and suction step was started for 0.4 s. After this process, IL-phase was introduced to the 15 μL micro-

cell. This step was applied for 1 s. In order to apply a delay time, the rotation of peristaltic pump was stopped. The stopped time was applied for 2 s, in order to obtain a stable experimental condition prior to quantitation. Fluorescence signal was recorded at 455 ± 5 nm. The excitation wavelength was fixed at 320 ± 5 nm. Schematic diagram of stopped-flow injection spectrofluorimetry applied in the present study is shown in Figure 1.

Preparation of pharmaceutical formulations and biological samples

In order to obtain analyzable pharmaceutical solution, six piroxicam capsules or powdered tablets were entirely mixed, and afterwards a proper amount of powder containing 10 mg of PXM was dissolved in 5 M NH_3. To prepare a clear solution, the resulting sample was filtered into a 100 ml volumetric flask by Whatman No. 42 filter paper, and made up to the mark using ultra pure water. Prior to quantitation, a proper dilution was performed, in order to ensure the concentration of the pharmaceutical solution was in the dynamic range.

In order to obtain analyzable human plasma samples, 1.0 ml of this real sample were spiked with PXM and deproteinized by addition of 5 ml acetonitrile. After this process, the resulting biological real sample was centrifuged at 4000 rpm for 15 min, and 2.0 ml of the clear upper pahse was diluted to 100 ml. Aliquot of 10 ml of this sample was utilized for each test. 10 ml of human urine samples were transferred into centrifuge tubes. Urine samples were centrifuged for 4 min at 4000 rpm. Afterwards, aliquots of 2 ml from clear upper phase were transferred into new centrifuge tubes, spiked with different concentrations of PXM and diluted to 20 ml. In order to determine the trace levels of PXM, aliquot of 10 ml of this solution was subjected to TCIL-DLPME-SFIS.

Results and discussion

In the recommend method, an efficient sample pretreatment method called temperature-controlled ionic liquid dispersive liquid phase microextraction (TCIL-DLPME) was followed by stopped-flow injection spectrofluorimetry (SFIS) for preconcentration and trace level determination of PXM in real samples. To achieve a proper efficiency and stability, different variables affecting the recommended method were studied and optimized. Pre-concentration factor (PF) was evaluated according to the following equation:

$$PF = \frac{C_{sed}}{C_0}$$

In this equation, C_{sed} and C_0 show the concentration of PXM in the enriched phase and initial concentration of PXM in the aqueous phase, respectively. C_{sed}, for extractor solvents and diluting agents, was measured using the calibration graph obtained from direct injection of PXM in enriched phase.

Spectrofluorimetric calibration curve and spectral characteristics

Since PXM has a cyclic conjugated structure, this compound shows considerable fluorescence signal. The emission spectra of 6 standard solutions of PXM with different concentrations in the range of 0.2-150 µg l^{-1} were recorded using TCIL-DLPME-SFIS (see Figure 2). Fluorescence signal was recorded at 455 ± 5 nm. The excitation wavelength was fixed at 320 ± 5 nm. To achieve stable, reproducible and accurate data, the reagent blank must have no measurable impact on the fluorescence signal of PXM. Hence, the sample enrichment procedure was applied for reagent blank using the mentioned excitation and emission wavelengths. The data obtained in this test shown no

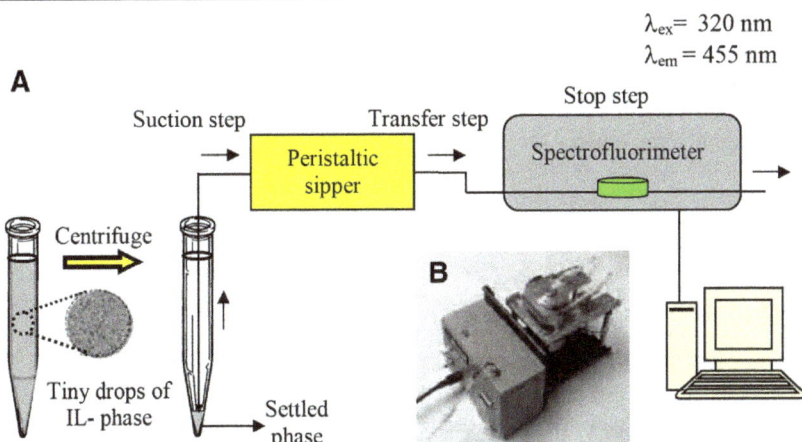

Figure 1 (A) Schematic diagram of SFIS (B) Structure of peristaltic sipper unit. Utilized experimental conditions: λ_{ex} 320 ± 5 nm; λ_{em} 455 ± 5 nm; suction time 0.4 s; transferring time 1 s; delay time 2 s.

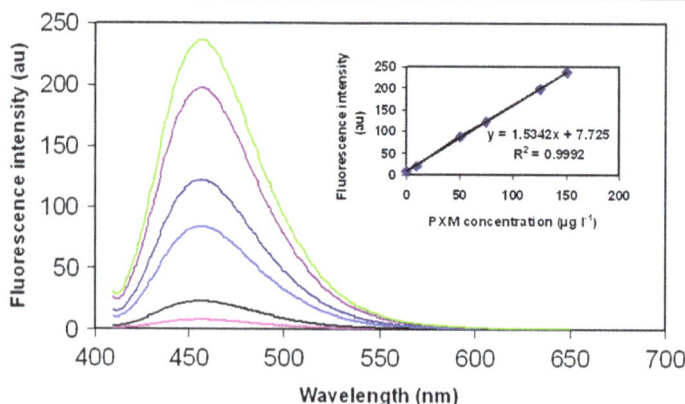

Figure 2 Fluorescence spectra obtained for 6 standard solutions of PXM with different concentrations (0.2, 10, 50, 75, 125, 150 µg l⁻¹). Utilized experimental conditions: Sample volume 10 ml; [Hmim][PF$_6$] 55 mg; NaPF$_6$ 180 mg; pH 3; temperature 40°C; centrifugation time 5 min. λ_{ex} 320 ± 5 nm; λ_{em} 455 ± 5 nm. Inset: Calibration curve and corresponding equation in the linear range of analytical signals.

significant impact. Hence, the mentioned wavelengths were selected for the rest of the work.

Selection of IL

Following consideration can ease the selection of IL: (a) the density of extractor must be higher than aqueous phase, (b) extractor must be liquid through the experiments, (c) IL must show proper hydrophobic manner and (d) IL must be certainly inexpensive. ILs containing $(CF_3SO_2)_2N^-$ are relatively expensive and those containing PF_6^- are relatively inexpensive. According to the mentioned points, [Hmim][PF$_6$] was selected as a microextraction solvent in all experiments.

Type of diluting agent

Kind of diluting agent is one the important factors in TCIL-DLPME. Since the density of ionic liquid is relatively high, this extractor must be diluted prior to transfer and quantitation. In the present test, some organic diluting agent involving methanol, ethanol, acetone and acetonitrile were investigated. Because of the better performance of ethanol and its better safety, this diluting material was utilized in all the tests.

Influence of IL amount

In this investigation, the influence of [Hmim][PF$_6$] amount on the TCIL-DLPME and subsequent analytical signals was tested. The influence of this factor was tested within the range of 10–120 mg (Figure 3). Stable data were achieved at 55 mg of IL. When a larger amount of extractor to be used, the volume of the enriched phase increases and the signal intensity decreases. As a result,

55 mg of extractor was selected as an optimum value and used in the following experiments.

Influence of common ion amount and ionic strength

Based on the results obtained in our previous works, dissolving a common ion of extractor can provide more stable dada. As it was described, this act can decrease the solubility of the extraction phase and provide better sensitivity. For this evaluation, NaPF$_6$ was applied in all tests a common ion source. The impact of this factor was tested in the range of 0–300 mg. Figure 4 show the obtained results in this experiment. A better stability was achieved at 180 mg. Therefore, this amount was applied for the rest of the work.

Based on the results obtained in our previous studies, in traditional sample enrichment methods based on ILs, the volume of remaining enriched phase depends on the value of the ionic strength. As it was explained above, in order to overcome this phenomenon, a common ion of extractor phase was dissolved in the sample under study. NaNO$_3$ was utilized as an electrolyte to test the impact of this factor. This factor was carefully evaluated over the range of 0–35% (w/v) and no measurable impact was observed in this range.

Influence of pH

The pH of the sample solution plays a critical role in the extraction of ionizable organic molecules such as PXM. The influence of this factor on the microextraction of PXM was evaluated within the range of 1–8 using HCl and NaOH. The best data is obtained at pH values where the uncharged condition of the compound of interest is prevalent. The reported acidic constants for PXM are pK_{a1} = 1.81 and pK_{a2} = 5.12 [20]. Figure 5 shows a possible

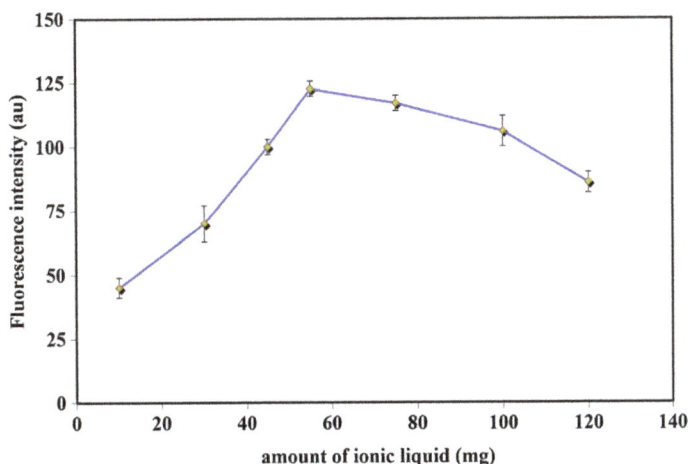

Figure 3 Effetc of IL amount. Utilized experimental conditions: Sample volume 10 ml; PXM concentration 75 µg l^{-1}; NaPF$_6$ 180 mg; pH 3; temperature 40°C; centrifugation time 5 min. λ_{ex} 320 ± 5 nm; λ_{em} 455 ± 5 nm.

equilibrium between the neutral molecule (LH^0) and the zwitterion (LH$^\pm$). The variation of analytical signals versus pH revealed that a better extraction was obtained at pH 3 (Figure 6). Thus, pH 3 was used in the following study.

Influence of temperature
Complete dispersion of IL-phase in the sample solution is occurred by applying a relatively high temperature. The obtained data revealed that the solubility of extractor at temperature above 30°C significantly increased. A series experiments were performed in order to optimize the temperature in the range of 30–70°C. A better stability and

sensitivity was obtained at 40°C, therefore this temperature was used an optimum value. In the next step, sample solutions were cooled in the temperature range of 0-25°C. By applying a low temperature, the analytical sensitivities improve which is due to the solubility decrease of extractor phase at low temperatures. Hence, a temperature of 0°C was utilized through the rest of the work.

Influence of centrifuge conditions
In this experiment, the impact of this factor on the sensitivity and reproducibility was tested in the range of 1000–6000 rpm. In order to settle the extractor phase,

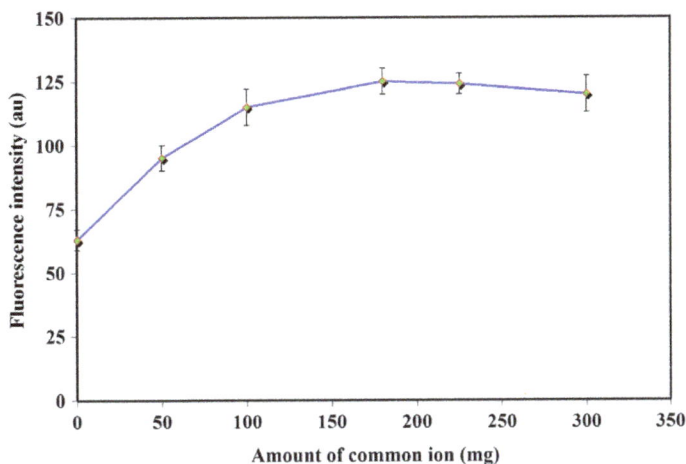

Figure 4 Effect of common ion. Utilized experimental conditions: Sample volume 10 ml; PXM concentration 75 µg l^{-1}; [Hmim][PF$_6$] 55 mg; pH 3; temperature 40°C; centrifugation time 5 min. λ_{ex} 320 ± 5 nm; λ_{em} 455 ± 5 nm.

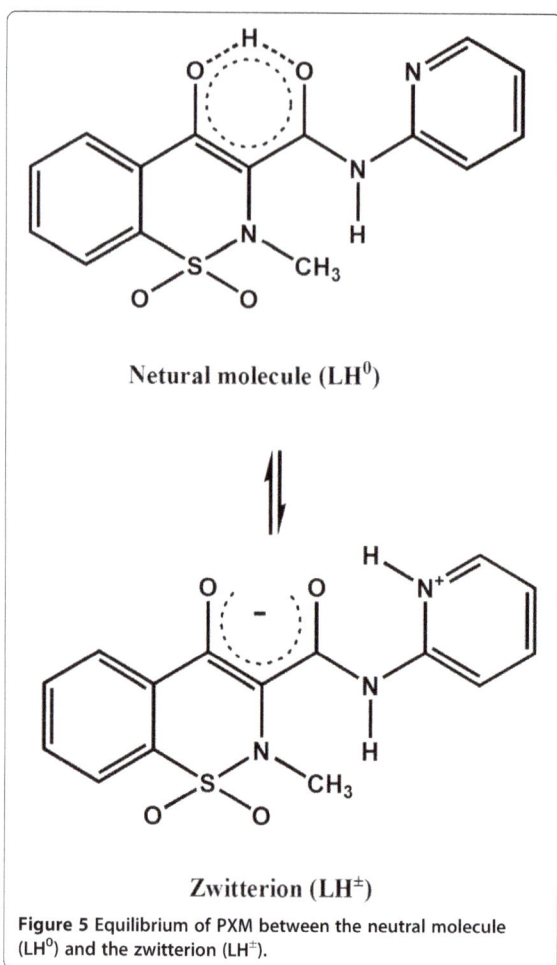

Figure 5 Equilibrium of PXM between the neutral molecule (LH⁰) and the zwitterion (LH±).

3500 was suitable. Hence, 4000 rpm was chosen as the optimum value. After this study, the impact of centrifugation time on the sensitivity and stability of signals was tested. After 4 min, no measurable change was observed. As a result, 5 min was selected as the centrifugation time. Table 1 shows the tested and selected experimental conditions.

Selectivity of the method

In the present study, in order to demonstrate the selectivity of the method, the impact of some possible interfering substances such as Na^+, Ca^{2+}, Zn^{2+}, Mg^{2+}, Cl^-, PO_4^{3-}, SO_4^{2-}, citric acid, starch, glucose, lactose, sucrose, ascorbic acid, uric acid, oxalic acid and lactic acid on the determination of PXM at 75 µg L^{-1} was tested. 100-fold the mentioned substances have no observable impact on the fluorescence responses (fluorescence response change below 5%).

Method evaluation

In order to obtain calibration graph and linear dynamic range, different concentrations of PXM standard solutions were subjected to TCIL-DLPME-SFIS. The designed method provided a linear dynamic range of 0.2-150 µg l^{-1} PXM. Analytical performance of the combined methodology is summarized in Table 2. The limit of detection (LOD) of TCIL-DLPME-SFIS was defined using the following equation:

$$LOD = ks_{bl}/m.$$

In the mentioned equation, the value of K is 3, s_{bl} shows the standard deviation of the blank signals and m

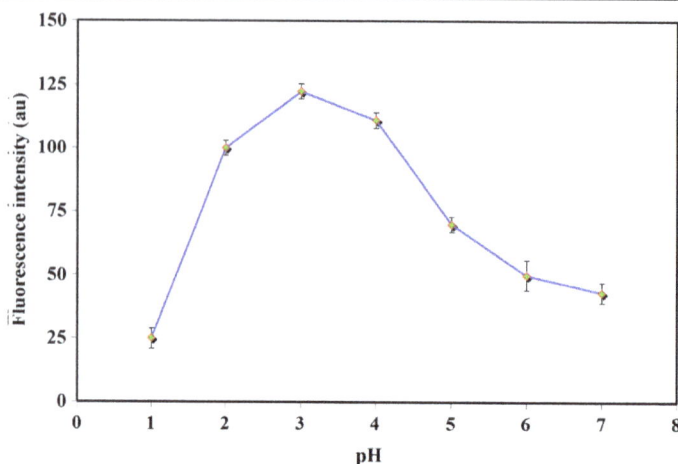

Figure 6 Effect of pH. Utilized experimental conditions: Sample volume 10 ml; PXM concentration 75 µg l^{-1}; [Hmim][PF$_6$] 55 mg; NaPF$_6$ 180 mg; temperature 40°C; centrifugation time 5 min. λ_{ex} 320 ± 5 nm; λ_{em} 455 ± 5 nm.

Table 1 Evaluated and optimized experimental conditions of TCIL-DLPME-SFIS

Microextraction factors	Evaluated range	Optimized value
Amount of [Hmim][PF$_6$] ionic liquid (mg)	10-120	55
Amount of common ion (NaPF$_6$) (mg)	0-300	180
pH	1-8	3
Temperature (°C)	30-70	40
Centrifugation rate (rpm)	1000-6000	4000
Centrifugation time (min)	> 2	5
Instrumental factors	**Evaluated range**	**Optimized value**
Suction time (s)	0.1-3	0.4
Transferring time (s)	0.1-3	1
Delay time (s)	0.1-4	2
Excitation wavelength (nm)	200-400	320 ± 5
Emission wavelength (nm)	410-700	455 ± 5
Excitation and emission slit widths (nm)	5-20	10

Table 3 Determination of PXM in real samples using TCIL-DLPME-SFIS[a]

Sample	Added (µg l^{-1})	Found (µg l^{-1})	Recovery (%)	RSD (%)
Human plasma	0.0	-	-	-
	5.0	4.8	96	4.0
	75.0	73.2	97.6	3.3
	150.0	148.3	98.9	3.9
Human urine	0.0	-	-	-
	5.0	5.2	104	3.0
	75.0	72.8	97.1	3.1
	150.0	144.0	96	4.3
Prioxicam capsule	0.0	9.6	-	-
	5.0	14.3	97.9	3.9
	75.0	80.6	95.3	3.2
	150.0	147.1	98.1	3.0
Prioxicam tablet	0.0	9.7	-	-
	5	14.0	95.2	4.2
	75.0	80.9	95.5	3.0
	150.0	146.3	97.5	4.7

[a] The illustrated results correspond to the average of three independent measurements.

shows the calibration slope. By this way, the LOD found was 0.046 µg l^{-1}. In order to define the repeatability of the designed system, four 75 µg l^{-1} standard solutions of PXM were analyzed and by this way the relative standard deviation (RSD) was 3.1%.

Analysis of PXM in real samples

The analytical applicability of the designed TCIL-DLPME-SFIS was tested by the quantitation of PXM in the spiked human urine and spiked human plasma. These data are summarized in Table 3. These tests revealed that the mean recoveries of PXM in studied real biological samples were in the range of 96–103% and 95.2-104% for plasma and urine samples, respectively. The obtained data demonstrated the acceptable accuracy and precision of the designed methodology. In the next experiments, the proposed technique was utilized for the

Table 2 Analytical performance of the proposed methodology

Analytical parameter	Performance
Dynamic range (µg L^{-1})	0.2-150
Correlation coefficient (R^2)	0.9992
LOD[a] (µg L^{-1})	0.046
RSD[b] (%) (n = 4) (C$_{PXM}$ = 75 µg L^{-1})	3.1
PF[c] (C$_{PXM}$ = 75 µg L^{-1})	31.2
Sample volume (mL)	10
Temperature (°C)	40

[a] Limit of detection.
[b] Relative standard deviation.
[c] Preconcentration factor.

quantitation of PXM in pharmaceutical formulations including tablets and capsules. The obtained data are shown in Table 3. The recent data show the validity of the designed TCIL-DLPME-SFIS for the determination of PXM in pharmaceutical formulations.

Conclusion

In this study, a benign and simple sample enrichment method called temperature- controlled ionic liquid dispersive liquid phase microextraction (TCIL-DLPME) was followed by stopped-flow injection spectrofluorimetry (SFIS) for quantitation of piroxicam in pharmaceutical and biological samples. Ionic liquid was used an extractor instead of toxic solvents, in order to protect the environment against harmful material and provide a better safety for chemists during the experiments. Traditional sample enrichment methods based on the application of ionic liquid suffer from some limitations such as the dependence of extraction efficiency on ionic strength values. To remove the latter problem, the microextraction procedure was assisted by a common ion of extractor. The application of stopped-flow injection mode makes it possible to increase the speed of quantitative measurements, decrease the required enriched phase and provide a better reproducibility and automation. Fluorimetry was applied as a determination technique because of some advantages including good selectivity and sensitivity, low cost of analysis and high response speed. For quality control of PXM, the present methodology is an efficient, benign, simple and inexpensive analytical tool.

Competing interests
The authors declare that they have no competing interests.

Authors' contributions
All authors contributed equally. All authors read and approved the final manuscript.

Acknowledgment
Support of this investigation by the Islamic Azad University Tehran south branch through grant is gratefully acknowledged.

Author details
[1]Department of Applied Chemistry, Faculty of science, Islamic Azad University, South Tehran Branch, Tehran, Iran. [2]Center of Excellence in Electrochemistry, Faculty of Chemistry, University of Tehran, Tehran, Iran.

References
1. Banerjee R, Chakraborty H, Sarkar M: Photophysical studies of oxicam group of NSAIDs: piroxicam, meloxicam and tenoxicam. *Spectrochim Acta Part A* 2003, **59**:1213–1222.
2. Kormosh ZA, Hunka IP, Bazel YR: Spectrophotometric determination of piroxicam. *J Anal Chem* 2011, **66**:378–383.
3. Gholivand MB, Karimian N: Development of piroxicam sensor based on molecular imprinted polymer modified carbon paste electrode. *Mat Sci Eng C* 2011, **31**:1844–1851.
4. Nakamura A, Nakashima MN, Wada M, Nakashima K: Semi-micro column HPLC of three oxicam non-steroidal anti-inflammatory drugs in human blood. *Bunseki Kagaku* 2005, **54**:755–760.
5. Chen ZL, Wu SM: Capillary zone electrophoresis for simultaneous determination of seven nonsteroidal anti-inflammatory drugs in pharmaceuticals. *Anal Bioanal Chem* 2005, **381**:907–912.
6. Ji HY, Lee HW, Kim YH, Jeong DW, Lee HS: Simultaneous determinations of piroxicam, meloxicam and tenoxicam in human plasma by liquid chromatography with tandem mass spectrometry. *J Chromatogr B* 2005, **826**:214–219.
7. Amin AS: Spectrophotometric determination of piroxicam and tenoxicam in pharmaceutical formulations using alizarin. *J Pharm Biomed Anal* 2002, **29**:729–736.
8. Kormosh Z, Hunka I, Bazel Y, Matviychuk O: Potentiometric determination of ketoprofen and piroxicam at a new PVC electrode based on ion associates of Rhodamine 6G. *Mat Sci Eng C* 2010, **30**:997–1002.
9. Pandey S: Analytical applications of room-temperature ionic liquids: a review of recent efforts. *Anal Chim Acta* 2006, **556**:38–45.
10. Berton P, Martinis EM, Martinezc LD, Wuilloud RG: Room temperature ionic liquid-based microextraction for vanadium species separation and determination in water samples by electrothermal atomic absorption spectrometry. *Anal Chim Acta* 2009, **640**:40–46.
11. Yao C, Anderson JL: Dispersive liquid-liquid microextraction using an in situ metathesis reaction to form an ionic liquid extraction phase for the preconcentration of aromatic compounds from water. *Anal Bioanal Chem* 2009, **395**:1491–1502.
12. Yao C, Li T, Wu P, Pitner WR, Anderson JL: Selective extraction of emerging contaminants from water samples by dispersive liquid-liquid microextraction using functionalized ionic liquids. *J Chromatogr A* 2011, **1218**:1556–1566.
13. Gharehbaghi M, Shemirani F, Baghdadi M: Dispersive liquid-liquid microextraction based on ionic liquid and spectrophotometric determination of mercury in water samples. *Int J Environ Anal Chem* 2009, **89**:21–33.
14. Baghdadi M, Shemirani F: Cold-induced aggregation microextraction: a novel sample preparation technique based on ionic liquids. *Anal Chim Acta* 2008, **613**:56–63.
15. Zhou QX, Bai HH, Xie GH, Xiao JP: Temperature-controlled ionic liquid dispersive liquid phase micro-extraction. *J Chromatogr A* 2008, **1177**:43–49.
16. Zeeb M, Ganjali MR, Norouzi P, Kalaei MR: Separation and preconcentration system based on microextraction with ionic liquid for determination of copper in water and food samples by stopped-flow injection spectrofluorimetry. *Food Chem Toxicol* 2011, **49**:1086–1091.
17. Zeeb M, Sadeghi M: Modified ionic liquid cold-induced aggregation dispersive liquid-liquid microextraction followed by atomic absorption spectrometry for trace determination of zinc in water and food samples. *Microchim Acta* 2011, **175**:159–165.
18. Zeeb M, Ganjali MR, Norouzi P: Modified ionic liquid cold-induced aggregation dispersive liquid-liquid microextraction combined with spectrofluorimetry for trace determination of ofloxacin in pharmaceutical and biological samples. *DARU* 2011, **19**:446–454.
19. Zeeb M, Ganjali MR, Norouzi P: Preconcentration and trace determination of chromium using modified ionic liquid cold-induced aggregation dispersive liquid-liquid microextraction: application to different water and food samples. *Food Anal Method.* in press.
20. Takacs-Novzk K, Tam KY: Multiwavelength spectrophotometric determination of acid dissociation constants-Part V: microconstants and tautomeric ratios of diprotic amphoteric drugs. *J Pharm Biomed Anal* 2000, **21**:1171.

Effects of rutin on acrylamide-induced neurotoxicity

Vahideh Sadat Motamedshariaty[1], Sara Amel Farzad[1], Marjan Nassiri-Asl[2] and Hossein Hosseinzadeh[3*]

Abstract

Background: Rutin is an important flavonoid that is consumed in the daily diet. The cytoprotective effects of rutin, including antioxidative, and neuroprotective have been shown in several studies. Neurotoxic effects of acrylamide (ACR) have been established in humans and animals. In this study, the protective effects of rutin in prevention and treatment of neural toxicity of ACR were studied.

Results: Rutin significantly reduced cell death induced by ACR (5.46 mM) in time- and dose-dependent manners. Rutin treatment decreased the ACR-induced cytotoxicity significantly in comparison to control (P <0.01, P < 0.001). Rutin (100 and 200 mg/kg) could prevent decrease of body weight in rats. In combination treatments with rutin (50, 100 and 200 mg/kg), vitamin E (200 mg/kg) and ACR, gait abnormalities significantly decreased in a dose-dependent manner (P < 0.01 and P < 0.001). The level of malondialdehyde significantly decreased in the brain tissue of rats in both preventive and therapeutic groups that received rutin (100 and 200 mg/kg).

Conclusion: It seems that rutin could be effective in reducing neurotoxicity and the neuroprotective effect of it might be mediated via antioxidant activity.

Keywords: Rutin, Acrylamide, MTT assay, Neural toxicity, Antioxidant

Introduction

Risk factors in food are either of chemical or microbiological origin, or a combination of both. Acrylamide (ACR), one such risk factor, is a possible human carcinogen [1]. It is an industrial chemical and has been known as an occupational hazard for decades [2,3]. However, in recent years, ACR has been found to form in fried and baked starchy foods during cooking [4,5]. This latter finding has greatly raised public concerns over ACR's potential health risk due to dietary exposure to people. ACR is a neurotoxic chemical and can cause peripheral and central neuropathy in humans and laboratory animals [6].

Early morphological studies suggested that both human and experimental neurotoxicities were mediated by cerebellar Purkinje cell injury and by degeneration of distal axons in the peripheral (PNS) and central nervous system (CNS) [7]. In addition to neurotoxicity, considerable experimental data from rodent studies has shown that ACR induces reproductive toxicity (e.g. reduced litter size) and genotoxic effects (e.g. DNA strand breaks, dominant lethal mutation) [3,8,9]. There are several reports that antioxidant agents could rescue neurotoxicity induced by ACR via increasing antioxidant activity [10-14].

Rutin (3, 3′, 4′, 5, 7 -pentahydroxyflavone-3-rhamnoglucoside) is a flavonoid of the flavonol type that is found in many typical plants, such as buckwheat, passion flower, apple and tea. It is also an important dietary constituent of foods and plant-based beverages [15]. Rutin has several pharmacological properties, including antioxidant, anticarcinogenic, cytoprotective, vasoprotective, cardioprotective and neuroprotective activities [16-23]. In humans, it attaches to the iron ion (Fe), preventing it from binding to hydrogen peroxide, which would otherwise create a highly reactive free radical that may damage cells [24].

The present study was therefore designed to investigate the protective effects of rutin in prevention and treatment of neural toxicity induced by ACR.

* Correspondence: hosseinzadehh@mums.ac.ir
[3]Pharmacodynamics and Toxicological Department, Pharmaceutical Research Center, School of Pharmacy, Mashhad University of Medical Sciences, Mashhad, Iran
Full list of author information is available at the end of the article

Materials and methods

Materials

RPMI 1640 and FBS were purchased from Gibco. (4,5-dimethylthiazol-2-yl)-2, 5-diphenyl tetrazolium (MTT), rutin hydrate ≥94% (HPLC), TBA (2-thiobarbituric acid), n-butanol, potassium chloride, phosphoric acid and ACR were obtained from Merck. Vitamin E was purchased in injectable form from Osveh Company, Iran.

Cell culture

PC12 cells were obtained from Pasteur Institute (Tehran, Iran). Cells were maintained at 37°C in a humidified atmosphere (90%) containing 5% CO_2. Cells were grown in RPMI 1640 medium supplemented with 10% (v/v) heat-inactivated foetal bovine serum, 100 U/ml penicillin and 100 μg /ml streptomycin.

Cell viability

The viability of cultured cells was determined by assaying the reduction of 3-(4,5-dimethyl thiazol-2-yl)-2,5- diphenyl tetrazolium bromide (MTT) to formazan [25]. Briefly, PC12 cells were cultured in a 96-well microliter plate at a density of 5000 cell/well. After pretreatment with rutin (0.5, 1, 1.5, 2.5, 5, 10, 20, 40, 80 and 160 μM/ml) for 24 h, ACR at concentration of 5.46 mM was added to each well. The cells were then incubated for 48 h and then treated with MTT solution (0.5 mg/ml PBS) for 1 h at 37°C. Upper mediate replaced with dimethyl sulfoxide (DMSO). The absorbance was measured at 570 nm (630 nm as reference) in a plate reader (TECAN infinit M200) [14].

Experimental animals

Male Wistar rats (200–270 g) were housed in colony rooms with 12/12 h light/dark cycle at 21 ± 2°C and had free access to food and water. All animal experiments were carried out in accordance with Mashhad University of Medical Sciences, Ethical committee Acts.

Experimental design

To induce neurotoxicity in rats, the animals were exposed to ACR at a daily dose of 50 mg/kg intraperitoneally (i.p.) [26]. All doses of rutin were selected as our previous work [18]. This daily dose and the corresponding route have been well characterized with respect to neuropathological expression and neurological deficits. For our study on the preventive effect, the rats were divided at random into 7 groups (n = 6 in each group) and treatment was given as follows:

1) Saline (negative control) for 14 days
2) ACR (50 mg/kg, i.p.) for 14 days
3) Rutin (50 mg/kg, i.p.) for 3 days alone and afterward rutin (50 mg/kg, i.p.) + ACR (50 mg/kg, i.p.) for 11 days

4) Rutin (100 mg/kg, i.p.) for 3 days alone and afterward rutin (100 mg/kg, i.p.) + ACR (50 mg/kg, i.p.) for 11 days
5) Rutin (200 mg/kg, i.p.) for 3 days alone and afterward rutin (200 mg/kg, i.p.) + ACR (50 mg/kg, i.p.) for 11 days
6) Rutin (200 mg/kg, i.p.) for 14 days
7) Vitamin E (200 mg/kg, i.p.) (positive control) for 3 days alone and afterward vitamin E (200 mg/kg, i.p.) + ACR (50 mg/kg, i.p.) for 11 days

Behavioural testing to assess preventive effects was performed on the 15th day [14].

After studying doses of rutin in preventing neurotoxicity, the most effective dose was used to assess its therapeutic effect. For our study, the rats were divided at random into 5 groups (n = 6 in each group) and treatment was given as follows:

1) Normal saline (negative control) for 14 days
2) ACR (50 mg/kg, i.p.) for 3 days alone and afterward ACR (50 mg/kg, i.p.) + rutin (200 mg/kg, i.p.) for 11 days
3) ACR (50 mg/kg, i.p.) for 3 days alone and afterward ACR (50 mg/kg, i.p.) + vitamin E (200 mg/kg, i.p.) for 11 days
4) ACR (50 mg/kg i.p.) for 7 days alone and afterward ACR (50 mg/kg, i.p.) + rutin (200 mg/kg i.p.) for 7 days
5) ACR (50 mg/kg i.p.) for 7 days alone and afterward ACR (50 mg/kg, i.p.) + vitamin E (200 mg/kg, i.p.) for 7 days

Behavioural testing was performed on the 15th day [14].

The behavioural index (gait scores) examination

After completion of treatment, the rats were placed in a clear plexiglass box and were observed for 3 min. Following observation, a gait score was assigned from 1 to 4, where 1 = a normal, unaffected gait; 2 = a slightly affected gait (foot splay, slight hind limb weakness and spread); 3 = a moderately affected gait (foot splay, moderate hind limb weakness, moderate limb spread during ambulation) and 4 = a severely affected gait (foot splay, severe hind limb weakness, dragging hind limbs, inability to rear) [27].

Biochemical assay

Furthermore, a test was conducted to determine lipid peroxidation by determining thiobarbituric acid reactive products (TBAR) of lipid peroxidation in brain tissue of rats [28,29]. Malondialdehyde (MDA) is the final product of lipid peroxidation and its complex with TBA is red and has maximum absorbance at 532 nm; MDA was assessed as the lipid peroxidation indicator. Briefly, the brain tissue was homogenized in cold KCl solution (1.5%) to obtain a homogenous suspension (10%). To a 10-ml tube, 0.5 ml of suspension was poured and 3 ml

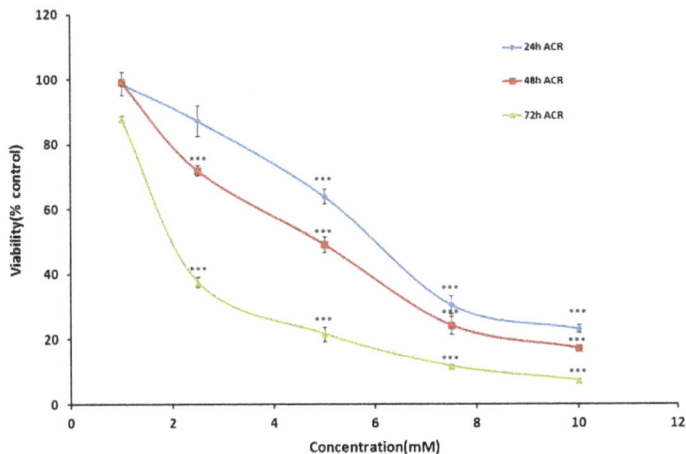

Figure 1 Cell viability of PC12 cells after exposure to different concentrations of acrylamide (ACR) for 24, 48 and 72 h. Cell viability was determined by MTT test. Data are expressed as mean ± SEM of 6 separate experiments. ACR was solubilised in PBS. For control cells PBS was used. ***$P < 0.001$ vs. control cells.

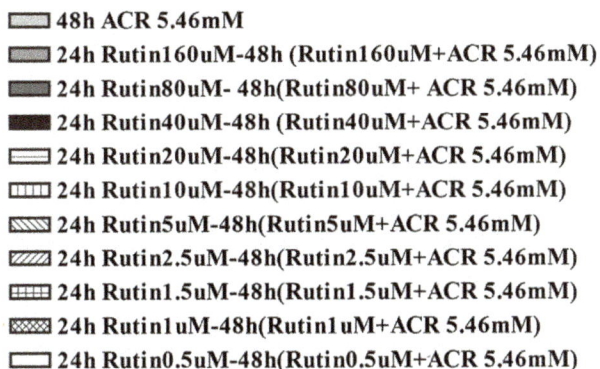

Figure 2 Effect of rutin on ACR-induced cytotoxicity in PC12 cells. Cells were pretreated with different concentration of rutin (0.5, 1, 1.5, 2.5, 5, 10, 20, 40, 80 and 160 μM/ml) for 24 h and ACR (5.46 mM) was added to each well later, followed by evaluation of cell viability using MTT assay. Data are expressed as the mean ± SEM of 6 separate experiments (n = 6). **$P < 0.01$, ***$P < 0.001$ vs. ACR-treated cells.

phosphoric acid (1%) and 1 ml TBA were added, following which the tube was placed in a boiling water bath for 45 min. Then, the suspension was cooled, 4 ml n-butanol added and the tube placed in vortex for complex mixing (1 min). Following this, the suspension was centrifuged (20000 rpm speed, 20 minutes) to separate the red-coloured upper phase and its absorbance was determined using the spectrophotometer. The standard curve for MDA (0–40 μM) was prepared [30].

Statistical analysis

Results are expressed as mean ± SEM. For in vitro assay, IC_{50} values were calculated using the method described by Litchfield and Wilcoxon method (PHARM/PCS software version 4). Statistical analyses were performed with ANOVA followed by the Tukey–Kramer test to compare the differences between means. Differences were considered statistically significant when P < 0.05.

Results

Effect of ACR in PC12 cells

The PC12 cells were treated with different concentration of ACR for 24, 48 and 72 h. Following this, the cell viability was measured using MTT test. Treatment of cells with ACR decreased viability in time- and dose-dependent manners, as shown in Figure 1. The IC_{50} (50% inhibitory concentration) value for treatment of PC12 cells with ACR for 48 h was 5.46 mM.

Effect of rutin on ACR-induced cytotoxicity in PC12 cells

PC12 cells were treated with different concentrations of rutin (0.5, 1, 1.5, 2.5, 5, 10, 20, 40, 80 and 160 μM/ml) for 24 h and then ACR (5.46 mM) was added to each well, followed by evaluation of cell viability using MTT assay. Rutin treatment decreased the ACR-induced cytotoxicity significantly in comparison to control (Figure 2).

Effect of ACR on rat body weight and the protective effect of rutin

The body weight of the ACR group decreased 33.6% after 14-day exposure to ACR (Figure 3). Treatment with rutin at a dose of 50 mg/kg failed to prevent weight loss caused by ACR. Therefore, body weight decreased after 14 days. However, rutin at doses of 100 and 200 mg/kg prevented decrease of body weight in rats. Vitamin E

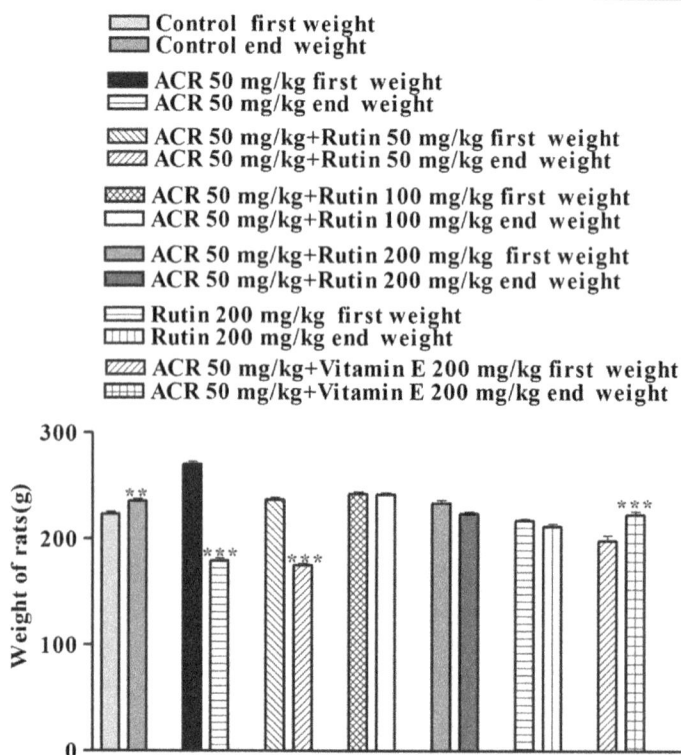

Figure 3 Protective effect of rutin (after 14 days of ACR exposure) by comparison between the initial and end weight of rats. Data are expressed as mean ± SEM, (n = 6), **P < 0.01, ***P < 0.001 vs. first weight of each group treated with drugs.

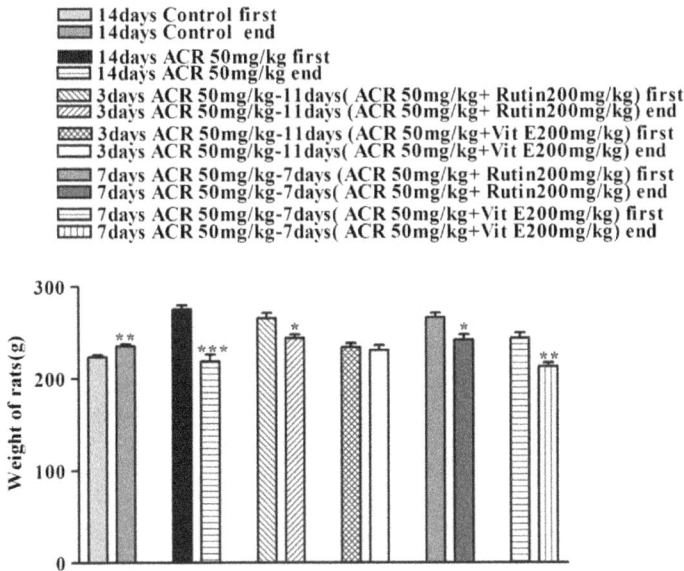

Figure 4 Therapeutic effect of rutin (after 14 days of ACR exposure) by comparison between the initial and end weight of rats.
Data are expressed as mean ± SEM, (n = 6). *P < 0.05, **P < 0.01, ***P < 0.001 vs. first weight of each group treated with drugs.

(200 mg/kg) increased the body weight in rats (P < 0.001) (Figure 3).

Effect of ACR on rat body weight and the therapeutic effect of rutin

In the control group, only the body weight increased after 14 days compared with the first weight (P < 0.01). In other groups, the body weight significantly decreased compared with the first weight. However, in the group administered vitamin E, there was no significant change in body weight after 3 days (Figure 4).

Effect of ACR on the behavioural index (gait scores) in rats and the protective effect of rutin

Exposure to ACR (50 mg/kg, i.p.) for 14 days led to progressive gait abnormalities in rats, as shown in Figure 5. In groups of rats that were treated with combination of rutin (50, 100 and 200 mg/kg), vitamin E (200 mg/kg)

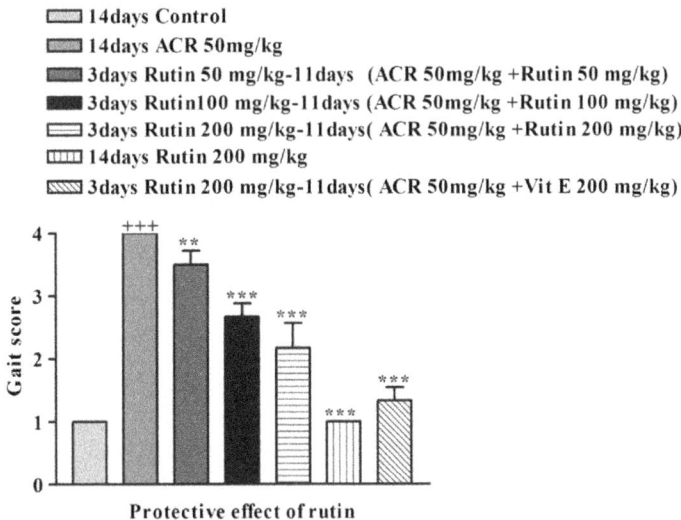

Figure 5 Protective effect of rutin on behavioural index (gait scores) in rats during treatment with ACR (50 mg/ kg, i.p.) for 14 days.
Data are expressed as the mean ± SEM, (n = 6). +++P < 0.001 vs. control, *P < 0.05 **P < 0.01, ***P < 0.001 vs. ACR-treated animals.

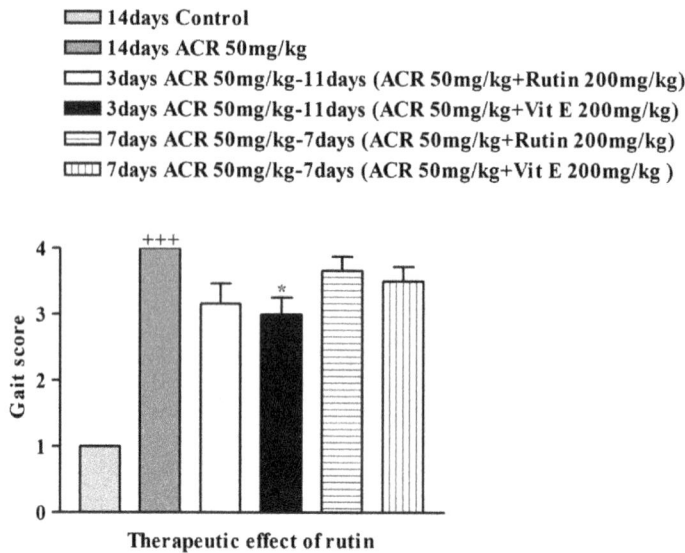

Figure 6 Therapeutic effect of rutin on behavioural index (gait scores) in rats during treatment with ACR (50 mg/ kg, i.p.) for 14 days. Data are expressed as the mean ± SEM, (n = 6). +++P < 0.001 vs. control, *P < 0.05 vs. ACR-treated animals.

and ACR, gait abnormalities significantly decreased in a dose-dependent manner (P < 0.01 and P < 0.001 vs. ACR-treated group) (Figure 5).

Effect of ACR on the behavioural index (gait scores) in rats and the therapeutic effect of rutin

The groups in which the therapeutic effect of rutin were evaluated, ACR was administered to the animals for 3 and 7 days and then treated 11 and 7 days with rutin and vitamin E with combination of ACR, respectively. In all groups, gait abnormalities decreased but the effect of vitamin E was only significant compared with ACR after 3 days treatment (P < 0.05) (Figure 6).

Effect of rutin in biochemical assay

There was an increase in the MDA levels following ACR administration compared with the control group (P < 0.001). The MDA levels significantly reduced dose dependently in all groups that were administrated rutin for preventive and therapeutic purposes (except on administration of 50 mg/kg rutin) (Tables 1 and 2).

Discussion

In this study, the neuroprotective effect of rutin on ACR-induced cytotoxicity in PC12 cells and ACR-induced neurotoxicity in rats was evaluated. Results showed that ACR could decrease cell viability in PC12 cells, which was

Table 1 Protective effect of rutin on lipid peroxidation following ACR administration

Groups	MDA concentration (nmol/g) tissue
14 days Control	45.75 ± 3.92
14 days ACR 50 mg/kg	92.58 ± 3.69+++
14 days Rutin 200 mg/kg	75.52 ± 2.55***
3 days Rutin 50 mg/kg-11 days (ACR 50 mg/kg + Rutin 50 mg/kg)	69.39 ± 4.26
3 days Rutin 100 mg/kg-11 days (ACR 50 mg/kg + Rutin 100 mg/kg)	49.7 ± 7.77*
3 days Rutin 200 mg/kg-11 days (ACR 50 mg/kg + Rutin 200 mg/kg)	47.76 ± 3.05***
3 days Vit E 200 mg/kg-11 days (ACR 50 mg/kg + Vit E 200 mg/kg)	52.67 ± 4.38***

Values are mean ± SEM (n = 6). +++P < 0.001 vs. control, *P < 0.05, ***P < 0.001 vs. ACR-treated animals.

Table 2 Therapeutic effect of rutin on lipid peroxidation following ACR administration

Groups	MDA concentration (nmol/g) tissue
14 days Control	45.75 ± 3.92
14 days ACR 50 mg/kg	92.58 ± 3.69+++
3 days ACR 50 mg/kg-11 days (ACR 50 mg/kg + Rutin 200 mg/kg)	65.10 ± 5.03**
3 days ACR 50 mg/kg-11 days (ACR 50 mg/kg + Vit E 200 mg/kg)	60.75 ± 3.46***
7 days ACR 50 mg/kg-7 days (ACR 50 mg/kg + Rurin 200 mg/kg)	69.67 ± 5.630*
7 days ACR 50 mg/kg-7 days (ACR 50 mg/kg + Vit E 200 mg/kg)	68.87 ± 5.14*

Values are mean ± SEM (n = 6). +++P < 0.001 vs. control, *P < 0.05, **P < 0.01, ***P < 0.001 vs. ACR-treated animals.

suppressed by administration of rutin. Also, rutin significantly inhibited behavioural index changes and body weight loss caused by ACR administration in rats. Also, the MDA levels significantly reduced in all groups of rutin.

ACR is known to induce apoptosis in time- and dose-dependent manners in neurons and astrocytes and significantly reduce the proliferation of neural progenitor cells and, in high concentrations [31]. In our study, ACR (5.46 mM) decreased cell viability in PC12 cells and pretreatment with rutin (0.5, 1, 1.5, 2.5, 5, 10, 20 and 40 µM/ml) increased the cell viability. According to previous studies, reactive oxygen species (ROS) have important role in the toxicity of ACR [31,32].

Antioxidant effects of rutin have been established in several studies [23,33]. Rutin and catechol-compounds are electron donors, and antioxidant activities of rutin and catechol and its derivatives indicate that they are potential antioxidants [34,35]. It seems that the protective effect of rutin in this model may be at least, in part, due to suppression of ROS generation because rutin has exhibited antioxidant effect in different studies [36].

ACR monomer is a potent neurotoxin and capable of inducing CNS and PNS damages in humans and animals. ACR induces ataxia, skeletal muscle weakness and weight loss in both occupationally exposed humans and experimental animal models [26,37]. Our results showed that treatment of animals with ACR (50 mg/kg, i.p.) for 11 days decreased body weight and caused gait abnormalities, and at the end of 14 days, ACR-exposed animals displayed severe abnormal gait (scores 4), but treatment of animals with rutin prevented the decrease in body weight and reduced abnormal gait.

In recent decades, there are several studies that have shown the neuroprotective effects of rutin [38-40]. Rutin has neuroprotective effect in brain ischemia and its administration attenuates ischemic neural apoptosis by inhibition of neurological deficit, lipid peroxidation, p53 expression and increase in endogenous antioxidant defence enzymes [41]. It was shown that the 4-oxo group and the 2,3 double bond in the C ring are common in rutin and that it may be related by its neuroprotective action [42]. Rutin has beneficial effects on hypoxic, glutamate and oxidative stress at concentrations as low as 1 nM on retinal ganglion cell. It appears that the sugar side chain of flavonoids may be important for neuroprotective activities [43].

The neuroprotective effect of vitamin E is related to its antioxidant activity [44,45]. For this reason, vitamin E was used was as a positive control in protection against ACR- induced neurotoxicity. As our results, vitamin E (200 mg/kg) increased the body weight compared to rutin as a preventive agent in rats.

It seems that the effect of vitamin E in the presence of ACR after 3 days treatment in inhibition of gait abnormalities is more than rutin (200 mg/kg). However, the protective and therapeutic effects of rutin (200 mg/kg) on lipid peroxidation following ACR administration are same as vitamin E (200 mg/kg).

It is possible that rutin by inhibiting neurological deficit could improve behavioral index of animals. Moreover, it was shown that rutin might be effective in treatment of tardive dyskinesia, an extrapyramidal movement disorder, through communicating the imbalance of dopaminergic transmission [46]. Pretreatment of rutin (100 and 200 mg/kg/day) for long-term caused behavioural and neurochemical changes in aged WAG male rats. It is possible that rutin may exert this effect by affecting brain dopaminergic and adrenergic systems [47]. Thus, there is another possibility that rutin could improve behavioral index of animals via modulating dopaminergic and adrenergic transmissions.

The results of the current study suggested that protective effect of rutin against ACR cytotoxicity in PC12 cells and rats was due to inhibition of ROS production in PC12 cells exposed to ACR or in the rat nervous system under ACR treatment.

Competing interests
The authors declare that they have no competing interests.

Authors' contribution
HH, designed the study, conducted, supervised experiment and prepared manuscript. SAF and VMS, conducted experiment and prepared manuscript. MNA, prepared manuscript. All authors read and approve the final manuscript.

Acknowledgments
The authors are thankful to the Vice Chancellor of Research, Mashhad University of Medical Sciences for financial support.

Author details
[1]Pharmaceutical Research Center, School of Pharmacy, Mashhad University of Medical Sciences, Mashhad, Iran. [2]Cellular and Molecular Research Centre, Department of Pharmacology, School of Medicine, Qazvin University of Medical Sciences, Qazvin, Iran. [3]Pharmacodynamics and Toxicological Department, Pharmaceutical Research Center, School of Pharmacy, Mashhad University of Medical Sciences, Mashhad, Iran.

References
1. Wenzl T, De La Calle MB, Anklam E: Analytical methods for the determination of acrylamide in food products: a review. *Food Addit Contam* 2003, 20:885–902.
2. Bull RA, Hansman GS, Clancy LE, Tanaka MM, Rawlinson WD, White PA: Norovirus recombination in ORF1/ORF2 overlap. *Emerg Infect Dis* 2005, 11:1079–1085.
3. Tyl RW, Friedman MA: Effects of acrylamide on rodent reproductive performance. *Reprod Toxicol* 2003, 17:1–13.
4. Rosén J, Hellenäs KE: Analysis of acrylamide in cooked foods by liquid chromatography tandem mass spectrometry. *Analyst* 2002, 127:880–882.
5. Tareke E, Rydberg P, Karlsson P, Eriksson S, Törnqvist M: Analysis of acrylamide, a carcinogen formed in heated foodstuffs. *J Agric Food Chem* 2002, 50:4998–5006.
6. Barber DS, LoPachin RM: Proteomic analysis of acrylamide-protein adduct formation in rat brain synaptosomes. *Toxicol Appl Pharmacol* 2004, 201:120–136.

7. Cavanagh J, Nolan CC: Selective loss of Purkinje cells from the rat cerebellum caused by acrylamide and the responses of β-glucuronidase and β-galactosidase. *Acta Neuropathol* 1982, 58:210–214.

8. Sega GA, Alcota RP, Tancongco CP, Brimer PA: Acrylamide binding to the DNA and protamine of spermiogenic stages in the mouse and its relationship to genetic damage. *Mutat Res* 1989, 216:221–230.

9. Working PK, Bentley KS, Hurtt ME, Mohr KL: Comparison of the dominant lethal effects of acrylonitrile and acrylamide in male Fischer 344 rats. *Mutagenesis* 1987, 2:215–220.

10. Xichun Z, Min'ai Z: Protective role of dark soy sauce against acrylamide-induced neurotoxicity in rats by antioxidative activity. *Toxicol Mech Methods* 2009, 19:369–374.

11. Alturfan AA, Tozan-Beceren A, Sehirli AO, Demiralp E, Sener G, Omurtag GZ: Resveratrol ameliorates oxidative DNA damage and protects against acrylamide-induced oxidative stress in rats. *Mol Biol Rep* 2012, 39:4589–4596.

12. Shinomol GK, Raghunath N, Bharath MM, Muralidhara M: Prophylaxis with Bacopa monnieri attenuates acrylamide induced neurotoxicity and oxidative damage via elevated antioxidant function. *Cent Nerv Syst Agents Med Chem* 2013, 13(1):3–12.

13. Mehri S, Abnous K, Mousavi SH, Shariaty VM, Hosseinzadeh H: Neuroprotective Effect of Crocin on Acrylamide-induced Cytotoxicity in PC12 cells. *Cell Mol Neurobiol* 2012, 32:227–235.

14. Hosseinzadeh H, Tabeshpur J, Mehri S: Effect of Saffron extract on Acrylamide- induced toxicity: In vitro and in vivo assessment. *Chin J Integr Med* 2014. In Press.

15. Kuntić V, Pejić N, Ivković B, Vujić Z, Ilić K, Mićić S, Vukojević V: Isocratic RP-HPLC method for rutin determination in solid oral dosage forms. *J Pharm Biomed Anal* 2007, 43:718–721.

16. Javed H, Khan MM, Ahmad A, Vaibhav K, Ahmad ME, Khan A, Ashafaq M, Islam F, Siddiqui MS, Safhi MM, Islam F: Rutin prevents cognitive impairments by ameliorating oxidative stress and neuroinflammation in rat model of sporadic dementia of Alzheimer type. *Neuroscience* 2012, 17:340–352.

17. Richetti SK, Blank M, Capiotti KM, Piato AL, Bogo MR, Vianna MR, Bonan CD: Quercetin and rutin prevent scopolamine-induced memory impairment in zebrafish. *Behav Brain Res* 2011, 217:10–15.

18. Nassiri-Asl M, Mortazavi SR, Samiee-Rad F, Zangivand AA, Safdari F, Saroukhani S, Abbasi E: The effects of rutin on the development of pentylenetetrazole kindling and memory retrieval in rats. *Epilepsy Behav* 2010, 18:50–53.

19. Mellou F, Loutrari H, Stamatis H, Roussos C, Kolisis FN: Enzymatic esterification of flavonoids with unsaturated fatty acids: effect of the novel esters on vascular endothelial growth factor release from K562 cells. *Process Biochem* 2006, 41:2029–3204.

20. Trumbeckaite S, Bernatoniene J, Majiene D, Jakstas V, Savickas A, Toleikis A: The effect of flavonoids on rat heart mitochondrial function. *Biomed Pharmacother* 2006, 60:245–248.

21. Schwedhelm E, Maas R, Troost R, Böger RH: Clinical pharmacokinetics of antioxidants and their impact on systemic oxidative stress. *Clin Pharmacokinet* 2003, 42:437–459.

22. Janbaz KH, Saeed SA, Gilani AH: Protective effect of rutin on paracetamol and CCl4-induced hepatotoxicity in rodents. *Fitoterapia* 2002, 73:557–563.

23. La Casa C, Villegas I, Alarcon de la Lastra C, Motilva V, Martin Calero MJ: Evidence for protective and antioxidant properties of rutin, a natural flavone, against ethanol induced gastric lesions. *J Ethnopharmacol* 2000, 71:45–53.

24. Afanas'ev IB, Dorozhko AI, Brodskii AV, Kostyuk VA, Potapovitch AI: Chelating and free radical scavenging mechanisms of inhibitory action of rutin and quercetin in lipid peroxidation. *Biochem Pharmacol* 1989, 38:1763–1769.

25. Mousavi SH, Tavakkol-Afshari J, Brook A, Jafari-Anarkooli I: Role of caspases and Bax protein in saffron-induced apoptosis in MCF-7 cells. *Food Chem Toxicol* 2009, 47:1909–1913.

26. LoPachin RM: Acrylamide neurotoxicity: Neurological, morphological and molecular endpoints in animal models, in advances in experimental medicine and biology. *Adv Exp Med Biol* 2005, 561:21–37.

27. LoPachin RM, Ross JF, Reid ML, Das S, Mansukhani S, Lehning EJ: Neurological evaluation of toxic axonopathies in rats: Acrylamide and 2,5-hexanedione. *Neurotoxicology* 2002, 23:95–110.

28. Hosseinzadeh H, Hosseini A, Nassiri-Asl M, Sadeghnia HR: Effect of *Salvia leriifolia* Benth. root extracts on ischemia-reperfusion in rat skeletal muscle. *BMC Complement Altern Med* 2007, 7:23.

29. Unal D, Yeni E, Erel O, Bitiren M, Vural H: Antioxidative effects of exogenous nitric oxide versus antioxidant vitamins on renal ischemia reperfusion injury. *Urol Res* 2002, 30:190–194.

30. Hosseinzadeh H, Sadeghnia HR, Ziaee T, Danaee A: Protective effect of aqueous saffron extract (*Crocus sativus* L.) and crocin, its active constituent, on renal ischemia-reperfusion-induced oxidative damage in rats. *J Pharm Pharm Sci* 2005, 8:387–393.

31. Park HR, Kim MS, Kim SJ, Park M, Kong KH, Kim HS, Kwack SJ, Kang TS, Kim SH, Kim HS, Lee J: Acrylamide induces cell death in neural progenitor cells and impairs hippocampal neurogenesis. *Toxicol Lett* 2009, 193:86–93.

32. Yousef MI, El-Demerdash FM: Acrylamide-induced oxidative stress and biochemical perturbations in rats. *Toxicology* 2006, 219:133–141.

33. Kamalakkannan N, Stanely Mainzen Prince P: Rutin improves the antioxidant status in streptozotocin-induced diabetic rat tissues. *Mol Cell Biochem* 2006, 293:211–219.

34. Anbazhagan V, Kalaiselvan A, Jaccob M, Venuvanalingam P, Renganathan R: Investigations on the fluorescence quenching of 2,3-diazabicyclo [2.2.2]oct-2-ene by certain flavonoids. *J Photochem Photobiol B* 2008, 91:143–150.

35. Manivannan C, Sundaram KM, Renganathan R, Sundararaman M: Investigations on photoinduced interaction of 9-aminoacridine with certain catechols and rutin. *J Fluoresc* 2012, 22:1113–1125.

36. Becker EM, Ntouma G, Skibsted LH: Synergism between and antagonism between quercetin and other chain-breaking antioxidants in lipid systems of increasing structural organization. *Food Chem* 2007, 103:1288–1296.

37. Shipp A, Lawrence G, Gentry R, McDonald T, Bartow H, Bounds J, Macdonald N, Clewell H, Allen B, Van Landingham C: Acrylamide: review of toxicity data and dose–response analyses for cancer and noncancer effects. *Crit Rev Toxicol* 2006, 36:481–608.

38. Javed H, Khan MM, Ahmad A, Vaibhav K, Ahmad ME, Khan A, Ashafaq M, Islam F, Siddiqui MS, Safhi MM, Islam F: Rutin prevents cognitive impairments by ameliorating oxidative stress and neuroinflammation in rat model of sporadic dementia of Alzheimer type. *Neuroscience* 2012, 210:340–352.

39. Tongjaroenbuangam W, Ruksee N, Chantiratikul P, Pakdeenarong N, Kongbuntad W, Govitrapong P: Neuroprotective effects of quercetin, rutin and okra (Abelmoschus esculentus Linn.) in dexamethasone-treated mice. *Neurochem Int* 2011, 59:677–685.

40. Yang YC, Lin HY, Su KY, Chen CH, Yu YL, Lin CC, Yu SL, Yan HY, Su KJ, Chen YL: Rutin, a flavonoid that is a main component of Saussurea involucrata, attenuates the senescence effect in D-Galactose aging mouse model. *Evid Based Complement Alternat Med* 2012, 2012:980276.

41. Khan MM, Ahmad A, Ishrat T, Khuwaja G, Srivastawa P, Khan MB, Raza SS, Javed H, Vaibhav K, Khan A, Islam F: Rutin protects the neural damage induced by transient focal ischemia in rats. *Brain Res* 2009, 1292:123–135.

42. Pu F, Mishima K, Irie K, Motohashi K, Tanaka Y, Orito K, Egawa T, Kitamura Y, Egashira N, Iwasaki K, Fujiwara M: Neuroprotective effects of quercetin and rutin on spatial memory impairment in an 8-arm radial maze task and neuronal death induced by repeated cerebral ischemia in rats. *J Pharmacol Sci* 2007, 104:329–334.

43. Nakayama T, Yamada M, Osawa T, Kawakishi S: Suppression of active oxygen-induced cytotoxicity by flavonoids. *Biochem Pharmacol* 1993, 45:265–267.

44. Yun JS, Na HK, Park KS, Lee YH, Kim EY, Lee SY, Kim JI, Kang JH, Kim DS, Choi KH: Protective effects of vitamin E on endocrine disruptors, PCB-induced dopaminergic neurotoxicity. *Toxicology* 2005, 216:140–146.

45. Gümüştaş K, Meta Güzeyli FM, Atükeren P, Sanus GZ, Kemerdere R, Tanrıverdi T, Kaynar MY: The effect of vitamin E on lipid peroxidation, nitric oxide production and superoxide dismutase expression in hyperglycemic rats with ceberal ischemia- reperfusion injury. *Turk Neurosurg* 2007, 17:78–82.

46. Bishnoi M, Chopra K, Kulkarni SK: Protective effect of rutin, a polyphenolic flavonoid against haloperidol-induced orofacial dyskinesia and associated

behavioural, biochemical and neurochemical changes. *Fundam Clin Pharmacol* 2007, **21**:521–529.

47. Pyrzanowska J, Piechal A, Blecharz-Klin K, Joniec-Maciejak I, Zobel A, Widy-Tyszkiewicz E: Influence of long-term administration of rutin on spatial memory as well as the concentration of brain neurotransmitters in aged rats. *Pharmacol Rep* 2012, **64**:808–816.

Amitriptyline, clomipramine, and doxepin adsorption onto sodium polystyrene sulfonate

Akram Jamshidzadeh[1,2*], Fatemeh Vahedi[2], Omid Farshad[3], Hassan Seradj[4], Asma Najibi[2] and Gholamreza Dehghanzadeh[5]

Abstract

Purpose of the study: Comparative in vitro studies were carried out to determine the adsorption characteristics of 3 drugs on activated charcoal (AC) and sodium polystyrene sulfonate (SPS). Activated charcoal (AC) has been long used as gastric decontamination agent for tricyclic antidepressants (TCA).

Methods: Solutions containing drugs (amitriptyline, clomipramine, or doxepin) and variable amount of AC or SPS were incubated for 30 minutes.

Results: At pH 1.2 the adsorbent: drug mass ratio varied from 2 : 1 to 40 : 1 for AC, and from 0.4 : 1 to 8 : 1 for SPS. UV–VIS spectrophotometer was used for the determination of free drug concentrations. The qmax of amitriptyline was 0.055 mg/mg AC and 0.574 mg/mg SPS, qmax of clomipramine was 0.053 mg/mg AC and 0.572 mg/mg SPS, and qmax of doxepin was 0.045 mg/mg AC and 0.556 mg/mg SPS. The results of adsorption experiments with SPS revealed higher values for the qmax parameters in comparison with AC.

Conclusion: In vitro gastric decontamination experiments for antidepressant amitriptyline, clomipramine, and doxepin showed that SPS has higher qmax values than the corresponding experiments with AC. Therefore, we suggest SPS is a better gastric decontaminating agent for the management of acute TCA intoxication.

Keywords: Adsorption, Tricyclic antidepressants, Activated charcoal, Sodium polystyrene sulfonate

Introduction

Tricyclic antidepressant (TCA) drug poisoning is a common cause of death from prescription drug overdose. Treatment includes aggressive supportive care, activated charcoal oral administration, alkalinization therapy, and management of arrhythmias, hypotension and seizures [1,2]. Activated charcoal (AC) has been used for gastric decontamination over the last century. It prevents absorption of substances in the gastrointestinal tract; thereby decreasing systemic absorption of potentially toxic agents [3]. Large reductions in drug absorption occur when AC is administered soon after drug ingestion [4]. AC is recommended for the treatment of TCA poisoning [5-7].

Sodium polystyrene sulfonate (SPS) is a potassium-binding resin used for the treatment of hyperkalemia [8].

SPS is not absorbed from the gastrointestinal tract. As the resin passes through the gastrointestinal tract, the resin removes the potassium ions by exchanging it for sodium ions. In clinical practice, SPS is often mixed with cathartics such as sorbitol to prevent constipation, which is sometimes seen with SPS [9-11].

The purpose of this in vitro investigation is: (a) to determine whether SPS is effective for the adsorption of amitriptyline, clomipramine, and doxepin; (b) to show whether SPS is better than AC in decreasing the free drug concentrations of TCAs; and (c) to determine the time needed for the complete adsorption process.

Materials and methods
Apparatus
A Cecil, UV–VIS spectrophotometer (England) with 1 cm quartz cells was used for all absorbance measurements.

* Correspondence: ajamshid@sums.ac.ir
[1]Pharmaceutical Sciences Research Center, Shiraz University of Medical Sciences, Shiraz, Iran
[2]Department of Pharmacology and Toxicology, Faculty of pharmacy, Shiraz University of Medical Sciences, Shiraz, Iran
Full list of author information is available at the end of the article

Table 1 Adsorption parameters (qmax, affinity constant K and R²) of amitriptyline, clomipramine and doxepin onto activated charcoal (AC) and sodium polystyrene sulfonate (SPS)

		Langmuir isotherm method		
		qmax	K	R^2
	Amitriptyline	0.055	3.469	0.972
AC	Clomipramine	0.053	3.464	0.945
	Doxepin	0.045	0.777	0.956
	Amitriptyline	0.574	0.702	0.904
SPS	Clomipramine	0.572	0.492	0.975
	Doxepin	0.556	0.225	0.914

Chemicals and reagents

Amitriptyline and doxepin were obtained from Darou Pakhsh Pharmaceutical Company (Iran) and clomipramine was obtained from Shahre Darou Pharmaceutical Company (Iran). AC (Asche ~ 5%; Fe < 0.3%; Particle size 75% < 40 μ; Loss on drying ~ 10%) and SPS were obtained from Modava Pharmaceutical Company (Iran). All other chemicals were of analytical reagent grade purchased from Merck (Germany) unless otherwise specified. Distilled water was used to prepare all solutions. Acidic medium pH 1.2, simulating gastric environment was prepared by adding 12 M hydrochloric acid to water. The final pH was checked by pH meter and kept at 1.2 during the experiments.

Standards for calibration curve

Standard stock solutions of amitriptyline, clomipramine, and doxepin were prepared in distilled water at the concentration of 0.25 mg/ml. Working standard solutions were prepared by suitable dilution of standard stock solution with distilled water.

Solutions for adsorption experiments

The sixteen working standard stock solutions of 0.25 mg/ml of drugs (amitriptyline, clomipramine, and doxepin) were prepared in the acidic medium pH 1.2 in 100 ml volumetric flasks, then 50–1000 mg AC was added to 100 ml of each working standard solution. Similarly, The fifteen working standard stock solution of 0.25 mg/ml of drugs

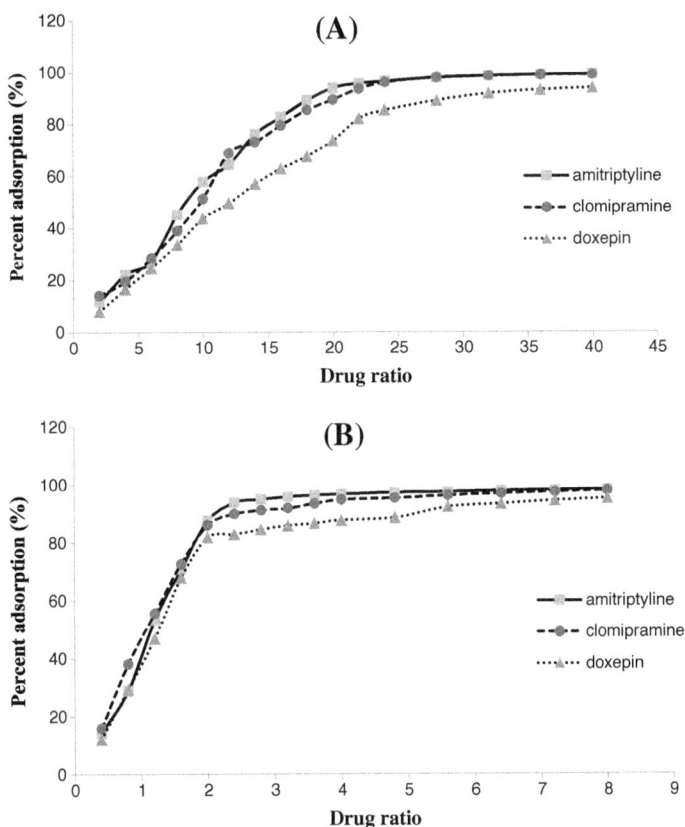

Figure 1 Amount of drug adsorbed onto A: activated charcoal (AC) and B: sodium polystyrene sulfonate (SPS).

(amitriptyline, clomipramine, and doxepin) were prepared in the acidic medium pH 1.2 in 100 ml volumetric flasks, and 10–200 mg SPS was added to 100 ml of each working standard solution. SPS was first washed carefully with distilled water to remove interference materials and then dried in oven at 80°C for 24 hours.

The suspensions were shaken at 37°C for 30 minutes to establish equilibrium. Each sample was filtered through a paper filter. 1 ml of the resulting filtrate was transferred to a tube and diluted with 9 ml hydrochloric acid (pH 1.2). The values of absorbance were measured at 239 nm for amitriptyline, 252 nm for clomipramine and 292 nm for doxepin. This process was repeated 3 times for each sample.

In order to study the kinetic profile of the adsorption process of each drug (amitriptyline, clomipramine and doxepin) onto AC and SPS, various incubation times were tried. 25 mg of each drug (amitriptyline, clomipramine and doxepin) were separately transferred to a 100 ml volumetric flask and 500 mg AC or 50 mg SPS were added. The suspensions were shaken at 37°C with different incubation times (20, 40, 60, 80, 100 and 120 min).

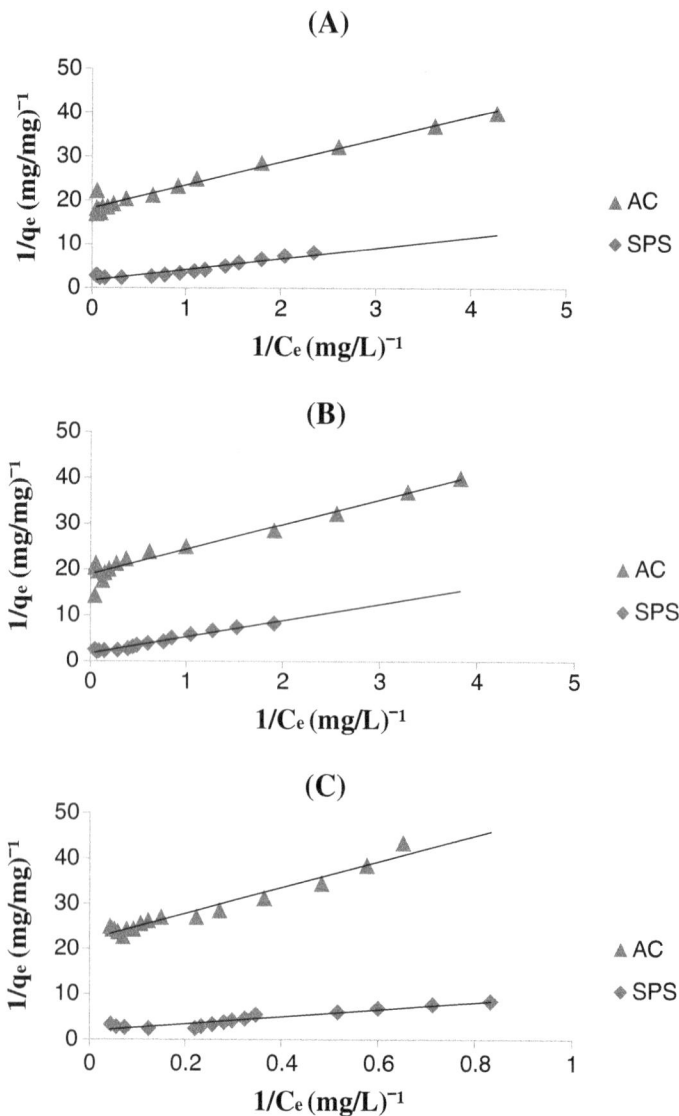

Figure 2 Langmuir plots of the adsorption of amitriptyline (A), clomipramine (B) and doxepin (C) onto activated charcoal (AC) and sodium polystyrene sulfonate (SPS).

Estimation of drug adsorption parameters (data analysis)
Several isotherm equations have been used for the equilibrium modeling of adsorption systems. Among these, the most widely used are the Langmuir and Freundlich isotherm equations. In our study, the Langmuir adsorption isotherm was used to estimate adsorption parameters: qmax was defined as the maximum quantity (mg) of drug adsorbed per mg AC or SPS. The affinity constant (K) in L/mg quantifies the interaction between drug and AC or SPS. The adsorption parameters were calculated by linear least-squares fitting of the following expression of the Langmuir model to the experimental data (Equation 1): [12].

$$\frac{1}{qe} = \frac{1}{qmax} + \frac{1}{Kqmax}\frac{1}{Ce}$$

qe = amount of drug adsorbed by AC or SPS (mg/mg)
Ce = drug concentration in the solution at equilibrium (mg/L)

Results

Drug adsorption onto AC and SPS
The results of adsorption experiments with SPS revealed higher values for the qmax parameters in comparison with AC. This defines a strong binding of amitriptyline, clomipramine, and doxepin onto SPS in comparison with AC (Table 1).

Figure 1A-B presents the amount of drug adsorbed onto AC and SPS. For AC, a minimum of 90% drug adsorption onto the adsorbent was reached when the adsorbent: drug ratios were 18: 1, 20: 1 and 28: 1 for amitriptyline, clomipramine, and doxepin, respectively. For SPS, a minimum of 90% drug adsorption to the adsorbent was reached when the adsorbent: drug ratios were 2: 1, 2.4: 1, and 4.8: 1 for amitriptyline, clomipramine, and doxepin, respectively.

Figure 2 shows Langmuir plots of the adsorption of amitriptyline (A), clomipramine (B) and doxepin (C) onto AC and SPS. These plots were used to determine the K and qmax values.

Effect of contact time
As shown in Figure 3, for an adsorption experiment with an AC: drug mass ratio of 20:1 and SPS: drug mass ratio of 2:1, the maximum adsorptions were established after 60 minutes. The plots indicate that the rate of drug adsorption increases rapidly in the beginning, but become very slow at the end.

Discussion
The Initial treatment of an acute overdose includes gastric decontamination of the patient [13]. AC has the capacity to adsorb a wide range of substances and organisms [14]. AC can bind with many drugs such as amitriptyline, clomipramine, and doxepin, and it is not absorbed in the gut. In our study, SPS, a cation-exchange resin, showed an effective adsorption of amitriptyline, clomipramine, and doxepin presumably based on their cationic properties.

Previous reports indicated that molecular structures of drugs are important factors in the adsorption mechanism. Higher adsorption is usually seen in aromatic compounds compared to aliphatic compounds of similar molecular size, and in branched-chain molecules compared to straight-chain molecules. Tricyclic antidepressants, having an aromatic containing tricyclic structure and a branched-chain structure, have been described to be well adsorbed to AC in vitro [15]. Most drugs are weak acids or bases. Weak acids and bases are weak electrolytes meaning that they are only ionized to a small extent (less than 1%) in neutral solution. The final pH of the drug solution will depend upon the pK_a. At pH 1.2 and 7.2, the amine group of amitriptyline (pK_a 9.4), clomipramine (pK_a 9.4), and

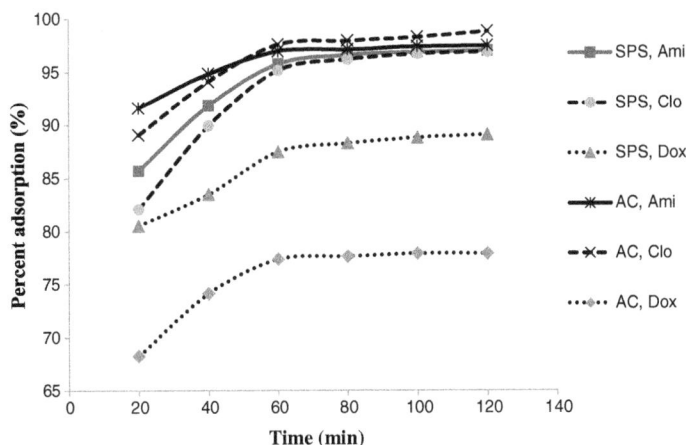

Figure 3 Drug mass ratio of activated charcoal (AC) and sodium polystyrene sulfonate (SPS).

doxepin (pK$_a$ 9.0) becomes protonated and these ionized substances adsorb poorly [16,17].

In its ionized form, adjacent molecules will repel each other when adsorbed on the AC surface because they carry the same electrical charge. The result is a lower density of drug packed together on the surface; therefore, the maximum adsorption capacity will be reduced compared to a non-ionized drug [15].

Ion exchange resins (IER) are insoluble polymers that contain acidic or basic functional groups and have the ability to exchange counter-ions within aqueous solutions surrounding them. Based on the nature of the exchangeable ion of the resin as a cation or anion form, it is classified as cationic or anionic exchange resins, respectively. Cation exchange resins contain covalently bound negatively charged functional groups and exchanges positively charged ions. SPS is a strongly acidic ion-exchange resin and is used to treat hyperkalemia [18]. SPS has been promising in animal and healthy human volunteers to reduce Li absorption and promote its elimination [19]. Previous studies showed that calcium polystyrene sulfonate, a cation-exchange resin, could adsorb imipramine, clomipramine, mianserin, trazodone, and ciprofloxacin based on their cationic properties [20].

The chemical behavior of this resin is similar to that of a strong acid. This resin is highly ionized in both the acid (R-SO$_3$H) and salt (RSO$_3$Na) forms of the sulfonic acid group (−SO$_3$H). The hydrogen and sodium forms of strong acid resins are highly dissociated, and the exchangeable Na$^+$ and H$^+$ are readily available for exchange over the entire pH range. Consequently, the exchange capacity of strong acid resins is independent of the solution pH [18].

In our study, SPS showed to effectively adsorb amitriptyline, clomipramine, and doxepin. This fact can be attributed to the adsorption of protonated amine groups of these drugs onto SPS surface after exchanging with sodium.

The initial faster rate of drug adsorption may be explained by the large number of sorption sites available for adsorption. For the initial bare surface, the sticking probability is large, and consequently adsorption proceeded with a high rate. The slower adsorption rate at the end is probably due to the saturation of active sites and attainment of equilibrium (Figure 3).

Conclusion

These adsorbents showed the adsorption characteristics by physical adsorption (AC) and complex formation of ion-exchange resin (SPS). In vitro experiments for antidepressant amitriptyline, clomipramine, and doxepin indicated that sodium polystyrene sulfonate (SPS) has higher qmax values than activated charcoal (AC). Therefore, we suggest SPS is a better gastric decontaminating agent for the management of acute TCA intoxication.

Competing interests

The authors declare that they have no competing interests.

Authors' contributions

AJ, FV, OF, HS, AN and GD carried out the amitriptyline, clomipramine, and doxepin adsorption onto sodium polystyrene sulfonate and drafted the manuscript. All authors read and approved the final manuscript.

Author details

[1]Pharmaceutical Sciences Research Center, Shiraz University of Medical Sciences, Shiraz, Iran. [2]Department of Pharmacology and Toxicology, Faculty of pharmacy, Shiraz University of Medical Sciences, Shiraz, Iran. [3]International Branch, Shiraz University of Medical Sciences, Shiraz, Iran. [4]Department of Pharmacognosy, Faculty of Pharmacy, Shiraz University of Medical Sciences, Shiraz, Iran. [5]Food and Drug Control Laboratory, Shiraz University of Medical Sciences, Shiraz, Iran.

References

1. Pimentel L, Trommer L: Cyclic antidepressant overdoses. A review. *Emreg Med Clin North Am* 1994, **12**(2):533–547.
2. Crome P: Poisoning due to tricyclic antidepressant overdosage. Clinical presentation and treatment. *Med Toxicol* 1986, **1**(4):261–285.
3. Lapus RM: Activated charcoal for pediatric poisonings: the universal antidote? *Curr Opin Pediatr* 2007, **19**(2):216–222.
4. Yeates PJ, Thomas SH: Effectiveness of delayed activated charcoal administration in simulated paracetamol (acetaminophen) overdose. *Br J Clin Pharmacol* 2000, **49**(1):11–14.
5. Crome P, Dawling S, Braithwaite RA, Masters J, Walkey R: Effect of activated charcoal on absorption of nortriptyline. *Lancet* 1977, **2**:1203–1205.
6. Neuvonen PJ, Olkkola KT, Alanen T: Effect of ethanol and pH on the adsorption of drugs to activated charcoal: studies in vitro and in man. *Acta Pharmacol Toxicol (Copenh)* 1984, **54**:1–7.
7. Sellers EM, Khouw V, Doman L: Comparative drug adsorption by activated charcoal. *J Pharm Sci* 1977, **66**:1640–1641.
8. Chernin G, Gal-Oz A, Ben-Assa E, Schwartz IF, Weinstein T, Schwatz D, et al: Secondary prevention of hyperkalemia with sodium polystyrene sulfonate in cardiac and kidney patients on renin-angiotensin-aldosterone system inhibition therapy. *Clin Cardiol* 2012, **35**(1):32–36.
9. Aschenbrenner DS, Venable SJ: *Drug Therapy In Nursing.* 3tdth edition. New York: Wolters Kluwer Health; 2009:589–592.
10. Sterns RH, Rojas M, Bernstein P, Chennupati S: Ion-exchange resins for the treatment of hyperkalemia: are they safe and effective? *J Am Soc Nephrol* 2010, **21**(5):733–735.
11. Watson M, Abbott KC, Yuan CM: Damned if you do, damned if you don't: potassium binding resins in hyperkalemia. *Clin J Am Soc Neohrol* 2010, **5**(10):1723–1726.
12. Tsitoura A, Atta-Politou J, Koupparis MA: In vitro adsorption study of fluoxetine onto Activated charcoal at gastric and intestinal pH using high performance liquid chromatography with fluorescence detector. *J Toxicol Clin Toxicol* 1997, **35**(3):269–276.
13. Bosse GM, Barefoot JA, Pfeifer MP, Rodgers GC: Comparison of three methods of gut decontamination in tricyclic antidepressant overdose. *J Emerg Med* 1995, **13**(2):203–209.
14. Rademaker CM, van Dijk A, de Vries MH, Kadir F, Glerum JH: A ready-to-use activated charcoal mixture. Adsorption studies in vitro and in dogs: its influence on the intestinal secretion of theophylline in a rat model. *Pharm Weekbl Sci* 1989, **11**(2):56–60.
15. Hoegberg LC, Groenlykke TB, Abildtrup U, Angelo HR: Combined paracetamol and amitriptyline adsorption to activated charcoal. *Clin Toxicol (Phila)* 2010, **48**(9):898–903.
16. Brenner GM, Stevens CW: *Pharmacology.* 3tdth edition. Philadelphia: Saunders Elsevier; 2010.
17. Flomenbaum NE, Goldfrank LR, Hoffman RS, Howland MA, Lewin NA, Nelson LS (Eds): *Goldfrank's Emergency Toxicology.* 8tdth edition. New York, NY: McGraw Hill; 2006.

18. Srikanth MV, Sunil SA, Rao NS, Uhumwangho MU, Ramana Murthy KV:
     Ion-Exchange Resins as Controlled Drug Delivery Carriers. *J Sci Res* 2010,
     2(3):597–611.
19. Ghannoum M, Lavergne V, Yue CS, Ayoub P, Perreault MM, Roy L:
     **Successful treatment of lithium toxicity with sodium polystyrene
     sulfonate: a retrospective cohort study.** *Clin Toxicol (Phila)* 2010,
     48(1):34–41.
20. Toyoguchi T, Ebihara M, Ojima F, Hosya J, Nakagawa Y: **In vitro study of the
     adsorption characteristics of drugs.** *Biol Pharma Bull* 2005, **28**(5):841–844.

Beneficial effects of pioglitazone and metformin in murine model of polycystic ovaries via improvement of chemerin gene up-regulation

Nahid Kabiri[1], Mohammad Reza Tabandeh[2*] and Seyed Reza Fatemi Tabatabaie[1]

Abstract

Background: Polycystic ovary syndrome (PCO) is recognized as the most common endocrinopathy in female. Chemerin is a novel adipocytokine that is expressed in ovary and upregulated in adipose tissue of obese, PCO patients. To date there is no report about the regulation of ovarian chemerin gene expression after PCO induction and treatment by insulin sensitizing drugs including pioglitazone and metformin.

Thirty female rats were divided into six experimental groups with five rats in each group including control group, PCO group (i.m injection of 4 mg estradiol benzoate for 40 days), metformin treated (200 mg/kg/day for 21 days), pioglitazone treated (20 mg/kg/day, for 21 days), PCO + metformin and PCO + pioglitazone. PCO was detected by microscopic observation of vaginal smear and treatment by metformin and pioglitazone was initiated one week after that. Ovarian chemerin expression was analyzed by real time PCR and western blotting.

Results: Our results demonstrated that PCO induction resulted in elevation of chemerin mRNA and protein levels in ovary in concomitant with incidence of insulin resistance and increasing androgen and progesterone production. We observed that metformin and pioglitazone attenuated ovarian chemerin expression and improved insulin resistance and abnormal steroid production in PCO rats.

Conclusion: Based on data presented here we concluded that alteration of ovarian chemerin expression may has important role in PCO development and manipulation of chemerin expression or signaling by pioglitazone or metformin can be a novel therapeutic mechanism in the treatment of PCO patients by these drugs.

Keywords: PCO, Chemerin, Gene expression, Ovary, Pioglitazone, Metformin

Background

Polycystic ovary syndrome (PCO) is recognized as the most common endocrinopathy in female during the reproductive age. PCO is characterized by reproductive dysfunction symptoms such as hyperandrogenic chronic anovulation due to excess androgen production, menstrual disturbances, infertility or subfertility and the presence of enlarged, sclerocystic ovaries. Obesity, insulin resistance, pancreatic-cell dysfunction and impaired glucose tolerance occur at least in 50% of women with PCO [1,2]. Previous reports have shown that hyperinsulinemia in these patients dysregulates LH secretion and promotes ovarian androgen secretion resulting in elevation of free androgen level [3].

Over the past decade it has been shown that adipocytes are secretory cells that produce a variety of proteins with hormonal actions, which collectively have been called adipocytokines. These cytokines have important roles in male and female reproductive physiology by regulation of carbohydrate and lipid metabolism in adipose or reproductive tissues such as hypothalamus-pituitary axis, ovary, uterus and embryo [4,5]. Among them, adiponectin, leptin, resistin and visfatin are the major adipocytokines which their changes in serum or adipose tissue have been identified in patients with obesity, insulin resistance and PCO [6,7]. Various secretion or gene expression patterns of adipocytokines or their receptors have been detected in adipose tissue or ovary of PCO patients [8,9].

* Correspondence: m.tabandeh@scu.ac.ir
[2]Department of Biochemistry and Molecular Biology, Faculty of Veterinary Medicine, Shahid Chamran University of Ahvaz, Ahvaz, Iran
Full list of author information is available at the end of the article

Chemerin is a novel adipocytokine which is predominantly expressed by adipocytes and its gene expression elevates in the adipose tissue of obese animals and human [7]. High correlations have been found between plasma chemerin level and different features of metabolic syndrome including body mass index, plasma triglycerides and blood pressure in human [10]. Chemerin knockdown animals demonstrate impaired adipocyte gene expression and unregulated glucose and carbohydrate metabolism [11]. Recent data demonstrate that recombinant chemerin promotes angiogenesis; a mechanism which is essential for adipose tissue expansion in obese patients [11,12]. Recently, inhibitory action of chemerin on FSH or IGF-1 induced steroidogenesis have been reported in granulosa cells [13-15]. Serum chemerin increases in women with PCO [16].

Insulin-sensitizing drugs (ISDs) such as metformin or thiazolidinediones (TZDs) ameliorate reproductive abnormalities, restore ovulation and regular estrous cycle, increase pregnancy rates and reduce androgenic symptoms in women with PCO [17,18]. The positive actions of these insulin-sensitizing agents on adipocytokine secretion or expression in adipose tissue or ovaries of PCO patients have been described. However the full mechanism of action of these two drugs in ovaries of PCO patient is still unraveled and further investigations remain to elucidate the precise mechanism of actions of these drugs at molecular levels.

To our knowledge, no study is available that identify the changes of chemerin gene expression in ovaries of animals or human with PCO and that compare the effects of pioglitazone and metformin on its gene expression in experimental model of PCO. Here for the first time we showed that ovarian chemerin gene expression changed after PCO induction and pioglitazone or metformin treatment.

Methods

Rat treatment regimes

Thirty Female Sprague-Dawley rats (3 month of age) weighing 150-180 g were housed in a temperature-controlled room (23 ± 1°C) with a 12 h light/dark cycle and were provided rat chow (Pars, Tehran, Iran) and water at libitum.

All animals used were cared for according to the Guide for the Care and Use of Laboratory Animals by the National Academy of Sciences (National Institutes of Health publication No. 86-23). The rats were allowed to acclimatize for 10 days before the beginning of the experiment. The estrous cyclicity was monitored by vaginal smears obtained between 08:00 and 12:00 hours and the rats with abnormal cyclicity were dismissed from the experiment.

The rats were divided into six experimental groups with five rats in each group: 1) healthy control (vehicle control), 2) PCO, 3) metformin treated 4) pioglitazone treated, 5) PCO and metformin treated and 6) PCO and pioglitazone treated. PCO was induced by a single i.m injection of 4 mg estradiol valerate (Loghman Pharmaceutical & Hygienic Co, Karaj, Iran) in 0.2 ml sesame oil (Barij Essense, Kashan, Iran) for 40 days [19] and detected by microscopic observation of vaginal smear. The presence of prolonged cornified cells for at least two consecutive estrous cycles was used as successful PCO induction. Treatment with metformin and pioglitazone was initiated one week after PCO induction.

Animals in metformin treated groups (groups 3 and 5) were received 200 mg/kg/day metformin (Loghman Pharmaceutical & Hygienic Co, Karaj, Iran) by gavage method for 21 days. Pioglitazone (Dorsa Pharmaceutical Co. Tehran, Iran) was daily used for the 21 days duration as the same method as metformin groups with dose of 20 mg/kg/day. Dosages of pioglitazone and metformin were chosen based on dosages that were clinically used in human patients (25-30 mg/kg/day for pioglitazone and 200-300 mg/kg/day for metformin).

Tissue and serum sampling

Animals were anesthetized by chloroform and serum samples were obtained by cardiac puncture, separated by centrifuging at 5,000 rpm for 5 minutes and stored at -20°C for the subsequent assays. Both ovaries were carefully trimmed of adhering fat and connective tissue, pooled and immediately frozen in liquid nitrogen at -80°C. The body weight and length (nose to anus lenght) of all rats were determined at the end of study and body mass index (BMI) was calculated by using following formula as described previously; body weight (g)/Length^2 (cm^2) [20]. Control ovaries were collected from rats at estrous or proestrous stages of cycle.

Ovarian morphology

Some ovary was removed, cleaned of adherent connective fat tissue, and fixed in 4% formaldehyde buffer for at least 24 hours. Thereafter the samples were dehydrated and imbedded in paraffin. The ovaries were partially longitudinally sectioned (4 μm, every tenth section mounted on the glass slide), stained with hematoxylin and eosin and the presence of healthy and atretic follicles, follicular cysts and corpora lutea was assayed. Antral follicles with pyknotic granulosa and theca layers, unhealthy, degenerative oocyte and filled in antral cavity with numerous apoptotic derbies were characterized as atretic follicles. Preantral follicles with degenerative oocyte and pyknotic granulosa layer were assigned as atretic follicles.

Hormone and glucose assays

Serum insulin levels were measured by using the Rat ELISA kits (Mercodia, Sweden) according to the manufacturer's recommendation. Insulin concentration was expressed as μg/L. The limit of detection of insulin was 0.01 μg/L and the intra-assay and interassay coefficients of variation were less than 4% and 8.13%, respectively. The calibrator ranges were between 0-10 μg/L (first calibrator at 0.01 μg/L).

The progesterone (P4) and testosterone (T) concentrations were determined by using a commercial radioimmunoassay kit (Immunotech, Radiová, Czech Republic). The limit of detection of P4 was 0.1 ng/ml, and the intra-assay and interassay coefficients of variation were less than 10% and 11%, respectively. The calibrator ranges were between 0 - 100 ng/mL (first calibrator at 0.1 ng/mL). The limit of detection of T was 0.1 ng/ml, and the intra-assay and interassay coefficients of variation were less than 12.1% and 11.2%, respectively. The calibrator ranges were between 0 – 25 ng/mL (first calibrator at 0.1 ng/mL). Blood glucose was determined by glucose oxidase method (Pars Azmoon, Tehran, Iran) as described by manufacturer.

HOMA-IR estimation
HOMA-IR was estimated through previously described formula (fasting glucose × fasting insulin/22.5) and represented by unit of mmol/L × μU/ml [21].

RNA preparation
Total RNA was extracted from ovaries using TriPure total RNA isolation kit according to the manufacturer's procedure (Roche Molecular System, USA), dissolved in dimethyl pyrocarbonate treated water and quantified at a wavelength of 260 nm by nanodrop spectrophotometry (Eppendorf, Hamburg, Germany). The RNA with optical density absorption ratio OD260 nm/OD280 nm between 1.8 and 2.0 was used for reverse transcription (RT) reaction. Genomic DNA was removed by treating 1 μg of isolated RNA with 2 units of DNase I (Fermentas Inc, Vilnius, Lithuania).

Reverse transcription – polymerase chain reaction
Reverse transcription was done in a total volume of 20-μl by using an AmpliSence cDNA synthesis kit (AmpliSens Enterovirus-Eph, Russia) as recommended by the manufacturer. The PCR reactions was performed in a 25-μl reaction using Taq DNA polymerase (Cinagen Co, Iran) and a thermal cycler (Eppendorf Mastercycler, Hamburg, Germany). Specific sets of primers (BIONEER, Seoul, South Korea) that used for amplification of rat chemerin were as follows; forward: 5′-ATG GCGGGCAACGGCGCCAT-3′ and reverse: 5′-CCAT CAACGTCGTCAACTAA-3′. Thermal conditions for amplification of chemerin were 35 cycles consisting of denaturing at 94°C for 1 min, annealing at 58°C for 1 min, extension at 72°C for 1 min, with an initial denaturing step at 95°C for 10 min and a final extension

step at 72°C for 10 min. cDNA from adipose tissue was used as positive control. Expression of chemerin in rat ovaries was confirmed by visualization of PCR product on agarose gel electrophoresis (1%).

Real time PCR
To evaluate the levels of chemerin gene expression in ovaries of different animals quantitative real-time PCR (qRT-PCR) was performed using the ABI Step One plus real-time PCR detection system (ABI plus; Applied Biosystems, USA), and qPCR™ Green master kit for SYBR Green I® (Applied Biosystems, USA). Relative expression level of chemerin transcript was compared to GAPDH as housekeeping gene. Specific sets of primers (Macrogen, Seoul, South Korea) that were used for amplification of rat GAPDH [GenBank: NM_017008.4] and chemerin [GenBank: NM_001013427] genes were designed using Beacon Designer 7.1. Sequences of primers for amplification of rat GAPDH and chemerin (BIONEER, Seoul, South Korea) were as follows; rat chemerin: 5′-TGTGGACAGTGCTGATGACCTGTT-3′ and 5′-CAGT TTGATGCAGGCCAGGCATTT-3′ and rat GAPDH: 5′-CTCATCTACCTCTCCATCGTCTG-3′ and 5′-CCTGC TCTTGTCTGCCGGTGCTTG-3′ Real time PCR reactions were performed with the following settings: 5 minutes of pre-incubation at 95°C followed by 40 cycles for 15 seconds at 95°C and 45 second at 60°C. Reactions were performed in triplicate. A reaction without cDNA was performed in parallel as negative control.

Relative quantification was performed according to the comparative $2^{-\Delta\Delta Ct}$. For analysis of qRT-PCR results based on $\Delta\Delta Ct$ method StepOne™ software was used. The result for the gene expression was given by a unitless value through the formula $2^{-\Delta\Delta Ct}$. Validation of assay to check that the primer for the GAPDH and chemerin had similar amplification efficiencies was performed as described previously [22].

Western blotting
Total protein from isolated ovaries was precipitated after RNA and DNA isolation using TriPure total RNA isolation kit according to the manufacturer's procedure (Roche Molecular System, USA) and its concentration was measured using Bradford method as described previously [23]. Twenty five μl of each protein sample (1 μg/μl) were mixed with 25 μl Laemmli sample buffer supplemented with 2-mercaptoethanol at a final concentration of 7.5% (vol/vol). The samples were heated for 15 min at 65°C, separated by 10% SDS-PAGE and electrophoretically transferred to a nitrocellulose membrane (Schleicher & Schuell, Inc., Keene, NH). The filters were blocked by incubation for 1 h in PBS with 5% nonfat milk. Blots were then washed in PBS-Tween and immunoblotted with primary antibody against mouse chemerin (Abcam,

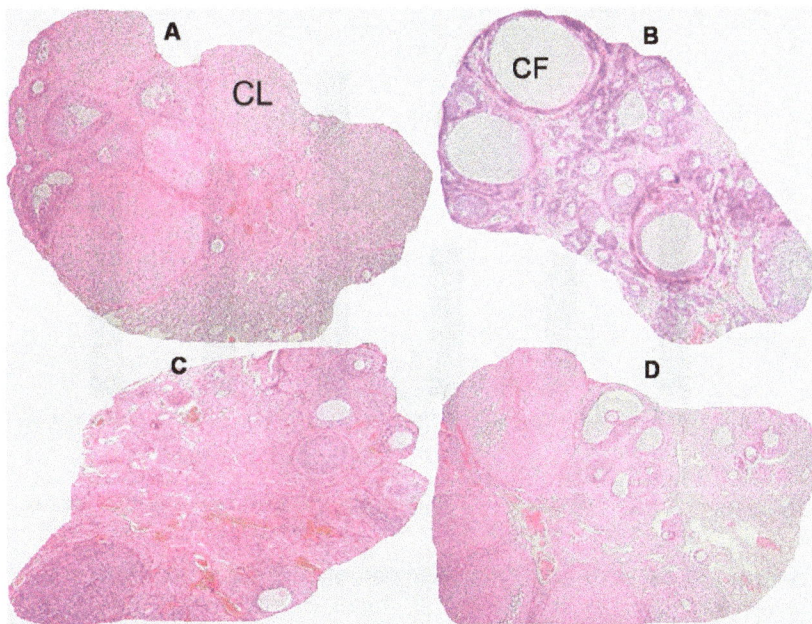

Figure 1 Ovarian features in normal rats **(A)**, estradiol induced PCO rats, **(B)** PCO rats treated with pioglitazone **(C)** and PCO rats treated with metformin **(D)**. Normal rats displayed follicles at different stages and the presence of corpora lutea (CL) **(A)**, while estradiol treatment resulted in formation of higher numbers of atretic and cystic follicles (CF) and the absence of CL **(B)**. Metformin and pioglitazone treated rats **(C and D)** exhibited lower numbers of CF, higher numbers of antral follicles and growing young CL. H & E staining (magnification × 40).

Cambridge, UK, Art No: ab112450) at 1:500 ratio. Detection of primary antibody was done using goat anti rabbit HRP-conjugated antibody (Abcam, Cambridge, UK, Art No; ab98467) at 1:1000 ratio and DAB reagent (Sigma Aldrich, Germany). Densitometric quantification of chemerin proteins in relation to GAPDH as calibrator was performed using Image J software (National Institutes of Health). Western blot was done in three independent experiments for each sample.

Statistical analyses

Data analyses were done using the SPSS 16.0 software package (SPSS Inc., Chicago, IL, USA). Two-way analysis of variance (ANOVA) and general linear model was fit to evaluate the effect of PCO status (PCO vs. control) and treatments (treatment with metformin or pioglitazon vs. no treatment) on each variable. The two-way ANOVA model is given by $Yijk = \mu + \alpha_i + \beta_j + (\alpha\beta)_{ij}$, where α_i and β_j represent the effects of PCO induction and treatment, and $(\alpha\beta)_{ij}$ represents the interaction of two factors. The Spearman rank correlation coefficient was used to estimate the correlation between chemerin gene expression and different parameters. All experimental data were presented as the mean ± SD. The level of significance for all tests was set at P < 0.05.

Result

The ovaries in the control group exhibited a typically normal appearance with small and medium sized antral follicles and corpora lutea (Figure 1A). The ovaries in the PCO group displayed typical PCO-like changes including presence of higher numbers of atretic and cystic follicles compared with the control group (Figure 1B). Metformin and pioglitazone treated rats exhibited lower numbers of atretic and cystic follicles, higher numbers of antral follicles and growing young corpora lutea compared with PCO group (Figure 1C-D). Restoration of normal follicular appearance was more pronounced in metformin treated rats compared with pioglitazon treated animals (Figure 1C-D).

The real time-PCR and western blot results demonstrated that chemerin mRNA and protein levels were elevated in ovaries of PCO rats when compared to that in healthy animals (*P < 0.05*) (Figure 2). The chemerin gene expression levels were decreased in ovaries of PCO rats in response to treatment with metformin and pioglitazone compared to untreated PCO rats (*p < 0.05*) (Figure 2). Metformin and pioglitazone had no effects on the levels of chemerin mRNA and protein in healthy treated rats in relation to healthy untreated animals regardless of PCO status (Figure 2) (*p > 0.05*).

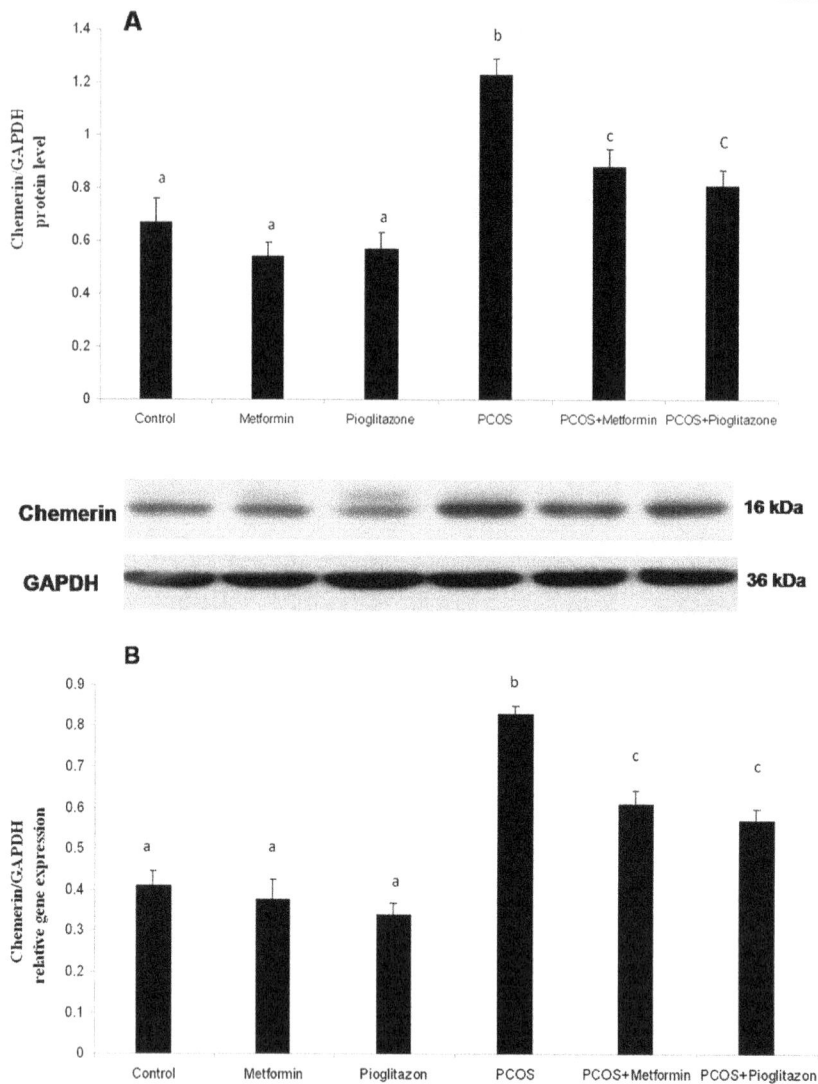

Figure 2 Chemerin protein (A) and mRNA levels (B) in rat ovaries after PCO induction and treatment with pioglitazone and metformin **(n = 5 in each group).** Chemerin was up-regulated in ovary of PCO rats compared with control animals, whereas its level decreased after treatment with metformin and pioglitazone. Data were presented as the mean ± SD. Different letters denote differences among groups at P < 0.05.

As shown in Figures 3 and 4 plasma glucose and insulin levels were higher in the PCO induced rats (1.92 ± 0.38 fold) when compared with normal untreated group (p <0.05) after controlling for the effect of treatment. Treatment of PCO rats with metformin and pioglitazone resulted in reduction of glucose (1.36 ± 0.27) and insulin (1.82 ± 0.36) levels in relation to PCO untreated rats (p < 0.05) (Figures 3 and 4). In healthy treated groups plasma insulin and glucose levels had no differences with healthy untreated animals (Figures 3 and 4), ($p > 0.05$) after controlling for PCO status.

The HOMA-IR index, which reflects whole body insulin resistance, was increased in PCO animals (3.63 ± 0.41 fold) (p < 0.05) (Figure 5) regardless of treatments. Metformin and pioglitazone induced reduction of HOMA-IR in PCO rats about 2.8 fold compared with untreated PCO animals (p < 0.05) (Figure 5). Healthy treated rats did not show clear changes in HOMA-IR level in relation to healthy untreated rats after controlling PCO status.

The plasma concentrations of T and P4 are shown in Figures 6 and 7 respectively. We found a 1.8 ± 0.3 fold increase of plasma T and a 6.9 ± 0.8 fold increase of P4

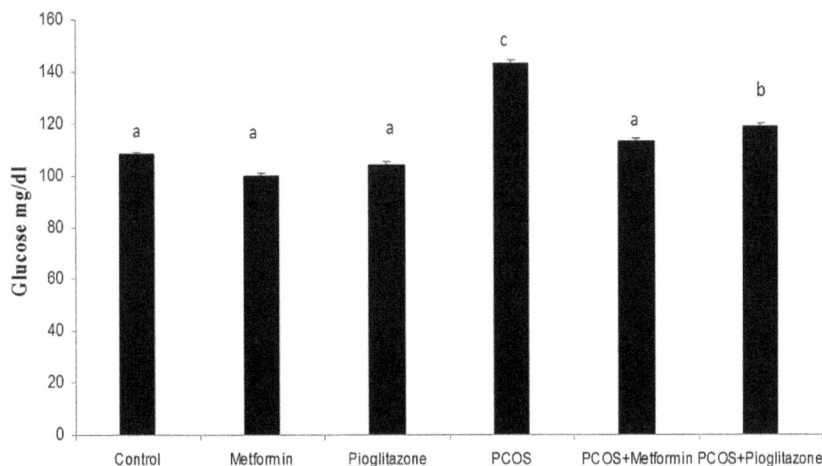

Figure 3 Serum glucose levels (mg/dl) in normal rats (n = 5), PCO induced rats (n = 5) and treated rats with metformin and pioglitazone (n = 5). Serum glucose was elevated in PCO rats compared with control animals. Treatment of PCO rats with metformin and pioglitazone resulted in reduction of glucose level in relation to PCO untreated rats. Data were presented as the mean ± SD. Different letters denote differences among groups at P < 0.05.

rats after induction of PCO ($p < 0.05$) (Figures 6 and 7) regardless of treatments. We found that in treated PCO rats, T concentrations were decreased by 1.2 ± 0.3 fold and 1.9 ± 0.5 fold after metformin and pioglitazone treatment respectively ($p < 0.05$) (Figure 6). The reduction of T level was more pronounced in PCO rats in the presence of pioglitazone compared with metformin ($p < 0.05$) (Figure 6), while metformin was more effective in reducing P4 concentration in this group ($p < 0.05$) (Figure 7).

Spearman Rank correlation analyses demonstrated that ovarian chemerin gene expression was positively associated with P4 ($p < 0.01$), HOMA-IR, BMI, insulin and glucose levels ($p < 0.05$) (Table 1). Δ chemerin gene expression in

treated PCO animals had positive correlation with Δ insulin, Δ HOMA-IR and Δ P4 ($p < 0.05$) (Table 1).

Discussion
PCO is a heterogeneous syndrome characterized by hyperandrogenism, insulin resistance and obesity [24]. The mechanism that is responsible for insulin resistance is unclear and several hypotheses have been suggested. Because obesity is linked to insulin resistance and many women with PCO are obese, it is possible that, at least in a subgroup of patients, insulin resistance is worsened by excessive adipose mass or abnormal secretion or action of adipocytokines [25]. Chemerin is a newly identified

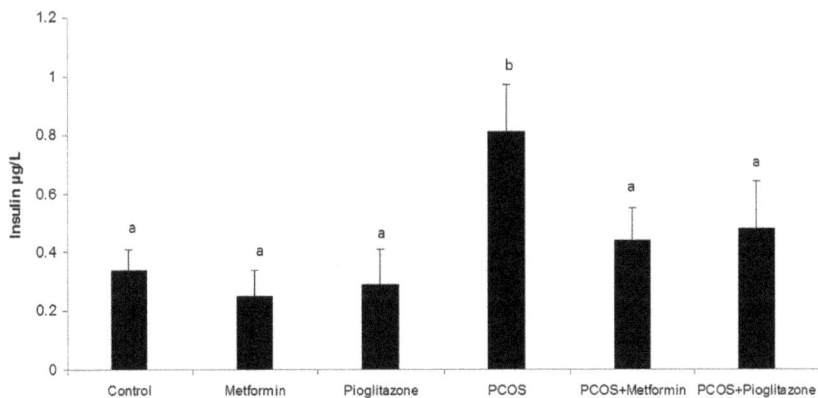

Figure 4 Serum insulin levels (ug/L) in normal rats (n = 5), PCO induced rats (n = 5) and treated rats with metformin and pioglitazone (n = 5). Serum insulin level was considerably higher in PCO rats compared with that in normal animals. Treatment of PCO rats with metformin and pioglitazone decreased the over-secretion of insulin in relation to PCO untreated rats. Data were presented as the mean ± SD. Different letters denote differences among groups at P < 0.05.

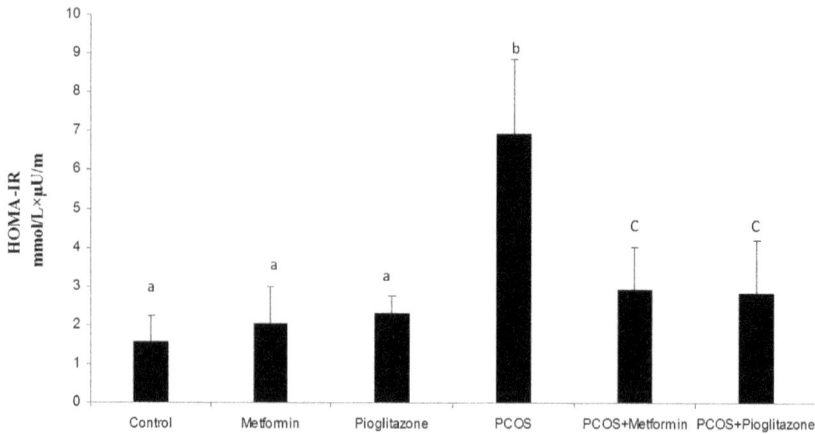

Figure 5 HOMA-IR index (mmol/L × uU/ml) in normal rats (n = 5), PCO induced rats (n = 5) and treated rats with metformin and pioglitazone (n = 5). Rats with PCO showed insulin resistance compared with normal rats, while treatment of those with metformin and pioglitazone attenuate insulin resistance in relation to PCO untreated rats. Data were presented as the mean ± SD. Different letters denote differences among groups at P < 0.05.

adipokine whose systemic levels are elevated in obesity and positively correlate with markers of the metabolic syndrome such as body mass index, triglycerides, high-sensitivity C-reactive protein [15,26]. Recently Tan et al demonstrated an increase of serum and subcutaneous and omental adipose tissue chemerin expression in women with PCO [10]. Chemerin is also expressed in ovary of animal and human, but few data exists on regulation of chemerin gene expression in polycystic ovaries [14,27]. Here we present novel data showing an increase of chemerin gene expression in rat ovary after induction of PCO. The animals in PCO group gained more weight, had higher plasma insulin and glucose levels and showed an elevation of HOMA-IR; an index of insulin resistance. Our findings

was in agreement with results of Wang et al which has shown the higher level of chemein expression in the ovary of dihydrotestosterone (DHT) induced PCO rats [15]. Several experiments have demonstrated that chemerin may play a role in pathophysiology of PCO in animal or human by direct action on ovary [10,13,14]. We know that formation of polycystic ovaries is critically associated with abnormal steroidogenesis. It has been found that chemerin decreases estradiol secretion and suppressed FSH-induced progesterone and estradiol secretion in preantral follicles and granulosa cells by inhibition of aromatase and p450scc expression [13].

It is also well recognized that development of polycystic ovaries is associated with new blood vessel formation

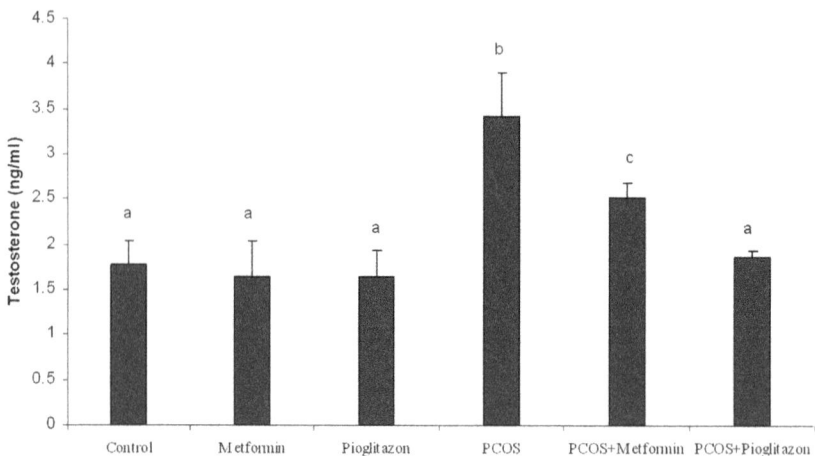

Figure 6 Serum testosterone (T) levels (ug/L) in normal rats (n = 5), PCO induced rats (n = 5) and treated rats with metformin and pioglitazone (n = 5). Induction of PCO caused an increasing the T level, while metformin and pioglitazone attenuated over secretion of T. Data were presented as the mean ± SD. Different letters denote differences among groups at P < 0.05.

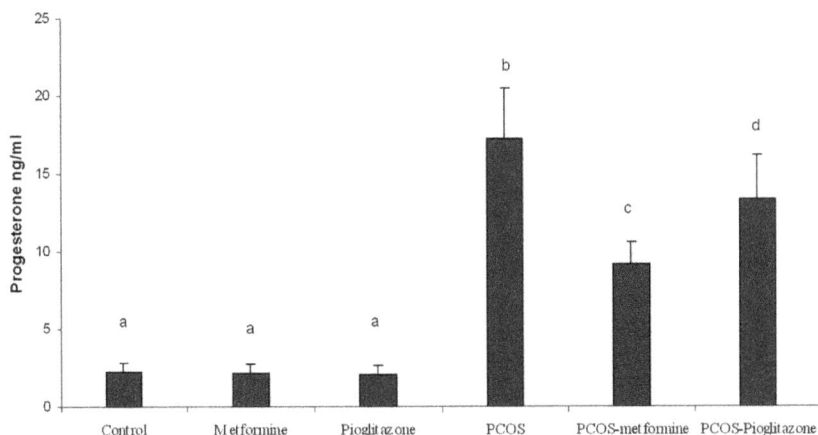

Figure 7 Serum progesterone (P) levels (ug/L) in normal rats (n = 5), PCO induced rats (n = 5) and treated rats with metformin and pioglitazone (n = 5). Induction of PCO caused an increasing the P level, while metformin and pioglitazone attenuated over secretion of T. Data were presented as the mean ± SD. Different letters denote differences among groups at P < 0.05.

[28]. Although there is no data about the effect of chemerin on ovarian angiogenesis, however it is plausible that chemerin may act as angiogenic factor. Recently Bozauglo et al using an *in vitro* angiogenesis assay has shown that chemerin induced the formation of capillary-like structures, a process which occur in obese patient and result in adipose tissue expansion [12]. These observations lead to the hypothesis that increasing the chemerin gene expression in ovary of PCO rats may alter ovarian steroidogenesis or angiogenesis and may play a role in the development and progression of this reproductive disorder.

It has been demonstrated that alteration of metabolic and endocrine function of adipocytes result in a higher secretion of proinflammatory substances including tumor necrosis factor alpha (TNF-α) and interleukin-6 (IL-6)

Table 1 Correlation between chemerin gene expression in ovaries of PCO rats with insulin, glucose, HOMA-IR index, testosterone, progesterone and body mass index (BMI) after PCO induction and treatment of PCO rats with pioglitazone and metformin

ΔChemerin mRNA (after treatment)		Chemerin mRNA (PCOS)		Variables
p	r	p	r	
0.0847	0.361	0.0327	0.661*	Glucose (mg/dl)
0.0432	0.578*	0.0087	0.754**	Insulin (µg/l)
0.0916	0.291	0.0414	0.523*	Testosterone (ng/ml)
0.0382	0.619*	0.0091	0.827**	Progesterone (ng/ml)
0.0478	0.564*	0.0276	0.678*	HOMA-IR
0.0739	0.378	0.0312	0.654*	BMI

*Correlation is significant at the 0.05 level.
**Correlation is significant at the 0.01 level.
Correlation coefficient (r) and statistical significance (P) are indicated.
(Δ) change in chemerin gene expression level after treatment.

[29]. Many reports have demonstrated that these potent inflammatory compounds alter normal physiology of ovary such as steroidogenesis and enhance the risk of PCO development [17,30]. Presence a positive association between increasing body weight and ovarian chemerin gene expression in this study raises the possibility that alteration of chemerin gene expression in ovary of PCO animals may be, in some part, due to increasing fat mass and releasing higher inflammatory mediators such as IL-6 and TNF-α. This hypothesis is supported by the fact that TNF-α increases adipocyte chemerin and elevation of serum TNF-α leads to higher systemic chemerin in mice [31].

We also found the higher plasma insulin level in animals with PCO compared with healthy rats and its positive association with ovarian chemerin gene expression. Interestingly, insulin elevates chemerin in human adipose tissue explants *in vitro*, and systemic chemerin increases after prolonged hyperinsulinemia in healthy individuals. This finding suggests that hyperinsulinemia which occur in our experiment may enhance the chemerin gene expression in polycystic ovaries and it may have role in progression of impaired steroid production [32].

Consistent with previous results, our study showed that chemerin has role in PCO development and manipulation of chemerin gene expression or its signaling may be a novel therapeutic approaches in the treatment of PCO patients. To clarify this hypothesis we test the effect of pioglitazone and metformin on the ovarian chemerin gene expression in normal and PCO animals. To our knowledge, this is the first report demonstrating that treatment of PCO rat with pioglitazone and metformin alter chemerin gene expression in the ovary. Here we reported for the first time that 21 days treatment of PCO rats with metformin and pioglitazone reduced ovarian chemerin mRNA and protein abundance with a concomitant decrease in insulin resistance in PCO animals. Reduction of chemerin gene expression was more pronounced in PCO rats in the presence of pioglitazone compared with metformin, while these drugs had no effects on the basal levels of ovarian chemerin mRNA and protein in healthy animals. We also found improvement of insulin resistance in animals treated with pioglitazone or metformin. Animals in these groups showed lower plasma insulin and glucose level and HOMA-IR compared with PCO animals.

Pioglitazone and metformin are the most important insulin-sensitizing agents currently used most often in clinical practice to improve insulin resistance of PCO patients via different mechanisms which are not thoroughly understood [33,34]. A diverse beneficial effect of pioglitazone and metformin on the treatment of PCO has been described in recent years [35]. Alteration of numerous genes involved in different ovarian functions such as cell proliferation, steroid production and new blood formation by these drugs have been detected and it demonstrate that their positive effects on ovarian function in PCO patients may be multifactorial [35,36]. Recently it has been found that troglitazone or metformin reduce the secretion of chemerin from adipoe tissue and metformin can also reduces chemerin blood levels in concomitant with improving insulin sensivity and decreasing BMI in women with PCO [10]. It has also been demonstrated that both drugs have anti-angiogenic actions, suppresses ovarian androgen production and reduce the secretion of proinflammatory factors including IL-6 and TNF-α [37-39]. Given our findings and those from other groups we hypothesized that these drugs may improve functional and endocrine disturbances of polycystic ovaries, in some part, by suppression of ovarian chemerin gene expression and attenuation of its adverse effect on normal functions of polycystic ovaries.

Conclusion

In conclusion, using a murine model of PCO, we provided novel evidence that chemerin is an important adipocytokine which may contribute to the dysregulation of ovarian function in PCO. Our study indicated that ovarian chemerin gene expression is associated with several key parameters of the metabolic syndrome in PCO status. Oral administration of pioglitazone and metformin to PCO rats altered the ovarian expression of chemerin genes. These results suggest that some therapeutic effects of metformin and pioglitazone in PCO may be due to their direct actions on ovarian chemerin gene expression.

Competing interests
The authors declare that they have no competing interests.

Authors' contributions
SRFT and MRT were the supervisors and designed the study. MRT carried out the molecular studies. SRFT carried out the hormone assays. All authors read and approved the final manuscript.

Acknowledgements
This work was funded by a Grant from Shahid Chamran University of Ahvaz research Council (Grant No: 636410, 1391.4.6).

Author details
[1]Department of Physiology, Faculty of Veterinary Medicine, Shahid Chamran University of Ahvaz, Ahvaz, Iran. [2]Department of Biochemistry and Molecular Biology, Faculty of Veterinary Medicine, Shahid Chamran University of Ahvaz, Ahvaz, Iran.

References
1. Kumar A, Woods KS, Bartolucci AA, Azziz R: Prevalence of adrenal androgen excess in patients with the polycystic ovary syndrome (PCO). Clin Endocrin 2005, 62:644–649.
2. David A, Ehrmann DM: Polycystic ovary syndrome. New Engl J Med 2005, 352:1223–1236.
3. Barnes RB, Rosenfield RL, Ehrmann DA, Cara JF, Cuttler L, Levitsky LL, Rosenthal IM: Ovarian hyperandrogenism as a result of congenital adrenal virilizing disorders: evidence for perinatal masculinization of neuroendocrine function in women. J Clin Endocrin Metabol 1994, 79:1328–1333.
4. Galic S, Oakhill JS, Steinberg GR: Adipose tissue as an endocrine organ. Mol Cell Endocrinol 2010, 316:129–139.
5. Mitchell M, Armstrong DT, Robker RL, Norman RJ: Adipokines: implications for female fertility and obesity. Reproduction 2005, 130(5):583–597.
6. Gnacińska M, Małgorzewicz S, Stojek M, Łysiak-Szydłowska W, Sworczak K: Role of adipokines in complications related to obesity. Adv Med Sci 2009, 54(2):150–157.
7. Goralski KB, McCarthy TC, Hanniman EA, Zabel BA, Butcher EC, Parlee SD, Muruganandan S, Sinal CJ: Chemerin, a novel adipokine that regulates adipogenesis and adipocyte metabolism. J Biol Chem 2007, 282:28175–28188.
8. Bideci A, Camurdan MO, Yeşilkaya E, Demirel F, Cinaz P: Serum ghrelin, leptin and resistin levels in adolescent girls with polycystic ovary syndrome. J Obstet Gynaecol Res 2008, 34:578–584.
9. Carmina E, Orio F, Palomba S, Cascella T, Longo RA, Colao AM, Lombardi G, Lobo RA: Evidence for altered adipocyte function in polycystic ovary syndrome. Eur J Endocrin 2005, 152:389–394.
10. Tang T, Lord JM, Norman RJ, Yasmin E, Balen AH: Insulin-sensitising drugs (metformin, rosiglitazone, pioglitazone, D-chiro-inositol) for women with polycystic ovary syndrome, oligo amenorrhoea and subfertility. Cochrane Database Syst Rev 2012, 16:5. CD003053.
11. Kaur J, Adya R, Tan BK, Chen J, Randeva HS: Identification of chemerin receptor (ChemR23) in human endothelial cells: Chemerin-induced endothelial angiogenesis. Biochem Biophys Res Commun 2010, 391:1762–1768.
12. Bozaoglu K, Joanne E, Curran Claire J, Mohamed S, Zaibi S, Segal D, Konstantopoulos N, Morrison S, Carless M, Dyer TD, Shelley A, Cole Harald HH, Eric G, Moses S: Chemerin, a Novel Adipokine in the Regulation of Angiogenesis. J Clin Endocrinol Metab 2010, 95:2476–2485.
13. Kim JY, Xue K, Cao M, Wang Q, Liu JY, Leader A, Han JY, Tsang BK: Chemerin Suppresses Ovarian Follicular Development and Its Potential Involvement in Follicular Arrest in Rats Treated Chronically with Dihydrotestosterone. Endocrinology 2013. doi:10.1210/en. 1001.
14. Tan BK, Chen J, Farhatullah S, Adya R, Kaur J, Heutling D, Lewandowski CK, Ohare PJ, Lehnert H, Randeva SH: Insulin and metformin regulate circulating and adipose tissue chemerin. Diabetes 2009, 58:1971–1978.
15. Wittamer V, Franssen JD, Vulcano M, Mirjolet JF, Le Poul E, Migeotte I, Brézillon S, Tyldesley R, Blanpain C, Detheux M, Mantovani A, Sozzani S, Vassart G, Parmentier M, Communi D: Specific recruitment of antigen-presenting cells by chemerin, a novel processed ligand from human inflammatory fluids. J Exp Med 2003, 198:977–985.
16. Haghighi N, Yaghmaei S, Hashemi P, Saadati F, Tehrani N, Ramezani F, Hedayati M: The association between serum chemerin concentration and polycystic ovarian syndrome. Tehran Univ Med J 2012, 70(5):320–324.
17. Checa MA, Requena A, Salvador C, Tur R, Callejo J, Espino JJ, Bregues FF, Herrero J: Insulin-sensitizing agenets: use in pregnancy as therapy in polycystic ovary syndrome. Hum Reprod Update 2005, 11(4):375–390.
18. Rezvanfar MA, Rezvanfar MA, Ahmadi A, Saadi HA, Baeeri M, Abdollahi M: Mechanistic links between oxidative/nitrosative stress and tumor necrosis

factor alpha in letrozole-induced murine polycystic ovary: biochemical and pathological evidences for beneficial effect of pioglitazone. *Hum Exp Toxicol* 2012, **31**:887–897.

19. Brawer JR, Munoz M, Farookhi R: Development of the polycystic ovarian condition (PCO) in the estradiol valerate-treated rat. *Biol Reprod* 1986, **35**:647–655.

20. Mani F, Fernandes AAH, Cicogna AC, Novelli Filho JLVB: Anthropometrical parameters and markers of obesity in rats. *Lab Anim* 2007, **41**:111–119.

21. Katsuki A, Sumida Y, Gabazza EC, Murashima S, Furuta M, Araki- Sasaki R, Hori Y, Yano Y, Adachi Y: Homeostasis model assessment is a reliable indicator of insulin resistance during follow-up of patients with type 2 diabetes. *Diabetes Care* 2001, **24**(2):362–365.

22. Livak K: *ABI Prism 7700 Sequence Detection System.* Foster City, CA: User Bulletin 2. PE. Applied Biosystems; 1997.

23. Bradford MM: A rapid and sensitive for the quantitation of microgram quantitites of protein utilizing the principle of protein-dye binding. *Anal Biochem* 1976, **72**:248–254.

24. Barber TM, McCarthy MI, Wass JAH, Franks S: Obesity and polycystic ovary syndrome. *Clin Endocrin* 2006, **65**:137–145.

25. Bozaoglu K, Segal D, Shields KA, Cummings N, Curran JE, Comuzzie AG, Mahaney MC, Rainwater DL, Vandeberg JL, MacCluer JW, Collier G, Blangero J, Walder K, Jowett JBM: Chemerin is associated with metabolic syndrome phenotypes in a Mexican-American population. *J Clin Endocrinol Metab* 2009, **95**:2476–2485.

26. Ernst MC, Sinal CJ: Chemerin: at the crossroads of inflammation and obesity. *Endocrin Metabol* 2010, **21**:660–667.

27. Bozaoglu K, Bolton K, McMillan J, Zimmet P, Jowett J, Collier G, Walder K, Segal L: Chemerin is a novel adipokine associated with obesity and metabolic syndrome. *Endocrinology* 2007, **148**(10):4687–4694.

28. Douglas NC, Nakhuda GS, Sauer MV, Zimmermann RC: Angiogenesis and Ovarian Function. *J Fertil Reprod* 2005, **13**(4):7–15.

29. González F, Rote NS, Minium J, Kirwan JP: Evidence of proatherogenic inflammation in polycystic ovary syndrome. *Metabolism* 2009, **58**(7):954–962.

30. González F: Inflammation in Polycystic Ovary Syndrome: underpinning of insulin resistance and ovarian dysfunction. *Steroids* 2010, **77**(4):300–305. 10.

31. Parlee SD, Ernst MC, Sinal CJ, Goralski KB: TNFα enhances the expression and secretion of chemerin from adipocytes. *FASEB J* 2009, **755**:5.

32. Rezvanfar MA, Saadi HAS, Gooshe M, Abdolghaffari AH, Baeeri MB, Abdollahi M: Ovarian aging-like phenotype in the hyperandrogenism-induced murine model of polycystic ovary. *Oxid Med Cell Long* 2014, **2014**:1–10.

33. Iuorno MJ, Nestler JE: Insulin-lowering drugs in polycystic ovary syndrome. *Obst Gynecol Clin North Am* 2001, **28**(1):153–164.

34. De Leo V, La Marca A, Petraglia F: Insulin-lowering agents in the management of polycystic ovary syndrome. *Endoc Rev* 2003, **24**(5):633–667.

35. Glueck CJ, Moreira A, Goldenberg N, Sieve L, Wang P: Pioglitazone and metformin in obese women with polycystic ovary syndrome not optimally responsive to metformin. *Human Reprod* 2003, **18**(8):1618–1625.

36. Wang Q, Leader A, Tsang BK: Inhibitory Roles of Prohibitin and Chemerin in FSH-Induced Rat Granulosa Cell Steroidogenesis. *Endocrinol* 2013. doi:10.1210/en.1836.

37. Angelidis G, Dafopoulos K, Messini KI, Valotassiou V, Tsikouras P, Vrachnis N, Psimadas D, Georgoulias P, Messinis IE: The Emerging Roles of Adiponectin in Female Reproductive System-Associated Disorders and Pregnancy. *Reprod Sci* 2013, **20**:872–881.

38. Libby P, Plutzky J: Inflammation in diabetes mellitus: role of peroxisome-proliferator-activated receptor-alpha and peroxisome-proliferator-activated receptor-gamma agonists. *Am J Cardiol* 2007, **99**:27–40.

39. Nestler JE, Jakubowicz DJ, Evans WS, Pasquali R: Effects of metformin on spontaneous and clomiphene-induced ovulation in the polycystic ovary syndrome. *N Engl J Med* 1998, **338**:1876–1880.

Unraveling the cytotoxic potential of Temozolomide loaded into PLGA nanoparticles

Darshana S Jain[1], Rajani B Athawale[1*], Amrita N Bajaj[2], Shruti S Shrikhande[1], Peeyush N Goel[3], Yuvraj Nikam[3] and Rajiv P Gude[3*]

Abstract

Background: Nanotechnology has received great attention since a decade for the treatment of different varieties of cancer. However, there is a limited data available on the cytotoxic potential of Temozolomide (TMZ) formulations. In the current research work, an attempt has been made to understand the anti-metastatic effect of the drug after loading into PLGA nanoparticles against C6 glioma cells.
Nanoparticles were prepared using solvent diffusion method and were characterized for size and morphology. Diffusion of the drug from the nanoparticles was studied by dialysis method. The designed nanoparticles were also assessed for cellular uptake using confocal microscopy and flow cytometry.

Results: PLGA nanoparticles caused a sustained release of the drug and showed a higher cellular uptake. The drug formulations also affected the cellular proliferation and motility.

Conclusion: PLGA coated nanoparticles prolong the activity of the loaded drug while retaining the anti-metastatic activity.

Keywords: C6 cell line, Gliomas, PLGA nanoparticles, Temozolomide

Background

Glioblastoma multiforme is WHO classified grade IV type of brain tumors depicting pleomorphism and atypical nuclei [1]. The current therapeutic modality for the treatment includes surgery followed by chemotherapy and radiation. Despite the progress in understanding of molecular basis in the gliomas, the prognosis of tumors remains dismal [2]. The main reason for the poor prognosis is the complexity of the brain and presence of Blood Brain Barrier (BBB). This comprises of endothelial cells that does not allow entry of exogenous material, bacteria, viruses and chemotherapeutic agents. Further, the expression of the efflux transporters adds to its complexity [3].

However, BBB allows the passage of small sized particles that are hydrophobic in nature [4]. Nanoparticles viz. solid lipid nanoparticles, polymeric nanoparticles, nano emulsions have been fabricated and used against gliomas

[5-7]. Small sized particles are better permeated though the barrier with the target ability to the cancerous cells. TMZ has been a drug of choice and is used as a first line agent for the treatment of gliomas after its surgical resection. However, due to a very short half life of 1.8 h and protein binding of 15% [8,9] repeated administration of the drug is required. In addition, less site specificity is demonstrated by the drug and thus the amount of the drug reaching the tumor site becomes limited. The probability of aiming the cancerous cells with sustained release of the loaded drugs/agents by nanoparticles prompted us to undertake the present work. Nanoparticles loaded with doxorubicin, daunorubicin, epirubicin, temozolomide, methotrexate and many other such chemotherapeutic agents have been prepared and characterized for various physico-chemical properties [10-14].

Polymeric nanoparticles are amongst the most preferred delivery system for treatment of cancers due to higher penetrability, sustainability, degradability and better payload. The reason for selecting PLGA is based on its tunable properties and biodegradability. Biodegradability leads to formation of lactic acid and glycolic acid that are readily cleared form the body as by products

* Correspondence: rajani.athawale@gmail.com; rgude@actrec.gov.in
[1]Department of Pharmaceutics, C.U. Shah College of Pharmacy, SNDT Women's University, Juhu Tara Road, Santacruz (West), Mumbai 400 049, India
[3]Gude Lab, Advanced Centre for Treatment, Research & Education in Cancer (ACTREC), Tata Memorial Centre, Kharghar, Navi Mumbai 410 210, India
Full list of author information is available at the end of the article

[15]. There are no reports for the *in vitro* performance of TMZ encapsulated in nanoparticulate formulations till date.

In this purview, we had decided to fabricate PLGA nanoparticles loaded with anti cancer agent TMZ for targeting glial cells. The prepared nanoparticles could thus reach the target cells by passage though the BBB and demonstrate better penetrability though the cancerous cells. Further, we have evaluated the performance index of both the free and encapsulated drug. The results clearly suggest the applicability of PLGA coated nanoparticles for the management of gliomas.

Methods
Cell lines
The C6 glioma cell line was procured from NCCS, Pune, India. It was maintained in HAM's 12 medium (GIBCO) supplemented with 10% heat inactivated fetal bovine serum, FBS (GIBCO) and primocin (100 µg/mL). Cultures were maintained at 37°C in 5% CO_2 humidified atmosphere.

Materials
Temozolomide was a generous gift sample from Cipla Pvt. Ltd. Vikhroli, Mumbai. PLGA was obtained as a gift sample from PURAC (PDLG 50:50 grade). Poloxamer 188 (Lutrol F 68) was obtained as a gift sample from BASF Ltd. Mumbai. All the other chemicals/reagents used were either of analytical grade or the highest purity commercially available.

Preparation of nanoparticles
PLGA nanoparticles were prepared by a method principally involving solvent diffusion technique [15]. Briefly, 50 mg of PLGA was solubilised in 4 mL of acetonitrile. To the same solution 30 mg of the drug was added and solubilised. The above solution was emulsified with an aqueous solution (4 mL) comprising of 0.5% poloxamer 188 using IKA -18 Ultraturrax. Emulsified organic solvent was carefully poured into 8 mL of prechilled 0.5% poloxamer 188 solution kept stirring over a magnetic stirrer. Solvent was allowed to slowly diffuse leaving behind homogenous nanoparticles. Particle size and zeta potential for the developed particles were noted using Malvern Zetasizer 90S.

Particle size analysis and polydispersity index measurements
Particle size and polydispersity index for the developed nanoparticles were noted using Malveren Zetasizer instrument 90S (Ver 6.12.). Particle size indicates the average size acquired by the nanoparticles when dispersed in water whereas the polydispersity index depicted the homogeneity in distribution of these particles. In our study, 20 µL of the nanoparticulate suspension was suitably diluted with HPLC grade water in the polystyrene cuvette. The cuvette was then placed in the pathway of scattered light to record the fluctuations in the intensity of the light due to the presence of the particles. The intensity of the scattered light was measured at 90° using Malvern software to give the hydrodynamic diameter and the polydispersity index [16].

Zeta potential and diffusion coefficient measurements
Zeta potential measurements enable to determine surface charge acquired by the particles in solution. Samples were diluted using the procedure discussed for particle size measurement. A dip cell with electrode was inserted into the cuvette and then placed in Malvern Zetasizer 90 S. Diffusion coefficients and the particle mobility was noted for each sample. An average of approximately 15 runs was measured at 90° at the stationery level in the cylindrical cell. Auto correlated software depicted the zeta potential values for each sample depending upon the mobility of the particles towards the electrode.

In- vitro dissolution study
Diffusion though dialysis membrane was assessed to determine the diffusion and further dissolution of the drug in the dissolution medium. Quantification of the drug from the withdrawn aliquots during *in-vitro* dissolution was performed using developed and prevalidated UV method (JASCO). Pure Drug and nanoparticle batches equivalent to 20 mg of drug were weighed and transferred to dialysis membrane {cut off 6-8 KDa and diameter of 21.5 mm (Hi media dialysis membrane no. 50) sealed at one end by thread. Approximately, 1 mL of dissolution medium (sodium acetate buffer pH 5) was added in these bags, and another end was sealed. Prepared dialysis bags were dialyzed by suspending in 500 mL of pH 5 sodium acetate buffer placed in dissolution flask (Apparatus: Dissolution tester: Electrolab 6 T). Dissolution was performed in pH 5 sodium acetate buffer dissolution medium at rotation speed of 100 rpm. Intermittently aliquots were withdrawn at prefixed time intervals. Each time 1 mL was withdrawn and replenished with the same amount of dissolution medium during the study. Volume of the aliquots was made to 10 mL with dissolution medium and absorbance was measured at λmax of 255 nm on a UV spectrophotometer. Calculation for % drug release was performed at each time point and graphs indicating % drug released vs. time were plotted and are represented in Figure 1.

Cellular proliferation using MTT cytotoxicity assay
Cytotoxicity was determined using MTT assay as previously reported [17,18]. Briefly, 2500 and 1500 cells/well were seeded in a 96-well plate respectively. After 24 h

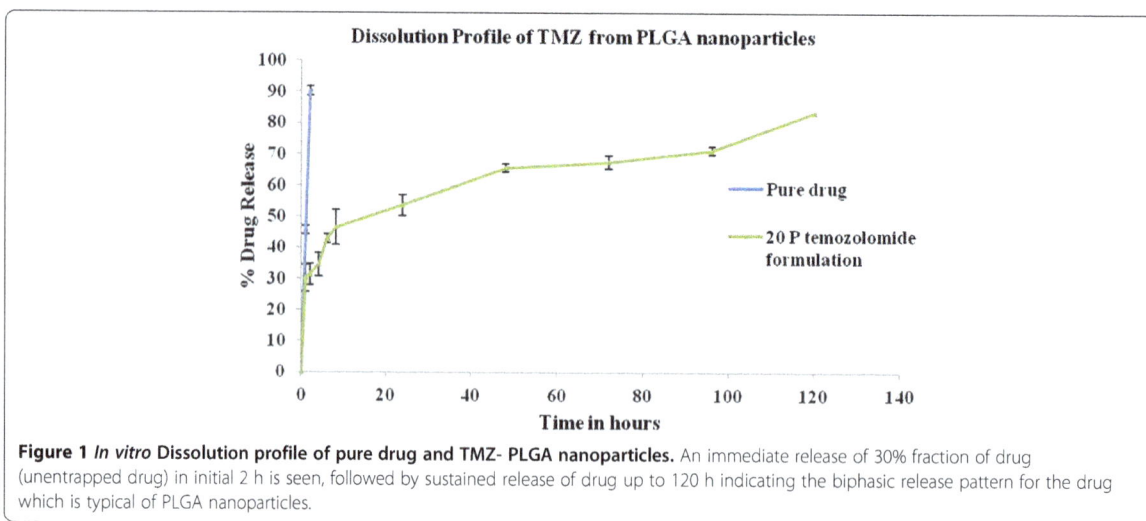

Figure 1 *In vitro* **Dissolution profile of pure drug and TMZ- PLGA nanoparticles.** An immediate release of 30% fraction of drug (unentrapped drug) in initial 2 h is seen, followed by sustained release of drug up to 120 h indicating the biphasic release pattern for the drug which is typical of PLGA nanoparticles.

cells were treated with pure drug TMZ, PLGA blank nanoparticles and PLGA nanoparticles loaded with TMZ at varying doses of (1,500-0.01 µg/mL). Plates were then incubated at 37°C for 72 h and 96 h in CO_2 incubator. The drug was discarded and the wells were washed twice with PBS at respective time points. MTT (1 mg/mL) was added to all the wells and incubated overnight. The plates were later centrifuged and the supernatant was finally discarded. The formazon crystals formed were dissolved in DMSO and the readings were taken using ELISA plate reader at dual wavelengths of 540/690 nm respectively. IC_{50}, the concentration required to kill 50% of the cells by TMZ was calculated. The graph was plotted on a logarithmic scale as percentage viability versus drug concentration and is represented in Figure 2.

Colony formation assay

Clonogenic assay was done to assess the long term cytotoxicity of different formulations. 600 cells were seeded in a 35 mm plate and after stabilization [19] treated with developed formulations: PLGA formulations (Drug loaded and blank) and pure drug. These were removed after an incubation period of 24 h, and the plates were washed with PBS to remove traces of the drug. Cells were later incubated in the presence of complete media for a period of 8–10 days. Fixation was done using 70% chilled methanol followed by staining using 1% crystal violet. Colonies containing 50 or more cells were counted and the results were plotted as number of colonies versus drug/formulation (Figure 3).

Wound scratch assay

Wound scratch assay was performed as per the earlier reports [18,20,21]. Approximately, 0.6 million cells were seeded into 35 mm plates. On the following day, cells were treated with 2 µg/mL mitomycin C for 1 h. The cells in the centre of the plates were later scraped using a sterile tip so as to form a wound. Sub-toxic doses of TMZ (75 µg/mL and 150 µg/mL), TMZ loaded formulations and PLGA formulations (equivalent to pure drug) were then added and incubated for 24 h. Drug formulations were removed and the plates were fixed using 70% methanol. The wound width was measured using the AxioVision Rel 4.8 imaging software, and the results were plotted as percent wound closure with respect to control. The controls were considered to be covered 100%. Results are represented in Figure 4.

Cellular morphology in presence of TMZ loaded in nanoparticulate formulation

Haematoxylin-Eosin (HE) staining was performed to observe the morphological changes upon drug treatment as described previously [17,18]. Sub-confluent cells were allowed to be grown on coverslips. Cells were then treated with TMZ, PLGA blank formulations and TMZ loaded into nanoparticulate formulations (concentration equivalent to 75 µg/mL) as done earlier and fixed using 70% chilled methanol. The cover slips were then stained using haematoxylin and eosin subsequently. Mounting was done on the glass slides using DPX mountant. Cells were later observed under Zeiss upright microscope. The results are shown in Figure 5.

Cellular uptake using confocal microscopy

The uptake of nanoparticles was performed using particles loaded with FITC, a hydrophilic dye. Sub-confluent cultures of C6 glioma were treated with only FITC and

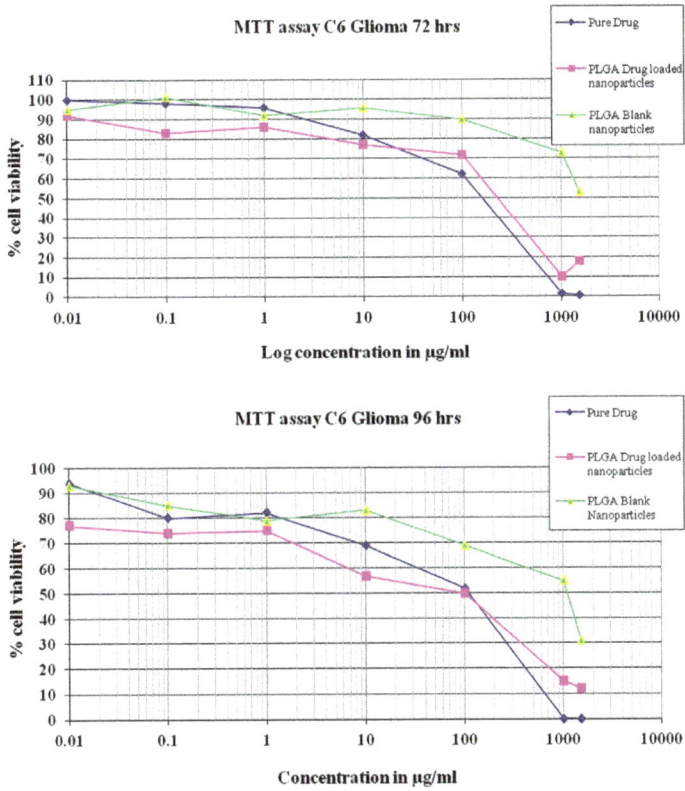

Figure 2 MTT assay performed for the pure drug and drug loaded PLGA nanoparticles. The observed IC_{50} was 150 μg/mL TMZ in pure form on C6 glioma irrespective of the time. However, the same drug when loaded into nanoparticles demonstrated an IC_{50} of 200 μg/mL and 150 μg/mL after 72 h and 96 h, respectively.

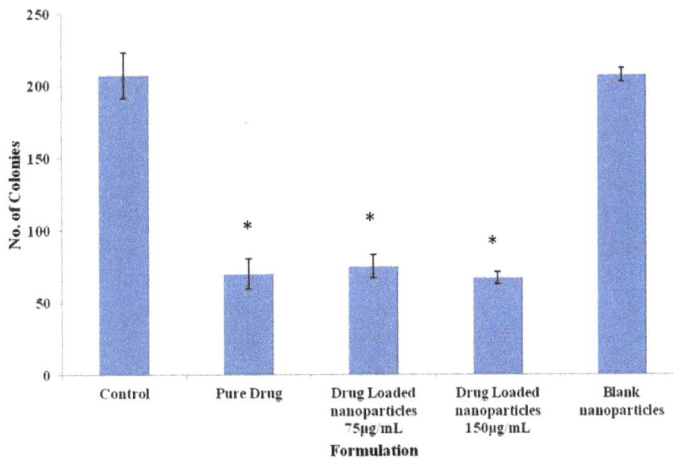

Figure 3 Clonogenic assay for pure drug, TMZ loaded PLGA nanoparticle formulations and placebo PLGA nanoparticles. The numbers of colonies for untreated and pure drug treated cells were found to be 221.00 ± 15.56 and 67.00 ± 10.26 respectively. However, in case of drug loaded nanoparticles the number of colonies were 75.00 ± 8.00, 70.66 ± 4.00 at concentrations of 75 μg/mL and 150 μg/mL respectively. (*$P < 0.05$).

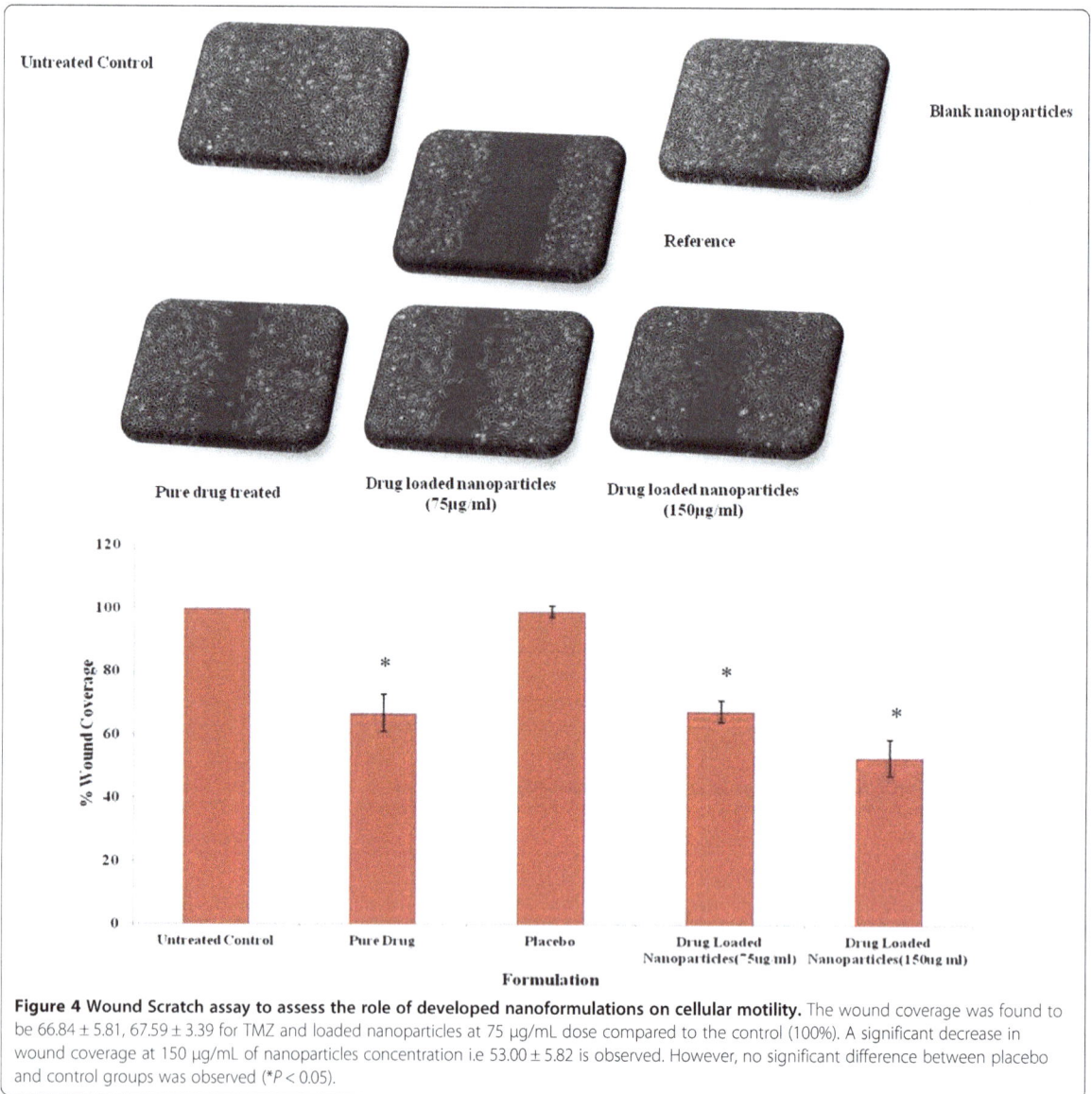

Figure 4 Wound Scratch assay to assess the role of developed nanoformulations on cellular motility. The wound coverage was found to be 66.84 ± 5.81, 67.59 ± 3.39 for TMZ and loaded nanoparticles at 75 μg/mL dose compared to the control (100%). A significant decrease in wound coverage at 150 μg/mL of nanoparticles concentration i.e 53.00 ± 5.82 is observed. However, no significant difference between placebo and control groups was observed (*P < 0.05).

FITC loaded nanoparticles for 2 h respectively. Cells were later washed with PBS and fixed using 1% paraformaldehyde (PFA). The cells were then treated with DAPI and then washing was done thrice with PBS. Mounting of coverslips was done using 2.5% DABCO on glass slides and then sealed with nail paint. Acquisition was done on LSM 510 confocal microscope from Zeiss at 63X. LSM image browser software was used for data analysis (Figure 6).

Cellular uptake using flow cytometry

Flow cytometric analysis was done to confirm our previous findings. Sub-confluent cultures of C6 glioma were treated with FITC and its loaded nanoparticles as done earlier [22]. Cells were thereafter harvested and fixed using 1% PFA. Cells were then washed using PBS and later suspended in the same. Acquisition was done using FACS Calibur and the results were analysed by CellQuest software (Figure 7).

Statistical analysis

All the experiments had been performed at least thrice. The results are indicated as Mean ± SD. One way ANOVA was used for the purpose of statistical significance. The results were considered to be statistically significant where *P < 0.05.

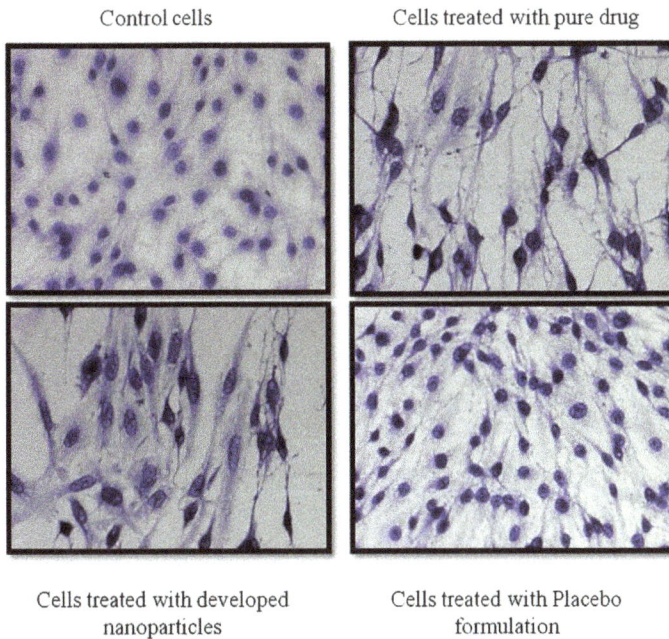

Figure 5 Changes in cellular morphology using HE staining. The spindle shape cells of C6 glioma is distorted after treatment with free TMZ and TMZ loaded formulations. Further, stress on the spindle fibres with further rounding up of the cells is being observed.

Results and discussion

Fabrication of nanoparticles

Solvent diffusion method was used for the fabrication of nanoparticles. Developed nanoparticles were subjected to particle size and zeta potential assessment. The particle size for the pure drug was found to be 1256 ± 82 nm (Approximately 1.3 μm crystalline structure particles). A size range of 150-160 nm was found for the developed nanoparticles with poly dispersity index values suggesting that the developed nanoparticles were monodisperse. The developed nanoparticles were then lyophilized and the assessment of the size was performed post lyophilisation. The developed lyophilized nanoparticulate formulation maintained the particle size even after reconstitution indicating stability and robustness of the developed nanoparticles. Zeta potential for the pure drug was found to be 17.40 ± 0.256 mV and for the developed nanoparticles was found to be -20.50 ± 0.069 mV.

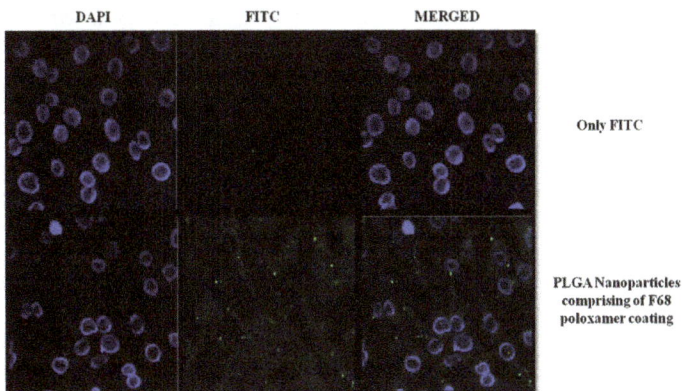

Figure 6 Immunofluorescence studies for cellular uptake of developed nanoparticles. Cells treated with FITC showed almost negligible fluorescence indicating absence of its uptake. However, cells treated with FITC loaded nanoparticles exhibited strong green fluorescence. Nucleus is stained with DAPI represented in dark blue colour.

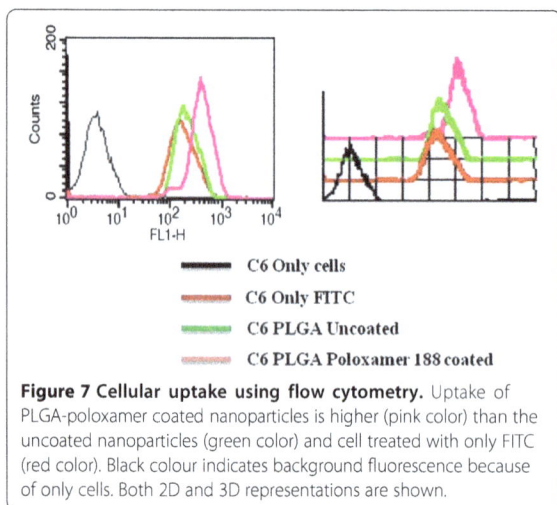

Figure 7 Cellular uptake using flow cytometry. Uptake of PLGA-poloxamer coated nanoparticles is higher (pink color) than the uncoated nanoparticles (green color) and cell treated with only FITC (red color). Black colour indicates background fluorescence because of only cells. Both 2D and 3D representations are shown.

There are numerous methods to design PLGA nanoparticles viz. solvent evaporation, microfluidisation, solvent diffusion, nanoprecipitation and salting out. The designed nanoparticles were developed successfully with solvent diffusion technique with acetonitrile as organic solvent. As the particles were designed for treatment of glioblastoma multiforme, the major obstacle to the delivery of particles would be passage though the BBB. However, BBB permit passage of small size entities (below 200 nm) which are hydrophobic in nature and hence particle size is an important parameter for entities aiming to pass the blood brain barrier. As the particle size range of our designed nanoparticles was below 200 nm better permeation can be expected though the barrier. The surface charge on the particle could be determined by the zeta potential. Negative values for the pure drug indicate that the charge on the surface is negative. The negatively charged drug particles are taken up the liver and further phagocytosized, thus only a small fraction of the drug remains in the circulation [23,24]. With the designed nanoparticles negative charge of the particles was maintained with the readings at the higher end of the negative charge. Higher values of the zeta potential determine the stability of the particle. Further, transmission electron microscopy images depicted formation of roughly round PLGA drug loaded nanoparticles. Poloxamer 188 layer with the thickness of around 6-10 nm was found using transmission electron microscopy [15].

In vitro dissolution profile

Dissolution was performed in sodium acetate buffer pH 5, considering the stability of the drug. TMZ is unstable at physiological pH and rapidly undergoes hydrolysis to form MTIC and AIC as metabolites. Pure drug diffuses out of the dialysis bag within 2 h as indicated in the graph plotted

for TMZ. This reading can be correlated with the half life of the drug being 1.8 h that means the drug is readily available for its action *in vivo*. However, the developed nanoparticles demonstrated a slow release pattern of the drug when loaded into PLGA nanoparticles. The half life of the drug is extended as indicated from dissolution profile. An immediate release of 30% fraction of drug (unentrapped drug) in initial 2 h is seen, followed by sustained release of drug up to 120 h indicating the biphasic release pattern for the drug which is typical of PLGA nanoparticles. The developed nanoparticles could sustain the drug release and extend the half life of drug. The data warrants the avoidance of repeated administration of TMZ and this would be of clinical significance because the developed formulation avoids repeated administration of the active component *in vivo*. This action was further confirmed and correlated with performed *in vitro* cell line study.

Nanoparticles exert anti-proliferative effects in a dose and time dependent manner

Time and dose-dependent based MTT studies were performed to determine the IC_{50} of TMZ (72 h and 96 h). The observed IC_{50} for pure TMZ was found out to be 150 µg/mL against C6 glioma irrespective of the time. However, the same drug when loaded into nanoparticles demonstrated an IC_{50} of 200 µg/mL and 150 µg/mL after 72 h and 96 h, respectively. As the time of exposure of formulations to the cells was increased, IC_{50} showed a significant decrease. This further correlated with the dose. As the dose of the pure drug and drug loaded formulation was increased IC_{50} of the compound decreased. However, for pure drug IC_{50} was concentration but not time dependent. The developed formulations released the drug at a very slow rate and hence a small proportion of drug is available to exhibit action each time (drug release profile in Figure 2). The obtained results can be correlated with the dissolution profile of the drug. The diffusion of the drug from the formulation continued for more than 120 h. Hence, even after 96 h IC_{50} for pure drug and drug loaded nanoparticles did not match, confirming slow release of the drug from the developed formulation, as well as time and concentration dependent cytotoxicity of developed formulations. Further, to confirm the absence of cytotoxic action of the excipients used in the developed formulation, MTT assay was also performed for the blank formulation. High IC_{50} (> 1000 µg/mL after 96 h exposure) value of the blank formulation depicts the safety of the polymer and other excipients used for fabricating the nanoparticles. Based on these observations, 75 µg/mL and 150 µg/mL of TMZ in free and loaded form were selected for performing the subsequent experiments with 24 h exposure.

Effect of nanoparticles on the clonogenic potential

Anti-proliferative activity of the cells was performed using clonogenic assay. The numbers of colonies for un-treated and pure drug treated cells were found to be 221.00 ± 15.56 and 67.00 ± 10.26. The number of col-onies for drug loaded nanoparticles was found to be 75.00 ± 80, 70.66 ± 40 at concentrations of 75 μg/mL and 150 μg/mL respectively ($P < 0.05$). Cancer cells show a self sufficiency towards growth signals [25]. These re-sults indicate that the cells lose the ability to replicate in the presence of drug and its formulations. The possible mechanism might be due to inhibition of EGFR and MAPK pathways by TMZ as reported earlier, that play key roles in the process of proliferation [26,27].

Nanoparticles affect motility of C6 glioma cells

Both pure TMZ and its nanoparticles formulations at dosage of 75 μg/mL showed a similar reduction in motility. The wound coverage was found out to be 66.84 ± 5.81, 67.59 ± 3.39 for pure and nanoparticles at 75 μg/mL dose compared to the control (100%). However, there was a sig-nificant decrease in wound coverage at 150 μg/mL of nanoparticles concentration i.e 53.00 ± 5.82 ($P < 0.05$). There was no significant difference between placebo and control groups respectively. The differences in migration between pure drug and drug loaded nanoparticles formu-lation (150 μg/mL) can be attributed to the slower diffu-sion of the drug from the nanoparticles. The effect of TMZ on Rho GTPase signaling might be the possible reason for hindering migration as earlier reported [27].

Changes in cellular morphology upon TMZ and PLGA nanoparticles treatment

C6 glioma cells exhibits atypical nuclei with pleomorph-ism characteristic of human glioma cancer. The spindle shape cells of C6 glioma is distorted after treatment with free TMZ and TMZ loaded formulation. Stress on the spindle fibres with further rounding up of the cells is being observed. Further, there is a decrease in cell volume and number with both the regimens, demonstrating equal effi-cacy of the developed drug loaded nanoparticles.

Immuno fluorescence showed a higher uptake of developed nanoparticles

C6 glioma cells were treated with FITC loaded into PLGA nanoparticles. Images for the uptake are depicted in Figure 6. Cells treated with pure dye showed almost negligible or background fluorescence indicating no up-take of the dye by the cells. However, cells treated with FITC loaded nanoparticles exhibited strong green fluor-escence. The nucleus of the cells is stained with DAPI represented in blue colour. These results indicated that the developed nanoparticles are able to modulate the uptake of hydrophilic dye after its encapsulation in

the particle. PLGA being a hydrophobic polymer with tunable properties masks the entity of FITC, a hydro-philic agent not readily permeating into the cells. Thus, it can be concluded that the uptake of hydrophilic/amphipathic agent will be enhanced by using PLGA de-signed nanoparticles.

Flow cytometric analysis showed an increase in uptake of developed nanoparticles

To further corroborate our earlier findings using confocal microscopy, we had performed the cellular uptake of the developed nano formulations in C6 glioma cells by flow cytometry. As can be seen in Figure 7, uptake of PLGA-poloxomer is high (pink color) than the uncoated (green color) and cell treated with only FITC (red color). These observations further substantiate our earlier findings.

Conclusions

The present study was performed to develop effective formulations targeting across the BBB. TMZ loaded nanoparticles were successfully prepared using solvent evaporation method. The developed nanoparticles exhib-ited slow release of the drug with prolongation of its half life. Further, cellular uptake of the nanoparticles was en-hanced as confirmed using confocal and flow cytometry. These properties certainly enhance the safety profile of the drug with reducing its toxicity. Hence, it may be con-cluded Poly Lactic glycolic acid (PLGA) nanoparticles sustain the cytotoxic action of TMZ in C6 Glioma cells.

Competing interests
The authors declare that they have no competing interests.

Authors' contributions
DJ collected data, performed experiments such as fabrication of nanoparticles and manuscript writing. RA, AB also helped in writing the manuscript and correcting the manuscript. SS helped in collecting the information and data related to nanoparticulate formulations. PG performed uptake studies, drafting manuscript and performing cell line experiments along with YN. RG is project collaborator and provided technical expertise in correcting and drafting the manuscript. All authors read and approved the final manuscript.

Acknowledgements
The authors are thankful to DST-INSPIRE and CSIR for providing financial assistance to Ms. Darshana S. Jain and Mr. Peeyush N Goel respectively. The authors are also thankful to Cipla Pvt. Ltd and BASF, Mumbai for providing gift sample of temozolomide and poloxamer 188 respectively financially support-ing the project. The authors also thank both the Confocal and flow cytometry facilities at ACTREC.

Author details
[1]Department of Pharmaceutics, C.U. Shah College of Pharmacy, SNDT Women's University, Juhu Tara Road, Santacruz (West), Mumbai 400 049, India. [2]SVKM's Dr. Bhanuben Nanavati College of Pharmacy, Vileparle, Mumbai 400 056, India. [3]Gude Lab, Advanced Centre for Treatment, Research & Education in Cancer (ACTREC), Tata Memorial Centre, Kharghar, Navi Mumbai 410 210, India.

References

1. Doolittle ND: **State of the science in brain tumor classification.** *Semin Oncol Nurs* 2004, **20**:224–230.
2. Gurney JG, Kadan-Lottick N: **Brain and other central nervous system tumors: rates, trends, and epidemiology.** *Curr Opin Oncol* 2001, **13**:160–166.
3. Laquintana V, Trapani A, Denora N, Wang F, Gallo JM, Trapani G: **New strategies to deliver anticancer drugs to brain tumors.** *Expert Opin Drug Deliv* 2009, **6**:1017–1032.
4. Begley DJ, Brightman MW: **Structural and functional aspects of the blood–brain barrier.** *Prog Drug Res* 2003, **61**:39–78.
5. Wang C-X, Huang L-S, Hou L-B, Jiang L, Yan Z-T, Wang Y-L, Chen Z-L: **Antitumor effects of polysorbate-80 coated gemcitabine polybutylcyanoacrylate nanoparticles *in vitro* and its pharmacodynamics *in vivo* on C6 glioma cells of a brain tumor model.** *Brain Res* 2009, **1261**:91–99.
6. Koziara JM, Lockman PR, Allen DD, Mumper RJ: **Paclitaxel nanoparticles for the potential treatment of brain tumors.** *J Control Release* 2004, **99**:259–269.
7. Sanchez De Juan B, Von Briesen H, Gelperina SE, Kreuter J: **Cytotoxicity of doxorubicin bound to poly (butyl cyanoacrylate) nanoparticles in rat glioma cell lines using different assays.** *J Drug Target* 2006, **14**:614–622.
8. Newlands E, Stevens M, Wedge S, Wheelhouse R, Brock C: **Temozolomide: a review of its discovery, chemical properties, pre-clinical development and clinical trials.** *Cancer Treat Rev* 1997, **23**:35–61.
9. Tentori L, Graziani G: **Recent approaches to improve the antitumor efficacy of temozolomide.** *Curr Med Chem* 2009, **16**:245–257.
10. Tian X-H, Lin X-N, Wei F, Feng W, Huang Z-C, Wang P, Ren L, Diao Y: **Enhanced brain targeting of temozolomide in polysorbate-80 coated polybutylcyanoacrylate nanoparticles.** *Int J Nanomedicine* 2011, **6**:445–452.
11. Gao K, Jiang X: **Influence of particle size on transport of methotrexate across blood brain barrier by polysorbate 80-coated polybutylcyanoacrylate nanoparticles.** *Int J Pharm* 2006, **310**:213–219.
12. Ying X, Wen H, Lu W-L, Du J, Guo J, Tian W, Men Y, Zhang Y, Li R-J, Yang T-Y: **Dual-targeting daunorubicin liposomes improve the therapeutic efficacy of brain glioma in animals.** *J Control Release* 2010, **141**:183–192.
13. Tian W, Ying X, Du J, Guo J, Men Y, Zhang Y, Li R-J, Yao H-J, Lou J-N, Zhang L-R: **Enhanced efficacy of functionalized epirubicin liposomes in treating brain glioma-bearing rats.** *Eur J Pharm Sci* 2010, **41**:232–243.
14. Friedman HS, Kerby T, Calvert H: **Temozolomide and treatment of malignant glioma.** *Clin Cancer Res* 2000, **6**:2585–2597.
15. Jain D, Athawale R, Bajaj A, Shrikhande S, Goel PN, Gude RP: **Studies on stabilization mechanism and stealth effect of Poloxamer 188 onto PLGA nanoparticles.** *Colloids Surf B Biointerfaces* 2013, **109**:59–67.
16. Nerkar N, Bajaj A, Shrikhande S, Jain D: **Fabrication of liposheres for paclitaxel and assessment of *in vitro* cytotoxicity against U373 cancer cell lines.** *Thai J Pharm Sci* 2012, **36**:117–130.
17. Dua P, Gude RP: **Antiproliferative and antiproteolytic activity of pentoxifylline in cultures of B16F10 melanoma cells.** *Cancer Chemother Pharmacol* 2006, **58**:195–202.
18. Goel PN, Gude R: **Unravelling the antimetastatic potential of pentoxifylline, a methylxanthine derivative in human MDA-MB-231 breast cancer cells.** *Mol Cell Biochem* 2011, **358**:141–151.
19. Franken NA, Rodermond HM, Stap J, Haveman J, Van Bree C: **Clonogenic assay of cells *in vitro*.** *Nat Protoc* 2006, **1**:2315–2319.
20. Pichot C, Hartig S, Xia L, Arvanitis C, Monisvais D, Lee F, Frost J, Corey S: **Dasatinib synergizes with doxorubicin to block growth, migration, and invasion of breast cancer cells.** *Br J Cancer* 2009, **101**:38–47.
21. Lee HS, Seo EY, Kang NE, Kim WK: **[6]-Gingerol inhibits metastasis of MDA-MB-231 human breast cancer cells.** *J Nutr Biochem* 2008, **19**:313–319.
22. Jain D, Athawale R, Bajaj A, Shrikhande S, Goel PN, Nikam Y, Gude RP: **Poly lactic acid (PLA) nanoparticles sustain the cytotoxic action of temozolomide in C6 Glioma cells.** *Biomed Aging Path* 2013. doi:10.1016/j.biomag.2013.08.003.
23. Chen H, Wang L, Yeh J, Wu X, Cao Z, Wang YA, Zhang M, Yang L, Mao H: **Reducing non-specific binding and uptake of nanoparticles and improving cell targeting with an antifouling PEO-b-PgammaMPS copolymer coating.** *Biomaterials* 2010, **31**:5397–5407.
24. Frohlich E: **The role of surface charge in cellular uptake and cytotoxicity of medical nanoparticles.** *Int J Nanomedicine* 2012, **7**:5577–5591.
25. Hanahan D, Weinberg RA: **Hallmarks of cancer: the next generation.** *Cell* 2011, **144**:646–674.
26. Ramis G, Thomas-Moya E, de Mattos SF, Rodriguez J, Villalonga P: **EGFR inhibition in glioma cells modulates rho signaling to inhibit cell motility and invasion and cooperates with temozolomide to reduce cell growth.** *PLoS One* 2012, **7**:e38770.
27. Chen M, Rose AE, Doudican N, Osman I, Orlow SJ: **Celastrol synergistically enhances temozolomide cytotoxicity in melanoma cells.** *Mol Cancer Res* 2009, **7**:1946–1953.

Study of the pharmacokinetic changes of Tramadol in diabetic rats

Hoda Lavasani[1], Behjat Sheikholeslami[1], Yalda H Ardakani[1], Mohammad Abdollahi[2,3], Lida Hakemi[1] and Mohammad-Reza Rouini[1,3]*

Abstract

Background: Besides the pathological states, diabetes mellitus may also alter the hepatic biotransformation of pharmaceutical agents. It is advantageous to understand the effect of diabetes on the pharmacokinetic of drugs. The objective of this study was to define the pharmacokinetic changes of tramadol and its main metabolites after *in vivo* intraperitoneal administration and *ex vivo* perfused liver study in diabetic rat model.

Tramadol (10 mg/kg) was administered to rats (diabetic and control groups of six) intraperitoneally and blood samples were collected at different time points up to 300 min. In a parallel study, isolated liver perfusion was done (in diabetic and control rats) by Krebs-Henseleit buffer (containing 500 ng/ml tramadol). Perfusate samples were collected at 10 min intervals up to 180 min. Concentration of tramadol and its metabolites were determined by HPLC.

Results: Tramadol reached higher concentrations after i.p. injection in diabetics (C_{max} of 1607.5 ± 335.9 ng/ml) compared with control group (C_{max} of 561.6 ± 111.4). M1 plasma concentrations were also higher in diabetic rats compared with control group. M2 showed also higher concentrations in diabetic rats. Comparing the concentration levels of M1 in diabetic and control perfused livers, showed that in contrast to intact animals, the metabolic ratios of M1 and M5 (M/T) were significantly higher in diabetic perfused liver compared to those of control group.

Conclusions: The pharmacokinetic of tramadol and its three metabolites are influenced by diabetes. As far as M1 is produced by Cyp2D6, its higher concentration in diabetic rats could be a result of induction in Cyp2D6 activity, while higher concentrations of tramadol can be explained by lower volume of distribution.

Introduction

The capacity of organisms to eliminate xenobiotics such as pharmaceutical drugs and environmental pollutants from their body is subject to change. One of the best-known effective factors is the genetic variation of drug metabolizing enzymes and transporters. Numerous genetic polymorphisms have been reported with cytochrome P450 (P450s) [1]. In addition to the genetic background, xenobiotic-induced transcriptional activation or deactivation (i.e. induction or inhibition) has been documented in large numbers and drawing many researchers' attention in order to avoid unfavorable drug–drug interactions and side effects of therapeutic drugs [2]. Physiological and

pathophysiological conditions also affect the activity of P450s and other enzymes. Obesity and diabetes are worldwide concerns as risk factors for metabolic syndromes in the liver [3].

Diabetes mellitus, a disease with wide prevalence in humans, involves many complications including micro- and macro angiopathy as well as neuropathy, which in turn leads to increase the incidence of many diseases. Besides these pathological states, it is believed that possible diabetes-induced alterations in the hepatic biotransformation of pharmaceutical agents could also pose additional health risk because of dangerous side effects due to drug toxicity [4]. Considering the number of diabetic patients and their increased opportunities for drug therapy compared to healthy subjects, it is of great interest to understand the effect of this disease on drug metabolism.

Several chemicals have been used for induction of insulin-dependent diabetes mellitus in animal models, principally alloxan, streptozotocin and zinc chelators [5].

* Correspondence: rouini@tums.ac.ir
[1]Biopharmaceutics and Pharmacokinetics Division, Department of Pharmaceutics, Faculty of Pharmacy, Tehran University of Medical Sciences, 14155-6451, Tehran, Iran
[3]Pharmaceutical Sciences Research Centre, Faculty of Pharmacy, Tehran University of Medical Sciences, 14155-6451, Tehran, Iran
Full list of author information is available at the end of the article

According to the literature, streptozotocin causes structural alterations in pancreatic beta cells (total degranulation) within 48 h after administration and last up to 4 months [5].

In rat models of diabetes mellitus induced by streptozotocin (DMIS) some physiological changes including a decrease in bile flow rate [6], hepatotoxicity [7], impaired renal function [8,9], disorders of the gastrointestinal tract and reductions in protein binding of drugs due to elevated plasma fatty acid level and/or glycosylation of plasma proteins [9], have been reported. Glucuronidation and sulfation were also strongly affected in DMIS rats [10]. Recently, it was shown that the expression of CYP1A1, 2A1, 2B1, 2C12, 2E1, 3A4, 4A1 and/or 4A2 were apparently increased in DMIS rats [11-14]. However, CYP2C11, 2C13, 2A2 and 3A2 were suppressed [12].

Tramadol hydrochloride (T) is a centrally acting analgesic with efficacy and potency ranging between weak opioids and morphine. The drug is mostly eliminated via biotransformation in the liver in two main pathways including O-demethylation to O-desmethyltramadol (M1) (the pharmacologically active metabolite) by isoenzyme cytochrome P450 2D6 (CYP2D6) and N-demethylation to N-desmethyltramadol (M2) by cytochromes P450 2B6 (CYP2B6) and 3A4 (CYP3A4) [15]. These primary metabolites may be further metabolized to three additional secondary metabolites namely, N, N-didemethyltramadol (M3), N, N, O-tridesmethyltramadol (M4) and N, O-desmethyltramadol (M5). The O-desmethylated metabolites are then further conjugated with glucuronic acid and sulfate before excretion in urine [15].

Recently, tramadol was suggested as an effective oral medication to alleviate pain in diabetic painful neuropathy (DPN) [16,17] and the dose-dependent lowering effect of tramadol on the plasma glucose levels of DMIS rats was also reported by Cheng et al. [18]. Although tramadol is known to be effective for the symptomatic relief of DPN, little definitive data is available concerning the effects of diabetes on hepatic drug metabolism and pharmacokinetics of this compound. Moreover, the results of those studies are not equivocal and are often contradictory.

The objective of this study was to investigate the pharmacokinetic changes of tramadol and its main metabolites after *in vivo* intraperitoneal administration and *ex vivo* perfused liver study in the DMIS rat model.

Materials and methods
Materials
The pure substances of tramadol, M1, M2, M5 and cis-tramadol as internal standard (Figure 1) were kindly supplied by Grünenthal (Achen, Germany). All other chemicals were supplied by Merck (Darmstadt, Germany). Water used in all experiments was of Direct-Q® quality (Millipore, France).

Animals
Male Sprague–Dawley rats of 7 weeks old (weighing 250–300 g) were maintained in a clean room with 12 h light–dark cycle, controlled temperature environment between 20 and 23°C, a relative humidity of 50% and free access to standard laboratory chow and water. The study was approved by the Institutional Review Board of Pharmaceutical Research Centre of Tehran University of Medical Sciences. The animals were randomly divided into two experimental groups including control and DMIS rats.

Induction of diabetes
The animals were made diabetic with a single intravenous injection of streptozotocin (Sigma, USA). Freshly prepared streptozotocin (60 mg/kg) in 0.9% saline containing 0.01 M sodium citrate (pH adjusted to 4.5) was administered once to the overnight- fasted rats via the tail vein [19]. An equal volume of a citrate buffer of pH 4.5 (0.3 ml) was injected to the control rats. On day 7 after intravenous administration of streptozotocin (rat models of DMIS) or a citrate buffer (controls for rat model of DMIS), non-fasting blood glucose levels of rats were measured using the Accu-Chek Active® (Roche Diagnostics, Basel, Switzerland). The diabetic state was confirmed by glucose levels exceeding 200 mg/dl.

Intact diabetic rat study
At seventh day after the beginning of treatment with streptozotocin (DMIS rats), the femoral vein of one leg of DMIS and control rats were cannulated with previously heparinized intravenous 16–18 gauge catheter while each rat was under ketamine anesthesia using an intraperitoneal injection of xylazine/ketamine (15/75 mg/kg). Tramadol was administered intraperitoneally as 10 mg/kg, diluted in normal saline. The animals were kept under anesthesia until the end of the experiment. Approximately, 200 μl of venous blood samples were collected in heparinized tubes at: 0 (blank); 7.5, 15, 30, 45, 60, 90, 120, 165, 210, 255 and 300 min after tramadol administration. Blood samples were immediately centrifuged for 20 min at 1800 g and the plasma samples were stored at -80°C until HPLC analysis. A 250 μl of heparinized normal saline (15 units/ml) was used to flush the cannula to prevent blood clotting. At the end of the study, animals were sacrificed by cervical dislocation.

Isolated liver perfusion study
The isolated liver perfusion study was also conducted in the DMIS and control rats. Animals were anesthetized using an intraperitoneal injection of xylazine/ketamine (15/75 mg/kg). The portal vein and superior vena cava were catheterized with an intravenous 16–18 gauge catheter, respectively. 500 units of heparin were injected into the inferior vena cava. Freshly prepared Krebs-Henseleit

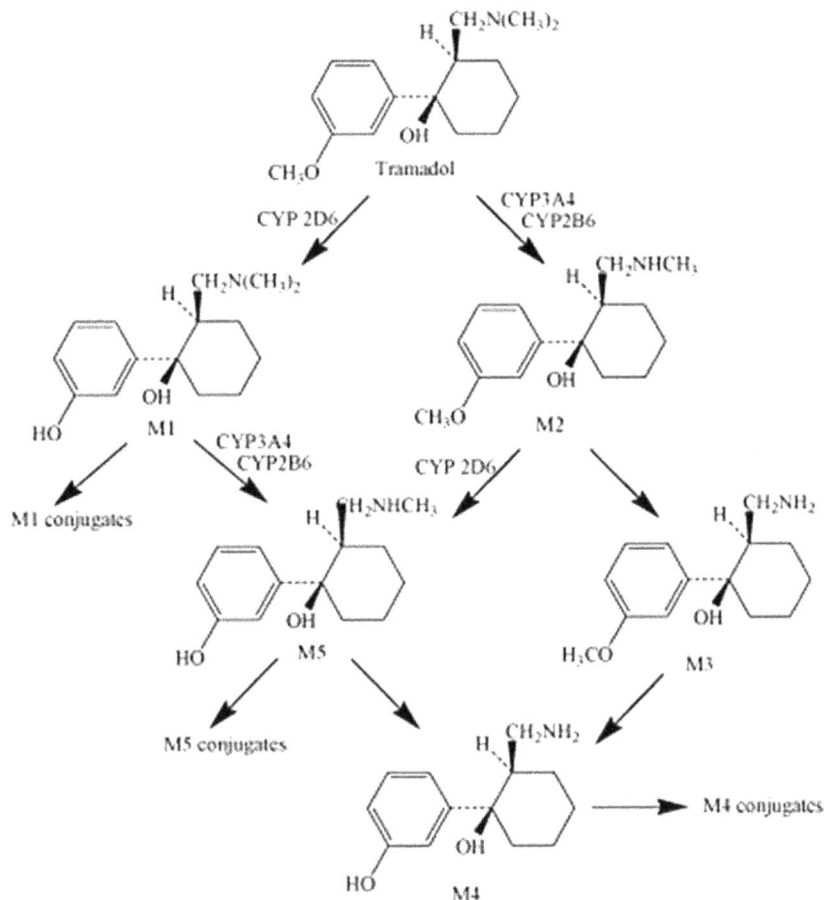

Figure 1 Metabolic pathway of tramadol.

buffer (118 mm NaCl, 4.5 mm KCl, 2.75 mm CaCl2, 1.19 mm KH2PO4, 1.18 mm MgSO4 and 25 mm Na HCO3, equilibrated with 95% O2/ 5% CO2, pH 7.4) (containing 500 ng/ml tramadol) was passed through the portal vein with a constant flow rate of 10 ml/min using a peristaltic pump. By this method, perfusion medium passed through the liver and then collected from the superior vena cava [20]. The total volume of the reservoir was 200 ml. The temperature (37°C), pH (7.4) and perfusion pressure (14 mmHg) were periodically monitored and kept unchanged through the study. Liver variability was proved by monitoring the liver enzymes activities (AST and ALT). Perfusate samples were collected at 10 min intervals up to 180 min.

Analytical method
Tramadol, M1, M2 and M5 concentration in rat plasma samples were determined by a previously described HPLC method [21]. Briefly, all analytes were extracted with ethylacetate and injected to a Knauer high-performance

liquid chromatography (Berlin, Germany), equipped with a low-pressure gradient HPLC pump, a fluorescence detector, a Rheodyne injector with a 100 μL loop and an online degasser. Excitation and emission wavelength were 200 nm and 301 nm respectively. Separation was achieved by a Chromolith™ Performance RP-18e 100 × 4.6 mm column (Merck, Darmastadt, Germany) protected by a Chromolith™ guard cartridge RP-18e 5 × 4.6 mm. A methanol: water (adjusted to pH of 2.5 by phosphoric acid) mixture (19:81, v/v) at flow rate of 2 ml/min was used as mobile phase. Data acquisition was carried out by using ChromGate chromatography software (Knauer, Berlin, Germany).

Pharmacokinetic analysis
The pharmacokinetics of tramadol and its metabolites were determined by non-compartmental analysis using Microsoft® EXCEL under Windows XP in both intact animal and isolated rat liver studies. Maximum plasma and perfusate concentrations (C_{max}) of analytes and their

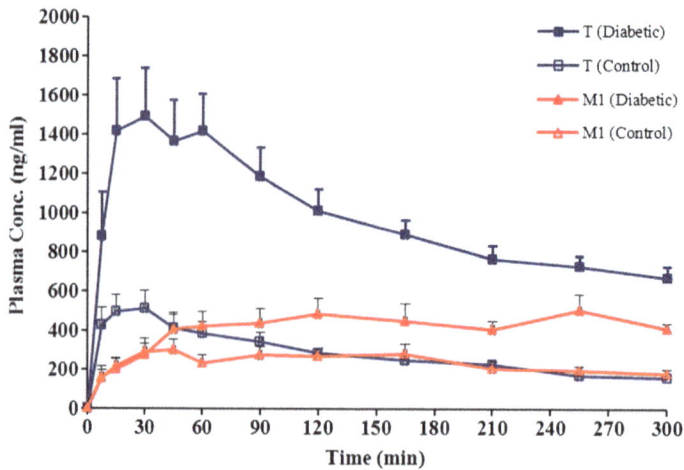

Figure 2 Plasma concentration-time profile of tramadol and M1 in intact control and diabetic rats after receiving a 10 mg/kg of tramadol intraperitoneally (n = 6 in each group, data are presented as mean ± SE).

corresponding times (Tmax) were recorded as observed. Elimination rate constant (β) was estimated as the absolute value of the slope of least-square linear regression of the terminal phase of the logarithmic concentration–time curves. The terminal half-life ($t_{1/2}$) was calculated as $0.693/\beta$. The area under the concentration versus time curve was calculated by the trapezoidal rule for the duration of sampling or last quantifiable concentration and extrapolated from the last point to infinity with β. Plasma clearance for tramadol (CL/F) was calculated as Dose/$AUC_{0-\infty}$. Metabolic ratios for AUCs or concentrations were calculated by dividing the AUC_{0-t} or concentrations of the metabolite by that of tramadol for plasma and perfusate samples.

Statistical evaluation

Data was expressed as mean ± SD. To compare the pharmacokinetic parameters of tramadol and its metabolites in DMIS rats and control group, an unpaired t-test was used for all parameters except T*max*, with which a nonparametric Wilcoxon two-sample test was used. A p-value of less than 0.05 was considered to be statistically significant.

Results and discussion

Studies showed that pharmacokinetic parameters of drugs can change by diabetes mellitus [22,23]. It has been suggested that plasma protein binding of drugs may change because of change in plasma fatty acid levels [9]. Moreover, an intracellular dehydration has been observed in

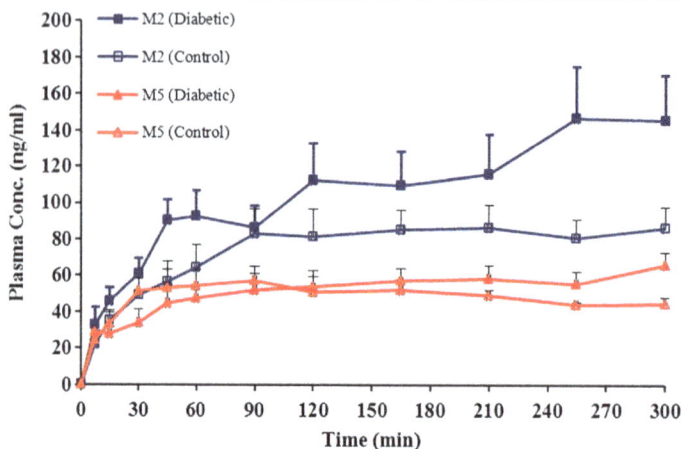

Figure 3 Plasma concentration-time profile of M2 and M5 in intact control and diabetic rats after receiving a 10 mg/kg of tramadol intraperitoneally (n = 6 in each group, data are presented as mean ± SE).

Table 1 Pharmacokinetic parameters of tramadol in diabetic and control rats

Parameter	AUC $_{0-300min}$ (ng.min/ml)		AUC $_{0-\infty}$ (ng.min/ml)		K_{el} (1/min)		App. Clearance (ml/min)	
	Control	Diabetic	Control	Diabetic	Control	Diabetic	Control	Diabetic
Mean	88879.2	292661.1	133344.4	548924.4	0.0036	0.0026	22.3	5.5
P Value	<0.05		<0.05		>0.05		<0.05	

male Sprague-Dawley DMIS rats [24]. Consequently both may affect the distribution of drugs in the body.

It has also been reported that cardiac index and the blood flow rate to the diaphragm, abdominal wall and kidney elevate in male Sprague-Dawley DMIS and Carworth Farms E (CFE) rats [25,26]. An increase in most cytochrome p450 isoenzymes activity has also been reported resulting in elevation of metabolites levels in diabetic rats [27].

Tramadol is quickly and almost entirely absorbed after an oral administration in human whereas its mean absolute bioavailability is reported to be only 65–70% as a result of the first-pass hepatic metabolism. The high total distribution volume of around 300 L after oral administration in human is caused by its high tissue affinity and distribution in fat tissues [28]. An enormous amount of tramadol is rapidly metabolized to three main metabolites in Liver. The principal metabolic pathways, O- and N-desmethylation, involve cytochrome P-450 isoenzyme 2D6, 2B6 and 3A4, respectively. The primary metabolites O-desmethyltramadol (M1) and N-desmethyltramadol (M2) may be further metabolized to N, O-didesmethyltramadol (M5). Ten to thirty percent of the parent drug is excreted unchanged in the urine. Tramadol and its metabolites are almost completely excreted via the kidneys and their biliary excretion is negligible [29].

Animal studies for diabetes especially in rats and mice have been commonly applied streptozocin to provide type 1 diabetes. It has been reported that intravenous administration of a dose ranging from 25 to 100 mg/kg STZ could successfully induce a dose dependent hyperglycemia in rats [30]. In this study, we used a single 60 mg/kg dose of STZ intravenously in order to induce the diabetes in rats.

Intact animals

Six rats completed the study in each group. Mean body weight of rats in two study groups were not statistically different at the beginning (285 ± 12 vs. 295 ± 16 grams in control and treatment groups respectively, p > 0.05). While

rats in treatment group showed a significant decrease in their body weight during 7 days of diabetes induction (295 ± 16 vs. 235 ± 11 grams respectively, p < 0.05), no significant changes was observed in body weight of control group animals during this period. Plasma glucose concentrations measured 7 days from the beginning of the study were significantly increased in animals given streptozotocin, 388.4 ± 164.4 mgdL^{-1} compared with the controls, 102.8 ± 31.1 mgdL^{-1} (P < 0.05). Animal in treatment group had much higher water consumption in comparison to control group. Plasma concentration-time profiles of tramadol and M1 are presented in Figure 2 and those of M2 and M5 in Figure 3 respectively. Calculated pharmacokinetic parameters for Tramadol and metabolites are presented in Tables 1 and 2 respectively.

After i.p. injection in intact rats, tramadol was absorbed rapidly in both groups and reached much higher concentrations in diabetic in comparison to control group with a C_{max} of 561.6 ± 111.4 and 1607.5 ± 335.9 ng/ml in control and diabetic rats respectively (p < 0.05). However the time to C_{max} (T_{max}) was longer in diabetics compared to control group (36.1 ± 17.1 min vs. 18.2 ± 11.4 min in diabetic and control rats respectively). Much higher area under plasma-concentration-time curve was also observed in diabetics in comparison to control group (292661.1 ± 49048.2 vs. 88879.2 ± 14483.4 ng.min.ml^{-1} respectively, p < 0.05). The terminal phase of tramadol plasma concentration-time profile in both groups showed no significant difference in elimination rate constant (0.0036 ± 0.0009 min^{-1} vs. 0.0026 ± 0.0008 min^{-1}) in control and diabetic groups respectively, (p > 0.05).

It has been assumed that tramadol is metabolized much more rapidly in animals than in humans, and M1, M2 and M5 are the main metabolites in all species [31]. Our study also confirms that M1, M2 and M5 are formed and M1 remains the major metabolite in rat. However it is not clear if the same enzymes in human and rat are responsible for metabolite formation in these two spices. In the present study, M1 remained the major metabolite of tramadol in both diabetic and non-diabetic intact rats.

Table 2 AUC $_{0-300min}$ (ng.min/ml) of tramadol metabolites; M1, M2, M5

Parameter	M1		M2		M5	
	Control	Diabetic	Control	Diabetic	Control	Diabetic
Mean	70835.2	124988.4	22447.3	31947.2	14486.2	15505.6
P Value	<0.05		>0.05		>0.05	

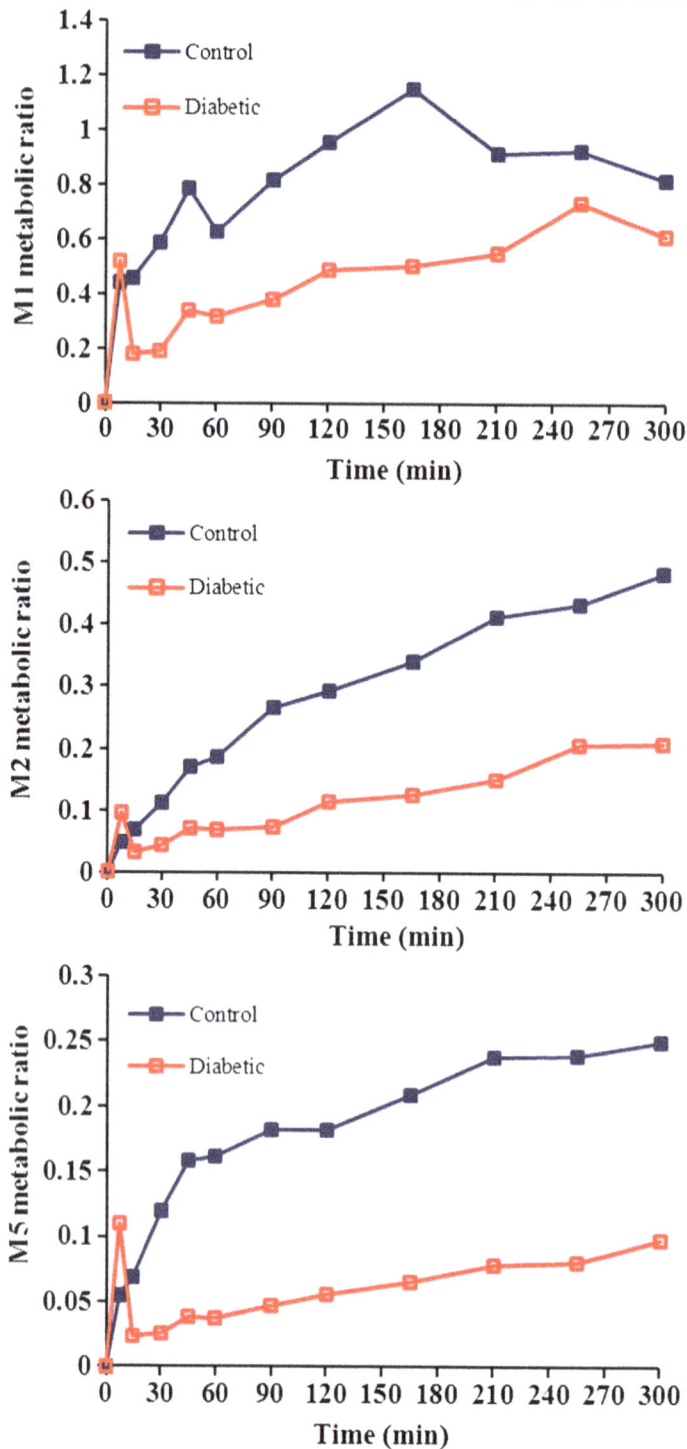

Figure 4 The metabolic ratio for M1, M2 and M5 in intact control and diabetic rats.

Similar to tramadol, the M1 plasma concentrations were higher in diabetic rats compared to control group which resulted in significantly higher AUCs in diabetics (124988.4 ± 33887.3 vs. 70835.2 ± 14341.5 ng.min.ml^{-1} in diabetic and control respectively). In both groups the concentration of M1 reached to an almost constant value in about 90 minutes after drug administration.

Similar to tramadol and M1, M2 showed higher concentrations in diabetics in comparison with control rats. The concentration of M2 in DMIS and control rats was increased up to last sampling point. However the increment trend in M2 concentration was much higher in diabetics resulted in marked increase in AUC of this metabolite in diabetics. As mentioned, diabetic group showed higher concentrations (almost 1.7 times in diabetic group after

300 min compared to control groups) and higher AUCs (31947.2 ± 9923.4 vs. 22447.3 ± 4871.6 ng.min.ml^{-1}) compared to control group. In contrast to M2 and similar to M1, the M5 concentrations reached to a plateau in both groups almost 60 minutes after drug administration and there was no significant differences between AUC of both groups (15505.6 ± 2433.2 vs. 14486.2 ± 2119.4 in diabetic and control respectively) ($p > 0.05$).

As it is clear from above explained data, the diabetes has markedly influenced pharmacokinetic of tramadol and its metabolites in rats. Figures 2 and 3 show that tramadol, M1 and M2 have higher concentrations in diabetic compared to control rats. Considering M1 as major metabolite and induction of its formation in diabetic rats, a reduction in plasma levels and AUC of tramadol

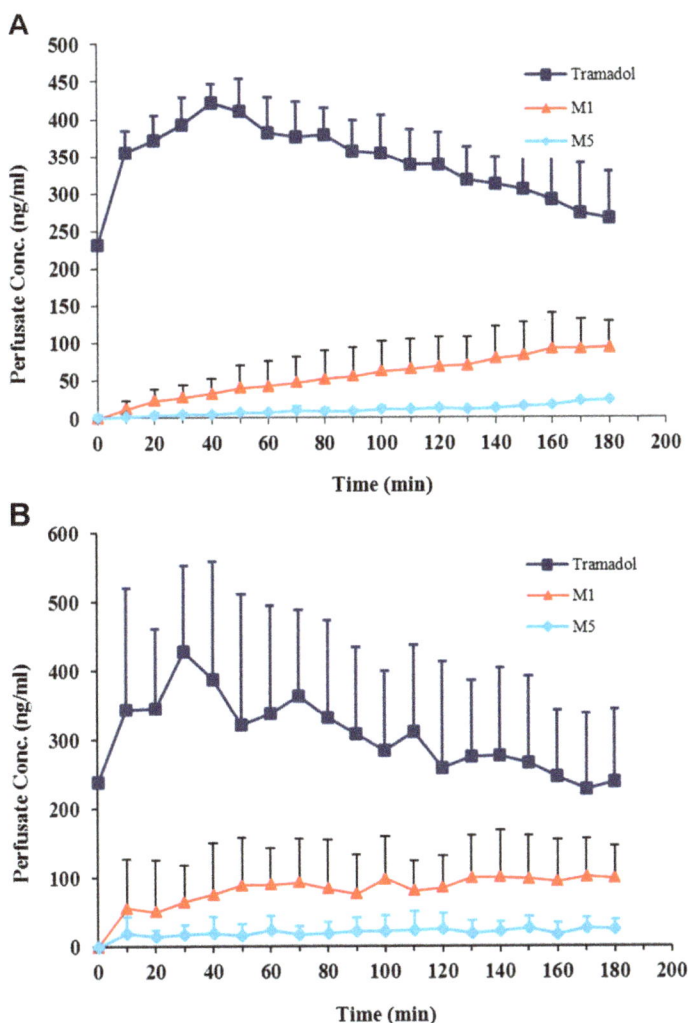

Figure 5 Perfusate concentration-time profile of tramadol, M1 and M5 in control (A) and diabetic (B) isolated rat liver (n = 6, data are presented as mean ± SE).

might be expected. Table 1 show that contrary to our expectation, both $AUC_{0-300min}$ and $AUC_{0-\infty}$ of tramadol are significantly higher in diabetic rats. To further pursue this argument, the metabolic ratios were studied for all three metabolites. Figure 4 shows that for all three metabolites, the metabolic ratio is higher in control in comparison to diabetic rats. These higher metabolic ratios in control rats may be caused by higher plasma levels of metabolites or lower tramadol plasma levels in control group. Lower plasma levels of tramadol could be resulted either from higher metabolism rate (contrary to our expectation) or higher distribution volume of the drug in control rats.

Diabetes may change the pattern of distribution of drugs in the body. Tramadol has a high volume of distribution in man [28]. Any reduction in fat tissue (which usually happens during diabetic state) may cause a reduction in volume of distribution of lipophilic drugs such as tramadol. Considering higher lipophilicity of tramadol compared to its metabolites and consequently higher distribution in fat tissue, such a phenomenon may also explain higher plasma concentration of tramadol in diabetic rats. In addition, the higher production level of alph1-acid glycoprotein, an acute-phase serum protein which is prominent in tramadol protein binding, in diabetic condition may further cause in decrease of volume of distribution and increase in plasma concentration of tramadol in diabetic rats. In isolated liver perfusion study, the metabolism of drugs could be investigated when to a high extent the effect of drug binding and distribution volume has been excluded. To further study the metabolic state of tramadol and clear the possible effect of distribution volume and protein binding on metabolite formation and metabolic ratios, an isolated rat liver study was performed in both normal and diabetic rat liver.

Isolated liver study

Six rats completed the study in each group. Similar to intact groups, the body weight and blood glucose levels between two groups were significantly different ($P < 0.05$). Perfusate sample concentrations of tramadol, M1 and M5 measured by HPLC in both groups. Similar to our previous study [20], M2 was not detected in isolated liver study samples. Figure 5 represents perfusate concentration-time profiles of tramadol, M1 and M5 in control and diabetic isolated livers respectively.

Similar to our previous study [20], M1 was the main metabolite formed in both diabetic and control livers and M2 metabolite was not seen (at least in concentrations higher than 2.5 ng/ml) in perfusion study. A comparison between concentration levels of M1 in diabetic and control livers showed that in contrast to intact animals, the metabolic ratios of M1 and M5 (M/T) are significantly higher in diabetic rats compared to those of control group (Figures 4 and 5). This higher metabolic

ratio in diabetic livers is the consequence of higher metabolite (M1 and M5) production, a result that could not easily be concluded in intact animal data. So it could be fulfilled that higher metabolic ratios in intact control rats in comparison to intact diabetic rats could be resulted from lower plasma levels of tramadol itself in control group (instead of higher metabolite production) which most possibly has been resulted from higher volume of distribution and lower protein binding of tramadol. To confirm the exact role of distribution volume and even protein binding on tramadol concentration and their effects on metabolic ratios in control and diabetic rats, the PK study of tramadol after iv administration and calculation of exact volume of distribution and clearance (instead of apparent Vd and Cl) is recommended.

Conclusion

In conclusion, the results of this study show that the pharmacokinetic of tramadol and its three metabolites has been influenced by diabetic condition. The higher concentration of M1 could be a result of induction of tramadol to M1 formation pathway, while higher concentrations of tramadol itself can be explained by its lower volume of distribution in diabetic rats.

Competing interests
The authors declare that they have no competing interests.

Authors' contributions
M-RR, YHA , MA, BSH and HL conceived the study. HL, BSH, YHA and LH performed the experimental work. All authors were involved in data analysis and interpretation. HL, BSH and YHA prepared the manuscript. All authors read and approved the final version.

Acknowledgments
This study was supported by a grant from Pharmaceutical Sciences research centre, Tehran University of Medical Sciences. Authors wish to Thank Dr. Hadi Esmaeeli for his technical assistance.

Author details
[1]Biopharmaceutics and Pharmacokinetics Division, Department of Pharmaceutics, Faculty of Pharmacy, Tehran University of Medical Sciences, 14155-6451, Tehran, Iran. [2]Department of Pharmacology and Toxicology, Faculty of Pharmacy, Tehran University of Medical Sciences, 14155-6451, Tehran, Iran. [3]Pharmaceutical Sciences Research Centre, Faculty of Pharmacy, Tehran University of Medical Sciences, 14155-6451, Tehran, Iran.

References
1. Nagata K, Yamazoe Y: Genetic polymorphism of human cytochrome p450 involved in drug metabolism. *Drug Metab Pharmacokinet* 2002, 17:167–189.
2. Waxman DJ: P450 gene induction by structurally diverse xenochemicals: central role of nuclear receptors CAR, PXR, and PPAR. *Arch Biochem Biophys* 1999, 369:11–23.
3. Cheng PY, Morgan ET: Hepatic cytochrome P450 regulation in disease states. *Curr Drug Metab* 2001, 2:165–183.
4. Gwilt PR, Nahhas RR, Tracewell WG: The effects of diabetes mellitus on pharmacokinetics and pharmacodynamics in humans. *Clin Pharmacokinet* 1991, 20:477–490.
5. Pickup JC, Williams G: *Textbook of Diabetes. Volume 1.* Oxford: Blackwell Scientific Publications; 1991:151–155.

6. Carnovale CE, Marinelli RA, Rodríguez Garay EA: Bile flow decrease and altered bile composition in streptozotocin-treated rats. *Biochem Pharmacol* 1986, **35**:2625–2628.

7. Watkins JB 3rd, Sherman SE: Long-term diabetes alters the hepatobiliary clearance of acetaminophen, bilirubin and digoxin. *J Pharmacol Exp Ther* 1992, **260**:1337–1343.

8. Park JM, Moon CH, Lee MG: Pharmacokinetic changes of methotrexate after intravenous administration to streptozotocin-induced diabetes mellitus rats. *Res Commun Mol Pathol Pharmacol* 1996, **93**:343–352.

9. Nadai M, Yoshizumi H, Kuzuya T, Hasegawa T, Johno I, Kitazawa S: Effect of diabetes on disposition and renal handling of cefazolin in rats. *Drug Metab Dispos* 1990, **18**:565–570.

10. Price VF, Schulte JM, Spaethe SM, Jollow DJ: Mechanism of fasting-induced suppression of acetaminophen glucuronidation in the rat. *Adv Exp Med Biol* 1986, **197**:697–706.

11. Dong ZG, Hong JY, Ma QA, Li DC, Bullock J, Gonzalez FJ, Park SS, Gelboin HV, Yang CS: Mechanism of induction of cytochrome P-450 ac (P-450j) in chemically induced and spontaneously diabetic rats. *Arch Biochem Biophys* 1988, **263**:29–35.

12. Thummel KE, Schenkman JB: Effects of testosterone and growth hormone treatment on hepatic microsomal P450 expression in the diabetic rat. *Mol Pharmacol* 1990, **37**:119–129.

13. Raza H, Ahmed I, Lakhani MS, Sharma AK, Pallot D, Montague W: Effect of bitter melon (Momordica charantia) fruit juice on the hepatic cytochrome P450-dependent monooxygenases and glutathione S-transferases in streptozotocin-induced diabetic rats. *Biochem Pharmacol* 1996, **52**:1639–1642.

14. Raza H, Ahmed I, John A, Sharma AK: Modulation of xenobiotic metabolism and oxidative stress in chronic streptozotocin-induced diabetic rats fed with Momordica charantia fruit extract. *J Biochem Mol Toxicol* 2000, **14**:131–139.

15. Wu WN, McKown LA, Liao S: Metabolism of the analgesic drug ULTRAM (Tramadol hydrochloride) in humans: API-MS and MS/MS characterization of metabolites. *Xenobiotica* 2002, **32**:411–425.

16. Chong MS, Hester J: Diabetic painful neuropathy: current and future treatment options. *Drugs* 2007, **67**:569–585.

17. Freeman R, Raskin P, Hewitt DJ, Vorsanger GJ, Jordan DM, Xiang J, Rosenthal NR: Randomized study of Tramadol/acetaminophen versus placebo in painful diabetic peripheral neuropathy. *Curr Med Res Opin* 2007, **23**:147–161.

18. Cheng JT, Liu IM, Chi TC, Tzeng TF, Lu FH, Chang CJ: Plasma glucose-lowering effect of Tramadol in streptozotocin-induced diabetic rats. *Diabetes* 2001, **50**:2815–2821.

19. Park JH, Lee WI, Yoon WH, Park YD, Lee JS, Lee MG: Pharmacokinetic and pharmacodynamic changes of furosemide after intravenous and oral administration to rats with alloxan-induced diabetes mellitus. *Biopharm Drug Dispos* 1998, **19**:357–364.

20. Rouini MR, Ghazi-Khansari M, Ardakani YH, Dasian Z, Lavasani H: A Disposition Kinetic Study in Rat perfused Liver. *Biopharm Drug Dispos* 2008, **29**:231–235.

21. Ardakani YH, Rouini MR: Improved liquid chromatographic method for the simultaneous determination of Tramadol and its three main metabolites in human plasma, urine and saliva. *J Pharm Biomed Anal* 2007, **44**:1168–1173.

22. Chang FY, Lee SD, Yeh GH, Wang PS: Hyperglycaemia is responsible for the Inhibited gastrointestinal transit in the early diabetic rat. *Acta Physiol Scand* 1995, **155**:457–462.

23. Xie W, Xing D, Zhao Y, Su H, Meng Z, Chen Y, Du L: A new tactic to treat postprandial hyperlipidemia in diabetic rats with gastroparesis by improving gastrointestinal transit. *Eur J Pharmacol* 2005, **510**:113–120.

24. Anwana AB, Garland HO: Intracellular dehydration in the rat made diabetic with streptozotocin: effects of infusion. *J Endocrinol* 1991, **128**:333–337.

25. Hill MA, Larkins RG: Alterations in distribution of cardiac output in experimental diabetes in rats. *Am J Physiol* 1989, **257**:H571–H580.

26. Lucas PD, Foy JM: Effects of experimental diabetes and genetic obesity on regional blood flow in the rat. *Diabetes* 1977, **26**:786–792.

27. Lee JH, Yang SH, Oh JM, Lee MG: Pharmacokinetics of drugs in rats with diabetes mellitus induced by alloxan or streptozotocin: comparison with those in patients with type I diabetes mellitus. *J Pharm Pharmacol* 2010, **62**:1–23.

28. Lewis KS, Han NH: Tramadol: a new centrally acting analgesic. *Am J Health Syst Pharm* 1999, **54**:643–652.

29. Budd K, Langford R: Tramadol revisited. *Br J Anaesth* 1999, **82**:493–495.

30. Hayashi K, Kojima R, Ito M: Strain differences in the diabetogenic activity of streptozotocin in mice. *Biol Pharmaceut Bull* 2006, **29**:1110–1119.

31. Lintz W, Erlacin S, Frankus E: Biotransformation of Tramadol in man and animal. *Arzneimittelforschung* 1981, **31**:1932–1943.

Formulation and optimization of itraconazole polymeric lipid hybrid nanoparticles (Lipomer) using box behnken design

Balaram Gajra[1*], Chintan Dalwadi[1] and Ravi Patel[2]

Abstract

Background: The objective of the study was to formulate and to investigate the combined influence of 3 independent variables in the optimization of Polymeric lipid hybrid nanoparticles (PLHNs) (Lipomer) containing hydrophobic antifungal drug Itraconazole and to improve intestinal permeability.

Method: The Polymeric lipid hybrid nanoparticle formulation was prepared by the emulsification solvent evaporation method and 3 factor 3 level Box Behnken statistical design was used to optimize and derive a second order polynomial equation and construct contour plots to predict responses. Biodegradable Polycaprolactone, soya lecithin and Poly vinyl alcohol were used to prepare PLHNs. The independent variables selected were lipid to polymer ratio (X_1) Concentration of surfactant (X_2) Concentration of the drug (X_3).

Result: The Box-Behnken design demonstrated the role of the derived equation and contour plots in predicting the values of dependent variables for the preparation and optimization of Itraconazole PLHNs. Itraconazole PLHNs revealed nano size (210 ± 1.8 nm) with an entrapment efficiency of $83 \pm 0.6\%$ and negative zeta potential of -11.7 mV and also enhance the permeability of itraconazole as the permeability coefficient (P_{app}) and the absorption enhancement ratio was higher.

Conclusion: The tunable particle size, surface charge, and favourable encapsulation efficiency with a sustained drug release profile of PLHNs suggesting that it could be promising system envisioned to increase the bioavailability by improving intestinal permeability through lymphatic uptake, M cell of payer's patch or paracellular pathway which was proven by confocal microscopy.

Keywords: Polymeric lipid hybrid nanoparticles, Box-behnken design, Entrapment efficiency, Drug loading, Optimization

Background

The frequency of acquiring bacterial, viral, or fungal infectious diseases increase each year due to the ease of transmission from person to person. From many forms of the infection, invasive fungal infections have become more common in recent years, with a nearly 500% growth in the incidence of blood stream infection with Candida spp. since the 1980 [1]. The azole antifungal agents represent a major drug class in the treatment of wide variety of fungal infections. These drugs can be divided in two main groups: the imidazoles and the triazoles [2].

Itraconazole (ITZ) is a potent triazole antifungal with broad spectrum of activity against fungal species and more efficacious for the treatment of both systemic and superficial fungal infections [3]. ITZ is widely clinically used for a variety of serious fungal infections in normal and immunocompromised hosts, including *Aspergillosis*, *Cryptococcus*, *Candida*, *Blastomyces*, disseminated *Penicillium mameffei* infections and *Histoplasma capsulatum var. capsulatum* and also it has less nephrotoxicity than Amphotericin B [4].

One of the problem with ITZ is its highly hydrophobic characteristics and extremely weak basicity with aqueous solubility of approximately 1 ng/ml at neutral pH [2].

* Correspondence: balaramgajra.ph@charusat.ac.in
[1]Department of Pharmaceutics & Pharmaceutical Technology, Ramanbhai Patel College of Pharmacy, Charotar University of Science and Technology, CHARUSAT Campus, Changa 388 421, Gujarat, India
Full list of author information is available at the end of the article

The Sporanox® marketed oral capsule and solution formulation of the ITZ are not allowed to be used in patients with impaired renal function and aged person. It is not because of the toxicity of the drug itself, but the adjuvant hydroxypropyl-β-cyclodextrin (HP-β-CD). Each milliliter of Sporanox® solution and capsule contains 10 mg of ITZ solubilised by 400 mg of HP-β-CD as an inclusion complex. Following a single intravenous dose of 200 mg Sporanox® to the subjects with severe renal impairment, clearance of HP-β-CD was 6-fold reduced compared with subjects with normal renal function [3]. Hence, a development of oral formulation of ITZ without HP-β-CD is very much important.

The classical polymer lipid hybrid nanoparticles (PLHN) are composed of liposomes and polymeric nanoparticles into a single delivery system. This type of nanoparticles are typically comprised of two distinct functional components: (i) a hydrophobic or hydrophilic polymeric core where poorly water-soluble or highly water soluble drugs are incorporated with high loading yields; (ii) a lipid layer surrounding the core that acts as a highly biocompatible shell and as a molecular fence to promote drug retention inside the polymeric core [5].

There are several pathways used by molecules to cross the epithelial cell barrier, which include transcellular (transport through the cell, with crossing of the cell membranes), paracellular (transport between adjacent cells), and transcytosis through enterocytes. Transcellular pathways through M cells is one of the mechanisms to transport nanoparticles across the intestinal barrier. M cells are associated with Peyer's Patches (PP), an organized component of the gut-associated lymphoid tissue (GALT) [6]. M cells have several properties that allow for adherence by NPs, such as reduced proteases, lack of mucus secretion, and a sparse glycocalyx [7]. A number of approaches have been used to target nanoparticles to M cells. Various nanoparticles like chitosan nanoparticle [8,9], solid lipid nanoparticle [10], polymeric nanoparticle [11-13] and nanoemulsion [14] are capable of enhancing intestinal absorption of poorly water soluble and permeable drugs.

The distinct advantage of this PLHNs have been demonstrated to include the unique advantages of both liposomes and polymeric nanoparticles while excluding some of their intrinsic limitations, thereby holding great promise as a delivery vehicle for various drugs [15]. In the present study emulsification solvent evaporation method was used to prepare PLHN and effect of different independent variables were checked on particle size and entrapment efficiency.

Material and methods
Materials
Poly (ε-caprolactone) (PCL) (Mw 70,000-90,000) was supplied as a gift sample from Sigma Aldrich, USA.

Itraconazole was provided as a gift sample from Intas Biopharmaceutical Ltd, Ahmedabad, India. Soya lecithin 30%, Polyvinyl alcohol and all other Materials like Dichloromethane (DCM), Tetrahydrofuran (THF) and Mannitol (PVA) were purchased from Himedia laboratories Pvt. Ltd, Mumbai, India. Double Distilled Water was used throughout the experiment.

Preparation of polymer lipid hybrid nanoparticles
PLHNs were prepared by the single emulsification evaporation method. In this method PCL and ITZ were dissolved into the DCM. Soya Lecithin with lipid to polymer ratio of 1:10 was dissolved into the aqueous phase [16]. In order to facilitate the solubilisation of the Soya Lecithin, water miscible organic solvent Tetrahydrofuran (4% v/v) was added into the aqueous solution. Polyvinyl Alcohol (PVA) was added as a stabilising agent (0.5 to 1.5% w/v) into the aqueous phase. The resulting PCL solution was then added into the aqueous solution drop wise with continuous stirring and kept aside for 1 to 2 hr to evaporate the DCM [17]. Then dispersion was centrifuged at 12,000 rpm for 30 min at room temperature and the pellet was redispersed in the double distilled water. The dispersion was sonicated and frozen at −90°C for 3 hr in a deep freezer and freeze dried (Benchtop K freeze dryer, Virtis, 4KBTZL/105, USA).

Optimization of PLHNs by box-behnken design
A Box-Behnken statistical design with 3 factors, 3 levels, and 15 runs was selected for the optimization study and the Design Expert® 8.0.6 software was used [18]. The independent variables selected were lipid to polymer ratio (X_1), concentration of surfactant (X_2) and concentration of drug (X_3) and dependent variables were particle size (Y_1) and entrapment efficiency (% EE) (Y_2) (Table 1) with high, medium and low level. A checkpoint analysis was performed to confirm the role of the derived polynomial equation and contour plots in predicting the responses [19]. Optimization was performed to find out the level of independent variables (X_1, X_2, and X_3) that would yield a minimum value of the particle size (Y_1) and maximum value of EE (Y_2).

Table 1 Variables and levels in Box-Behnken design

Independent variables		Level		
		−1	0	+1
X_1	Lipid to Polymer ratio	1:1	1:5	1:10
X_2	Concentration of surfactant (% w/v)	0.5%	1%	1.5%
X_3	Concentration of drug (% w/v)	0.06%	0.12%	0.18%
Dependent variables				
Y_1	Particle Size (nm)			
Y_2	% Entrapment Efficiency (nm)			

Table 2 Box-behnken experimental design with measured responses

Batch No	X₁	X₂	X₃	Particle size Y₁ (nm)	Entrapment efficiency Y₂ (%)
PLN1	−1	−1	0	251.0 ± 0.7	80.5 ± 0.3
PLN2	1	−1	0	353.0 ± 0.2	83.0 ± 0.2
PLN3	−1	1	0	214.0 ± 0.03	78.7 ± 0.07
PLN4	1	1	0	240.0 ± 1.2	83.0 ± 0.8
PLN5	−1	0	−1	244.0 ± 0.67	80.0 ± 0.64
PLN6	1	0	−1	248.0 ± 0.8	83.4 ± 0.4
PLN7	−1	0	1	234.0 ± 0.9	77.4 ± 0.04
PLN8	1	0	1	264.0 ± 1.31	81.2 ± 0.09
PLN9	0	−1	−1	319.0 ± 0.02	81.8 ± 0.8
PLN10	0	1	−1	223.0 ± 0.5	80.1 ± 0.32
PLN11	0	−1	1	344.0 ± 0.45	81.0 ± 0.34
PLN12	0	1	1	234.0 ± 0.51	78.0 ± 0.23
PLN13	0	0	0	245.0 ± 0.32	79.0 ± 1.02
PLN14	0	0	0	243.0 ± 0.08	79.9 ± 0.02
PLN15	0	0	0	240.0 ± 0.4	80.0 ± 0.05

Particle size

Particle size was measured by Dynamic light Scattering using the particle size Analyzer (Malvern Zetasizer S90, UK). All measurements were taken by scattering light at 90° and temperature of 25°C. Dispersion was centrifuged at 12,000 rpm for 30 min at room temperature. Supernant was discarded and the resultant pellet was redispersed in double distilled water. Dispersion was then appropriately diluted for the particle size measurement [20].

% Entrapment efficiency (% EE) and drug loading

Dispersion was centrifuged at 12,000 rpm for 30 min at room temperature, supernant was discarded, the obtained pellet was dissolved in DCM and drug concentration was analysed by UV/Visible Spectrophotometer at 264 nm [21]. Drug loading was determined by the direct method as described for the EE. Measured amount of final freeze dried formulation was dissolved into the DCM and analysed U.V.Visible Spectrophotometer at 264 nm. It was also calculated by the indirect method by the Equation 1.

$$Drug\ Loading = \frac{[Amount\ of\ ITZ\ entrapped]}{[Amount\ of\ ITZ\ Added + Amount\ of\ Excipients\ Added]} \tag{1}$$

Fourier transmission infrared spectroscopy (FTIR)

The samples were weighed approximately, homogenously dispersed in dried KBr in a mortar and pestle, and compressed under vacuum with compression force using round flat face punch for three minutes to produce pellet compact. The pellet was placed in the IR light path and the IR spectra were recorded using a FTIR spectrophotometer (NICOLET 6700, Thermo Scientific, USA). Spectrum was recorded in the wavelength region of 4000–400 cm − 1 [20].

Differential scanning calorimetry (DSC)

DSC Analysis was conducted using the Differential Scanning Calorimeter (DSC-60, Shimadzu, Japan). Sample curves were recorded at a scan rate of 10°C/min from 50 to 300°C. Each powder sample, 5–10 mg was analysed by same procedure. DSC of ITZ, PCL, soya lecithin, Mannitol, PVA, physical mixture and freeze dried final formulation was conducted to show the compatibility of drug with excipients and loading of the drug in to the polymeric matrix [22].

Powder x-ray diffraction (PXRD)

PXRD of various samples was recorded at room temperature with X-Ray Diffractometer (D2Phaser-brukker,

Table 3 Checkpoint batches with predicted and measured value

Batch code	X₁	X₂	X₃	Particle size(nm)		% Entrapment efficiency	
				Predicted	Measure	Predicted	Measure
CP1	0	−0.5	0.5	280.54	319 ± 0.4	79.77	77.79 ± 0.2
CP2	0	0.5	0.75	230.27	214 ± 0.8	78.48	80.57 ± 0.17
P-Value				1.00		0.995	

Table 4 Optimised formulation as per the design expert® 8.0.6 software

Independent variables	Criteria	Value	Desirability
Lipid: polymer	In range	0.96	
Concentration of surfactant	In range	0.81	
Concentration of drug	In range	−1	0.948
Dependent variables			
Particle size	Minimum	228.02	
% Entrapment efficiency	Maximum	83.87	

USA). The samples were scanned from the 5° to 50° (2θ) with a step size 0.02° and a step interval of 0.1 Sec [3].

Transmission electron microscopy (TEM)
TEM of PLHNs was performed following negative staining with Phosphotungstic acid (PTA) [5]. A drop of dispersion (1 mg/ml) was placed on copper grids followed by the addition of a drop of PTA. At the end of 3 min, excess liquid was removed, the grid air-dried and imaging conducted, using a transmission electron microscope (Holland Technai 20, Phillips, Holland) [15].

Zeta potential
The zeta potential of the dispersion was measured by determining the electrophoretic mobility using the Zetasizer (Malvern Zetasizer ZS90, UK). Dispersion was centrifuged at 12,000 rpm for 30 min at room temperature. Supernant was discarded and the resultant pellet was redispersed in double distilled water using ultrasonic probe system for 1 min with 50 s pulse at 200 v. Dispersion was then appropriately diluted and zeta potential was measured [5].

In-vitro drug release study
Drug release was performed by dialysis method. Dispersion was filled in dialysis tube (2.4 nm pore size, Himedia, India). Drug release was initiated by immersing the dialysis tube in 200 ml of release media on the magnetic stirrer at $37 \pm 5°C$ and 50 rpm [23]. Various release media were used for the release study like pH 7.4 phosphate buffer, 0.1 N HCL, pH 6.8 phosphate buffer with 3% SLS. Aliquots (5 ml) were withdrawn at specified time points and drug concentration was measured by UV/Visible Spectrophotometer at 264 nm. The release data was fitted with different kinetic models such as zero order, first order, Higuchi and Korsmeyer-Peppas model.

Ex-vivo permeation study
Male Wistar rats (250–320 gm) were sacrificed by the humane method. Permission for study was obtained from the institutional animal ethics committee (Protocol No. RPCP/IAEC/2011-2012/MPH-PT-13). All the procedures were followed as per guidelines of committee for the purpose of control and supervision of experiment on animals (CPCSEA), Division of Animal Welfare, Ministry of Forests and Environment, Government of India. After rats were sacrificed, the small intestine

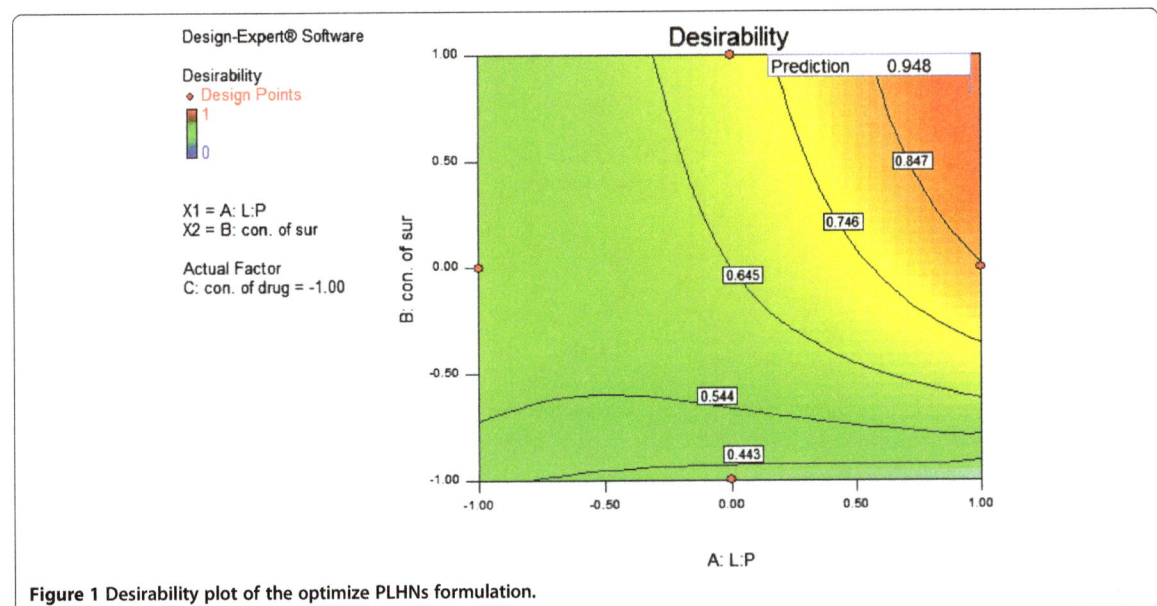

Figure 1 Desirability plot of the optimize PLHNs formulation.

was immediately excised and placed into ice-cold, bub-bled (carbogen, 95:5 O2/CO2) Ringer buffer. The je-junum, 20 cm distal from the pyloric sphincter was used. The tissue was rinsed with ice-cold standard Ringer buffer to remove luminal content and cut into segments. The freeze dried PLHN sample was reconstituted with one ml of phosphate buffer pH 6.8 [24]. Resultant sample was placed in lumen of intestine tied from one side and then tied from other side. The tissue was placed into organ bath filled with 40 mL of phosphate-buffer pH7.4. Continuous aeration and constant temperature of $37 \pm 0.5°C$ were maintained. Samples were taken from the receptor chamber at predetermined time interval and replaced with equal volume of buffer. Aliquots were assayed for the drug content using U.V. Visible Spectrophotometer at 264 nm [25]. It was compared with the simple drug solution in phosphate buffer pH 6.8.

Percentage drug permeation and permeability enhancement ratio was calculated from the Equation 2 and 3, respectively [26].

$$Papp = \frac{dQ}{dt} \times \frac{1}{ACo} \tag{2}$$

Where dQ/dt is the steady-state appearance rate on the acceptor side of the tissue, A is the area of the tissue (cm2) and Co is the initial concentration of the drug in the donor Compartment.

Permeability Enhancement ratio
$$= \frac{Papp\ of\ the\ nanoparticle\ formulation}{Papp\ of\ the\ drug\ solution} \tag{3}$$

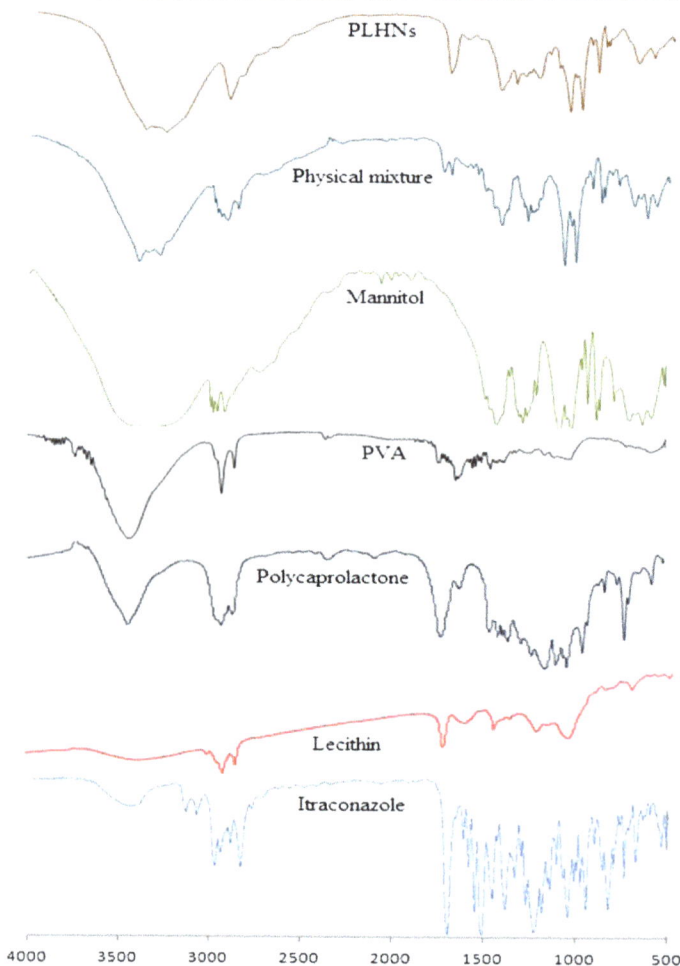

Figure 2 FTIR spectra of drug, excipients and formulation.

Formulation and optimization of itraconazole polymeric lipid hybrid nanoparticles (Lipomer) using...

97

In-vitro cellular uptake study with confocal laser scanning microscopy (CLSM)

For the cell uptake studies, PLHNs were labelled with fluorescent dye, Rhodamine B and placed into the lumen of the intestine, and kept for 1 hr into the phosphate buffer saline then the tissue was preserved in to the incubation media i.e. 10% formalin for the CLSM study [27]. The block was prepared using cryo-protectant embedding medium. The cross section of the intestinal tissue of 5 μm thickness was taken by cryomicrotome (CM1850, Leica) at –20°C. The section was placed on the slides coated with poly-L-lysine. The slides were incubated at 37°C for the 20 min for the fixation of the section. The slides were examined by CLSM (Zeiss LSM S10 META) through the z axis.

Optical excitation was carried out with 480 nm and fluorescence emission was detected above 520 nm for Rhodamine B [28].

Stability study

For stability study, freeze dried ITZ-PLHNs were stored at room temperature (~25°C), refrigerator (4° to 8°C) and accelerated condition (Temperature: $40 \pm 2°C$, Relative humidity: $75\% \pm 5$) over a period of 45 days in stopper glass vials. Samples were evaluated for particle size and drug content on 15th, 30th and 45th day. Chemical stability during the storage was checked by FTIR spectrophotometer after 45th day of storage [20].

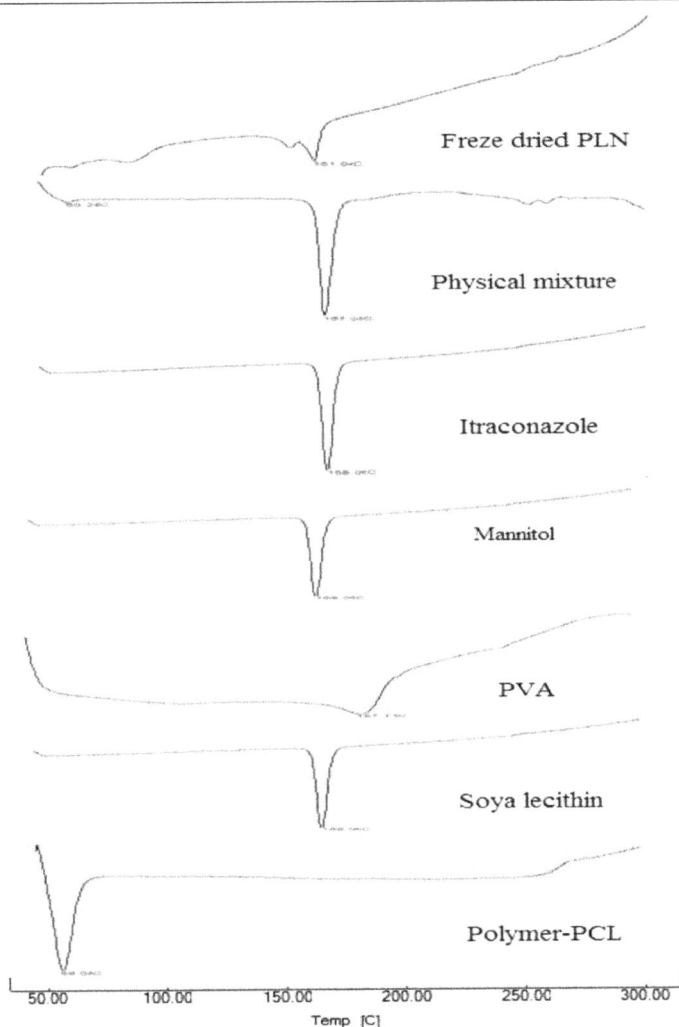

Figure 3 DSC thermograms of drug, excipients and formulation.

Results

Preparation of PLHN

In the method of preparation, DCM diffuses quickly into the aqueous solution, leaving PCL to precipitate and form nanoparticles. Soya lecithin was self-assemble on the surface of polymer nanoparticles through hydrophobic interactions to reduce the system's free energy. The hydrophobic tail of lipids was attached to the hydrophobic polymer core and the hydrophilic head group of lipids extend into the external aqueous environment [17].

Optimization of polymer lipid hybrid nanoparticle by box-behnken design

All the batches of PLHNs were evaluated for the particle size (Y1) and entrapment efficiency (Y2) and the results

are shown in the Table 2. Full model polynomial equations for the Particle size and entrapment efficiency are as follows:

For Particle Size,

$$
\begin{aligned}
Y_1 = {} & +242.67 + 13.87X_1(P = 0.0057) \\
& - 50.88X_2 (P = 0.0001) \\
& + 5.25X_3 (P = 0.1403) \\
& - 6.25X_1X_2 (P = 0.2005) \\
& + 6.50X_1X_3 (P = 0.1858) \\
& - 3.50X_2X_3 (P = 0.4466) \\
& + 1.04X_1^2 (P = 0.8227) \\
& + 33.54X_2^2 (P = 0.0006) \\
& + 3.79X_3^2 (P = 0.4294)(R^2 = 0.9869)
\end{aligned}
$$

$$(4)$$

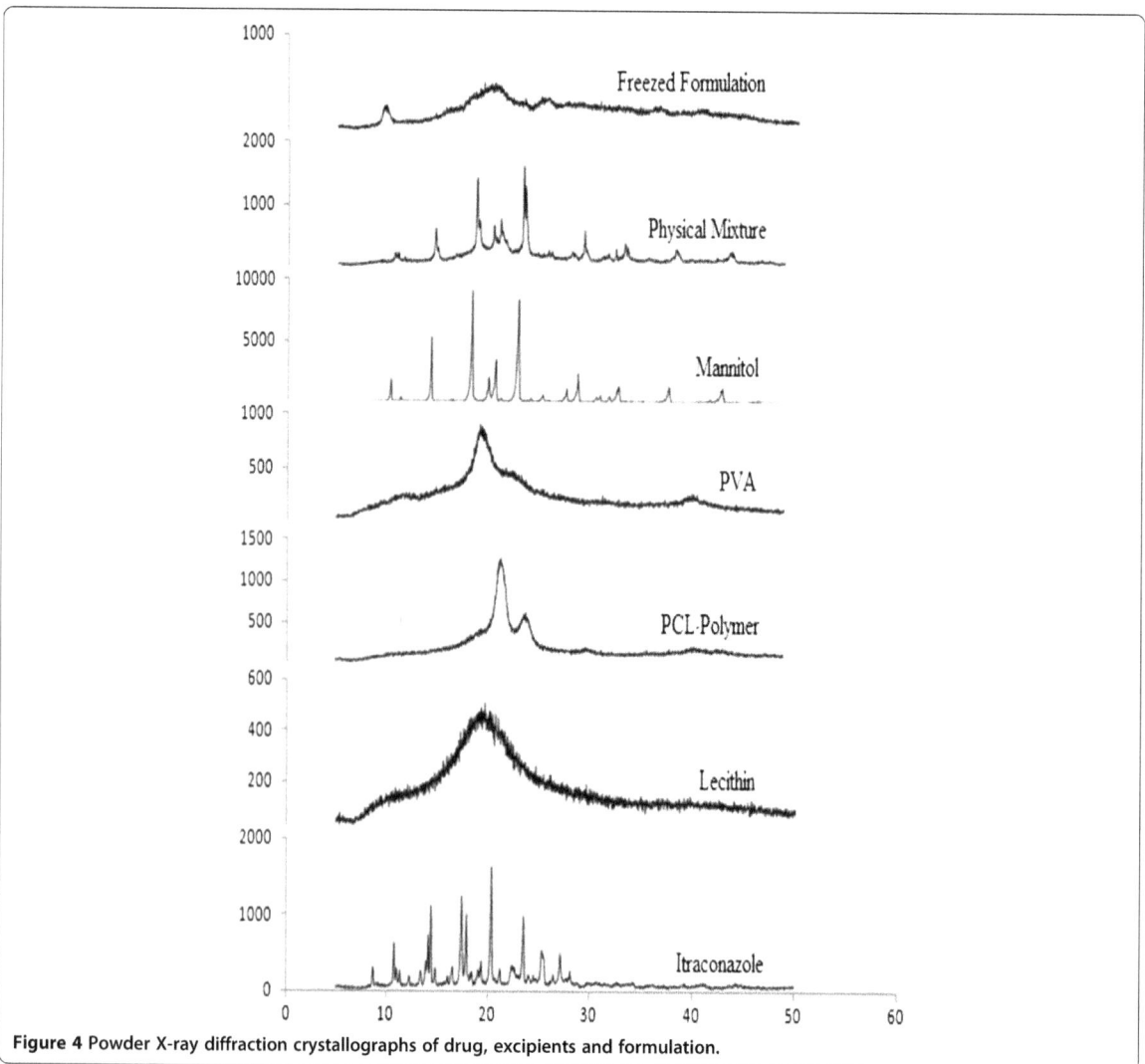

Figure 4 Powder X-ray diffraction crystallographs of drug, excipients and formulation.

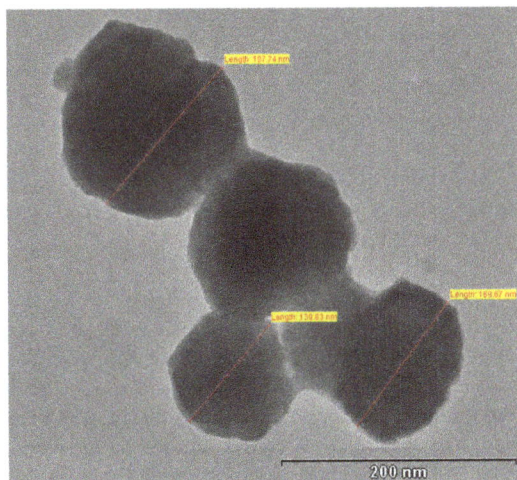

Figure 5 TEM image of ITZ-PLHNs.

$$Y_2 = + 79.63 + 1.75X_1 \ (P = 0.0006)$$
$$- 0.82X_2 (P = 0.0160)$$
$$- 0.96X_3 \ (P = 0.0085)$$
$$+ 0.46X_1X_2 (P = 0.2153)$$
$$+ 0.10X_1X_3 \ (P = 0.7647)$$
$$- 0.32X_2X_3 \ (P = 0.3657)$$
$$+ 0.96X_1{}^2 \ (P = 0.0361)$$
$$+ 0.70X_2{}^2 \ (P = 0.0928)$$
$$- 0.11X_3{}^2 \ (P = 0.7630) \ (R^2 = 0.9540)$$
$$(5)$$

Check point analysis

Two check point batches were prepared and evaluated for the particle size and EE as shown in Table 3. T-test was applied between actual and predicted values of dependent parameters and P-values are reported in

Table 3. At 5% significance, there was no significant difference between actual and predicted value of particle size and entrapment efficiency.

Optimization of formulation

After studying the effect of independent variables on the responses, the levels of these variables that give the optimum response were determined. Hence, all the variables were decided in range and the optimum formulation is one that gives lower value of particle size along with a high amount of drug entrapped. Values of the variables for the optimised batch are given in the Table 4. Desirability of the optimized batch was found to be 0.948 which is shown in Figure 1.

Particle size, entrapment efficiency and drug loading

Particle size was found to be in the range of 214.0 to 353.0 nm. Particle size of each batch is given in the Table 2. Particle size of the optimized batch was 210.7 ± 1.8 nm and PDI was 0.53 ± 0.67. Entrapment efficiency was found to be in the range of 77.4 to 83.4%. EE of each batch is given in the Table 2. Drug loading of the optimized batch determined by both direct and indirect method were 1.67% and 1.72%, respectively.

Freeze drying

The freeze dried formulation was found to be soft, white, and amorphous in nature. There was no significant increase in particle size observed (at 5% significant level) after freeze drying as compared to freshly prepared formulation.

FTIR spectroscopy

FTIR spectra of the drug, polymer, lipid, Mannitol, physical mixture and freeze dried formulation are shown in Figure 2. FTIR spectra of freeze dried formulation shows all the characteristic peak of the all components and not shown any additional new peak. The spectra of PLHN

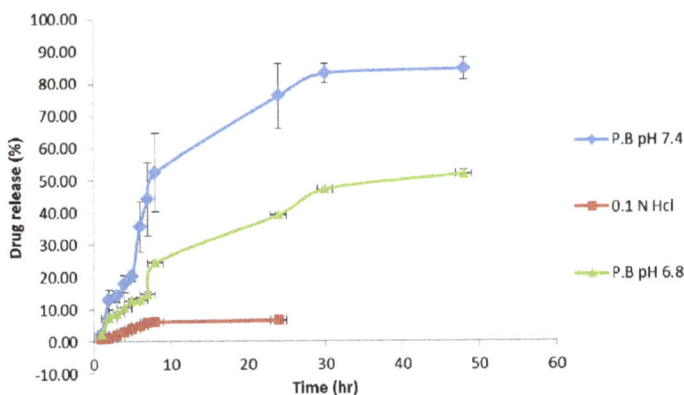

Figure 6 Drug release profile for ITZ-PLHNs formulation in Phosphate buffer pH 7.4, 0.1 N Hydrochloric acid and Phosphate buffer pH 6.8.

Table 5 Kinetic release parameter of ITZ-PLHNs

Release media	Zero order		First order		Higuchi		Koresmayer-Pepas	
	R^2	k_0 (h^{-1})	R^2	k_1(h^{-1})	R^2	k_H (h$^{-1/2}$)	R^2	n value
P.B pH 7.4	0.786	1.77	0.966	−0.01	0.975	15.16	0.9732	0.79

shows the characteristic peak of ITZ at 3421.55, 1378.15, 1052.01, 1378.15 cm^{-1} [29], PCL at 2925.28 cm^{-1} and peak of the Soya lecithin at 2925.28, 1437.68 cm^{-1}, PVA at 1735.73, 1652.65 cm^{-1} Mannitol at 1247.40 cm^{-1}. Thus this result indicates that there was no formation of the new peak, so drug and excipients are compatible with each other and also revealed that ITZ was successfully incorporated into the PLHNs.

Differential scanning calorimetry (DSC)
DSC thermograms of the Formulation, Physical mixture, ITZ, PCL, Soya lecithin, PVA and Mannitol are shown in Figure 3. DSC spectra of formulation and physical mixture gives the sharp peak at 161.0°C and 167.0°C, respectively which is the peak of mannitol and it does not show any new peak or additional peak. So, it is revealed that the excipients are compatible with the drug and there is no any reaction between the drug and excipients [3]. The melting endothermic peak of ITZ was observed at 168.04°C while the thermogram of the lyophilized ITZ incorporated PLHNs does not show the endothermic peak for ITZ [20].

Powder x-ray diffraction (PXRD)
The diffractograms shown in Figure 4 further confirmed the results of DSC thermal analysis. ITZ powder showed strong typical peaks of crystalline ITZ at 2θ scattered angles 14.49°, 17.53°, 20.38°, 23.5° and 25.29°. The presence of sharp peaks indicates crystalline nature of ITZ. The characteristic peak of ITZ was not observed in PLHNs at corresponding 2θ scattered angles indicating that the drug was encapsulated in the polymer and lipid carrier and also confirms that amorphous form of the formulation [3,20].

Transmission electron microscopy (TEM) morphology and zeta potential
The TEM image of ITZ-PLHNs is shown in Figure 5. The particles were spherical in shape and show the dim ring of lipid coat surrounding the polymeric core. The particle size was observed between 160–200 nm and is comparable to the results of particle size by particle size analyzer [15]. Zeta potential of the optimized ITZ-PLHNs was found to be −11.7 mV which is attributed to the non-ionic nature of the surfactant PVA as opposed to the anionic nature of the soya lecithin. Because of the negative zeta potential, it produces repulsion between

the nanoparticles and prevents the aggregation which gives the long-time stability [5,16].

In-vitro drug release
With the selection of lipid and polymer ratio, the release kinetics of PLHNs showed some unique features. There was absence of initial burst release observed, may be due to the uniform distribution of ITZ in the PLHNs matrix rather than just on the PLHNs surface. Drug released from the PLHN generally occurs through the drug diffusion and the polymer erosion mechanism. Sustained ITZ release from the PLHNs is attributed to the lipid matrix imparting a barrier to drug release [17].

Drug release profile of the ITZ-PLHNs in phosphate buffer pH 7.4, 0.1 N HCl and phosphate buffer pH 6.8 is shown in the Figure 6. The release profiles were fitted to various kinetic models such as zero-order, first-order, Higuchi equation and Korsmeyer–Peppas equation. ITZ release profile followed Higuchi model in the release media phosphate buffer pH 7.4 ($R^2 = 0.98$) as shown in Table 5 [30,31]. All the kinetic data were fitted to the Korsmeyer-Peppas Equation. Here n > 0.79, the drug is released from polymeric matrix system followed anomalous diffusion mechanism.

Ex-vivo permeability
Ex-vivo permeability studies are relevant approaches to evaluate the absorption enhancing effect of a colloidal drug carrier system on the intestinal tissue. Table 6 shows the comparison of the *ex-vivo* permeability of ITZ solution and ITZ-PLHN formulation. Figure 7 shows the % permeability of ITZ formulation after 240 min is 30%. Measurement of the apparent permeability coefficient (Papp) and the absorption enhancement ratio of PLHNs indicated that there is an increase in the permeability of ITZ from the ITZ-PLHN formulation [25,32].

In-vitro cellular uptake study with CLSM
The cellular uptake of the PLHNs was examined to demonstrate the penetration of the nanoparticles across

Table 6 P$_{app}$ and permeability enhancement ratio of the ITZ solution and formulation

Type of formula	P$_{app}$(cm/sec)	Permeability enhancement ratio
PLHNs Formulation	2.39×10^{-3}	1.476
ITZ Solution	1.61×10^{-3}	1

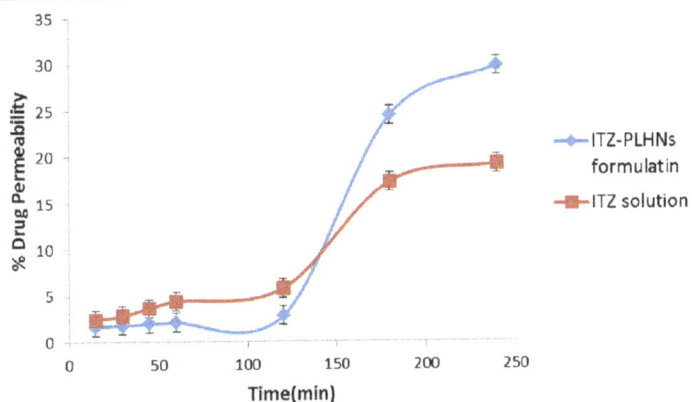

Figure 7 % cumulative ITZ Permeability of the ITZ solution and formulation.

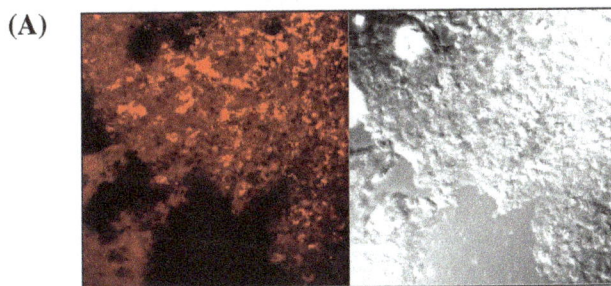

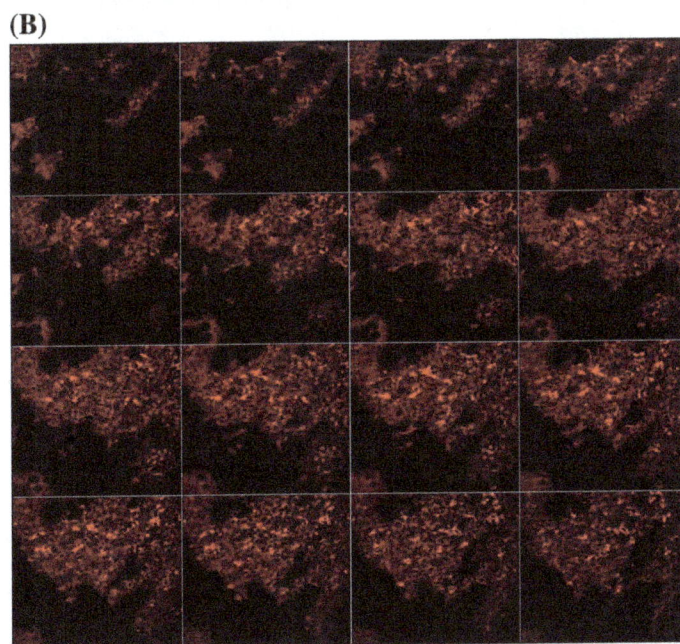

Figure 8 CLSM images of Rhodamine B labelled ITZ PLHNs A. combined three dimensional images, B. images of intestinal villi optically sectioned in the x-y plane at regularly spaced distances along the z-axis.

the intestinal barrier and also to study the mechanism of increase in the intestinal permeability of ITZ. The internalization of Rhodamine B loaded NPs incubated for 1 hr was visualized by CLSM. Figure 8(B) shows CLSM images of Rhodamine B labelled PLHNs treated intestinal villi optically sectioned in the x-y plane at regularly spaced distances along the z-axis whereas Figure 8(A) shows combined image containing Rhodamine labelled PLHNs internalized and distributed in the small intestinal mucosal cross-sections. The CLSM images show strong red fluorescent spherical particles in the intestinal villi of rat both on the surface of the intestinal enterocyte and on the M- cells [22]. Villi and microvillus of the intestinal tissue was stained red with the dye and Rhodamine B labelled nanoparticles are highlighted with red fluorescence [28].

Stability study

Stability study was carried out to know the chemical changes that may occur in the formulations. Table 7 shows the stability study data of particle size and drug content of ITZ-PLHNs formulation. Particle size of the formulation was increased slightly in accelerated, room temperature and refrigeration condition and drug content was decreased slightly from 96% to 95% for all the condition. No significant change in the particle size and drug content was revealed. FTIR spectra of the formulation after 45 days at room temperature, accelerated condition and refrigerated condition are shown in the Figure 9. It was revealed that there is no change as it shows the main peak of the drug intact at 2934.76, 1459.52, 1376.81, 1193.64 cm^{-1}.

Discussion

Effects of independent variables on particle size

For the particle size value of the correlation coefficient (R^2) of the polynomial equation (Equation 4) was found

Table 7 Stability study data for ITZ-PLHNs formulation

Day	Particle size (nm)	Assay (%)
First	232.8 ± 0.21	96.38 ± 0.02
Accelerated condition		
15	245.3 ± 0.35	96.29 ± 0.04
30	249.5 ± 0.61	95.50 ± 0.03
45	249.9 ± 0.32	95.39 ± 0.02
Room condition		
15	230.3 ± 0.31	96.30 ± 0.04
30	230.8 ± 0.34	96.28 ± 0.05
45	231.4 ± 0.41	96.25 ± 0.021
Refrigerator condition		
15	248.6 ± 0.32	96.12 ± 0.023
30	250.3 ± 0.23	95.43 ± 0.034
45	256.7 ± 0.36	95.28 ± 0.04

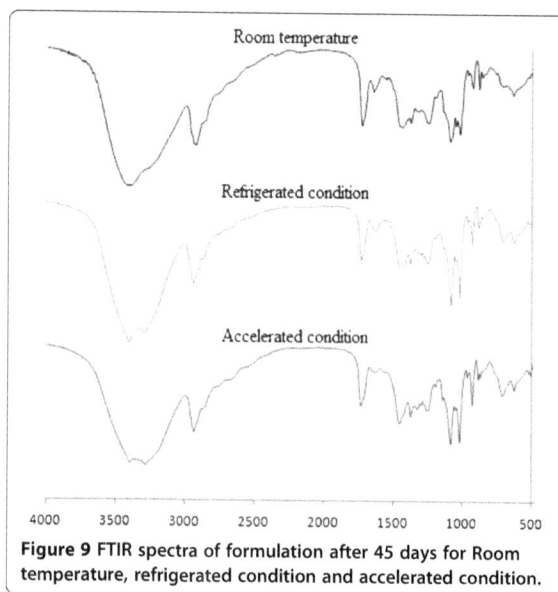

Figure 9 FTIR spectra of formulation after 45 days for Room temperature, refrigerated condition and accelerated condition.

to be 0.9869, indicating good fit of the model. Among the independent variable selected, X_1, X_2, X_2^2; lipid to polymer ratio, concentration of surfactant and square of the concentration of surfactant, respectively, are significant model terms (P < 0.05).

Here, variable X_1 and X_2^2 have positive effect on particle size as revealed by positive value of coefficient in the equation, it means that as lipid to polymer ratio (X_1) increases, particle size increases and X_2 has negative effect on particle size as revealed by negative value of coefficient in the Equation 4 it means that as the concentration of surfactant (X_2) increases particle size decreases.

From the response surface 3D plot for the particle size (Figure 10A), it was observed that as the concentration of surfactant increases, particle size decreases. This may be due to the reason that at lower concentration of PVA, it exists as a single molecule layer at surface of particle and at higher concentration it exists as an aggregated form and has an enhanced surfactant activity. It may also be due to effective reduction in the interfacial tension between aqueous and organic phase [33]. As the lipid to polymer ratio increases, particle size increases. This increase in the particle size may be because of increase in the viscosity of the inner polymeric phase that affects the shearing capacity of the mechanical stirrer [15,34].

Thus, the effect of the lipid to polymer ratio and the concentration of surfactant were significant, as it is evident from their high coefficients and the fact that the bars corresponding to variables X_1, X_2 and X_2^2 extend beyond the reference line in Pareto chart (Figure 10B).

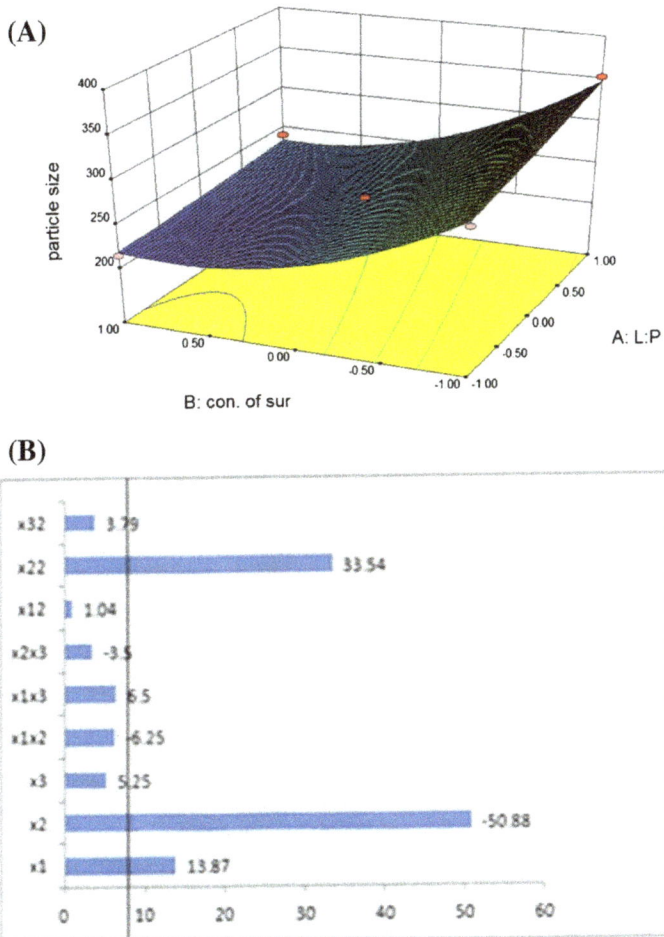

Figure 10 Response surface 3D plot (A) showing the effect of different variables on particle size and Pareto chart (B) showing the variables having P value greater than 0.05.

P value greater than 0.05 indicates that model terms were not significant so they were removed from the equation to generate the reduced model Equation 6 [19].

$$\text{Reduced model equation for particle size } (Y_1) = + 242.67 + 13.87X_1 - 50.88X_2 + 33.54X_2{}^2 \tag{6}$$

Effects of independent variables on entrapment efficiency (EE)

For Entrapment efficiency, the value of the correlation coefficient (R^2) of the Equation 5 was found to be 0.9540, indicating good fit of the model. Among all the independent variables X_1, X_2, X_3, $X_1{}^2$; lipid to polymer ratio, concentration of surfactant, concentration of the drug and square of the concentration of drug, respectively, are significant model terms ($P < 0.05$).

Here, variables X_1 has positive effect on EE as revealed by the positive value of coefficient in the Equation 5, means as lipid to polymer ratio increases, EE increases and X_2 and X_3 has negative effect on EE as revealed by the negative value of coefficient in the Equation 5, it means that as concentration of surfactant and concentration of the drug increases, EE decreases.

From the response surface 3D plot for the EE (Figure 11A), it shows that as the concentration of surfactant increases, EE decreases. This may be due to decrease in the particle size. It may also be due to increases the partition of the drug from internal to external phase of the medium at the high concentration of surfactant [34]. Figure 11B shows that as the lipid-polymer ratio increases, EE increases. This may be due to increase in the

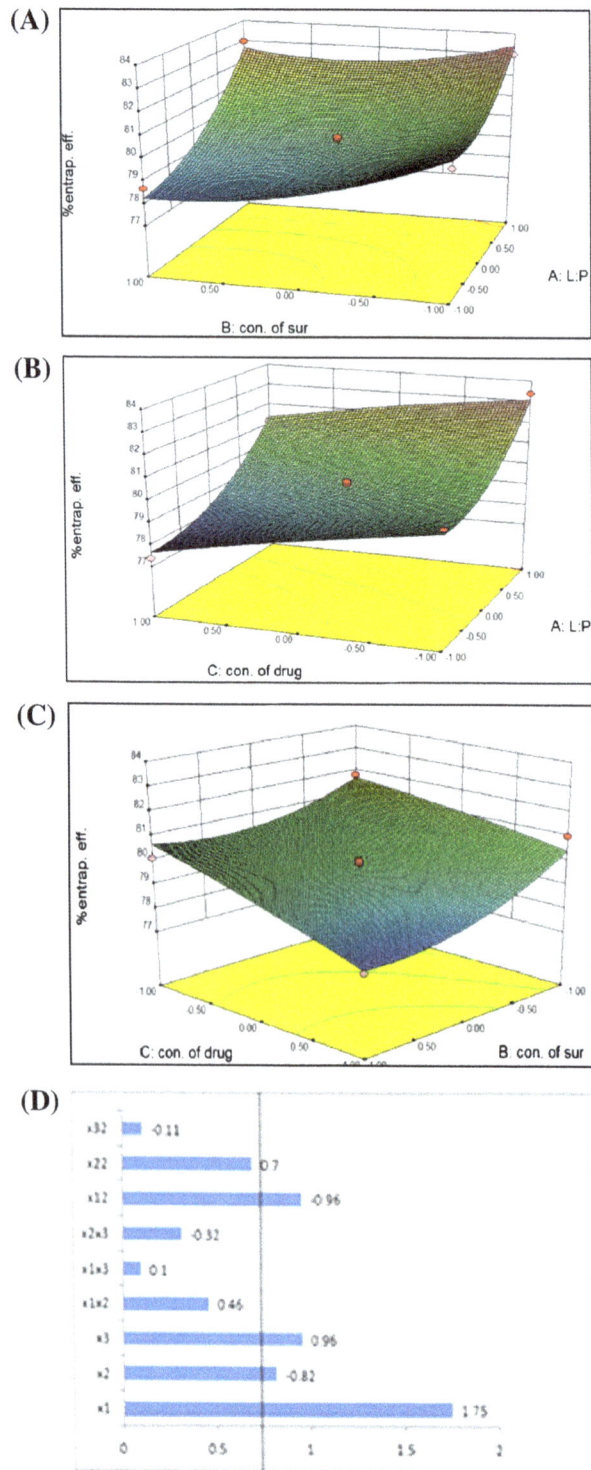

Figure 11 Response surface graphs (A,B,C) showing effect of different variables on % entrapment efficiency and Pareto chart (D) showing variables having P value greater than 0.05.

amount of the polymer provides more space to incorporate the drug and lipid layer at the surface of the polymer matrix and also reduces the escaping of the drug into external phase. Figure 11C shows that as the concentration of the drug increases, EE decreases. It may be due to reason that because ITZ is insoluble in water so at high concentration some amount of the drug may precipitate out.

Thus, the effect of the lipid to polymer ratio, the concentration of surfactant and concentration of drug were significant, as it is evident from their high coefficients and the fact that the bars corresponding to variables X_1, X_2, X_3 and X_1^2 extend beyond the reference line in Pareto chart (Figure 11D) for the EE. P value greater than 0.05 indicates that the model terms were not significant so they were removed from the equation to generate the reduced model Equation as:

$$\text{Entrapment efficiency } (Y_2) = \\ + 79.63 + 1.75X_1 - 0.82X_2 - 0.96X_3 + 0.96X_1^2 \tag{7}$$

In this study, the model was checked for lack of fit for both the responses; Particle size and EE. For lack of fit P values obtained for particle size and EE were 0.0524 and 0.3965, respectively and hence the current model provided a satisfactory fit to the data (P > 0.05) and has no lack of fit [19].

The derived polynomial equations and contour plots from the Box Behnken experimental design aid in predicting the values of selected independent variables for preparation of optimized PLHN formulations with desired properties. Factorial design was validated by check point analysis. From the result of the check point analysis P value calculated was greater than 0.05 so the model was validated. Optimized batch was selected based on overall desirability factor and having less particle size and high entrapment efficiency.

Optimized formulation was freeze dried to white, amorphous powder which was readily redispersed in to the water. FTIR and DSC of the freeze dried formulation indicate that the drug was satisfactorily incorporated in to the nanoparticles. XRD study revealed that ITZ loaded PLHNs were amorphous in nature. Morphology of PLHNs indicates that it has lipid surrounding the polymeric core and particles were spherical in shape. Optimized formulation was followed the Higuchi model for the drug release which indicates diffusion type of drug release from the matrix. Ex vivo permeability study indicates higher apparent permeability coefficient (Papp) for the ITZ-PLHNs formulation in comparison to the drug solution which confirms increase in drug permeability. This is also indicated by high permeability enhancement ratio.

The NPs absorption occurs in rat follicular mucosa (Peyer's patches) as well as non-follicular mucosa (normal enterocyte) as visualized in CLSM images. Interaction of NPs with M-cells of the Peyer's patches would suggest that NPs were concentrated on the follicle associated epithelium promoting the absorption through M cells. The red coloured particles clearly show internalization of the ITZ loaded PLHNs in the intestinal villi. From the results it could be concluded that no single mechanism appears dominant in ITZ loaded PLHNs uptake. Transcellular, Paracellular transport and endocytosis through M-cells of Peyer's patches may be the mechanisms by which the PLHNs facilitate ITZ absorption.

Stability study of the final optimized formulation revealed that there is no any major change in the particle size and drug content during the time period of 45 days. FTIR spectra of the formulation after 45 days revealed that the drug was in the stable form as the main peak of the drug was present unchanged into the spectra. Thus, Formulation does not give any physical and chemical changes at various environmental conditions for the period of 45 days.

Conclusion

In the present work, ITZ-PLHNs consisting of the polymeric core and lipid layer at the interface of the core were easily prepared by single emulsification evaporation method with tunable particle size and high entrapment efficiency. Box Behnken design was successfully applied to optimize the effect of lipid to polymer ratio, concentration of surfactant and concentration of drug on particle size and EE. The derived polynomial equations and contour plots aid in predicting the values of selected independent variables for preparation of optimum ITZ formulations with desired properties. Thus, PLHNs may help to improve the oral bioavailability as they directly penetrate in to the systemic circulation by lymphatic uptake, M cells of payer's patch and paracellular pathway that may reduce the effect of food and hepatic first pass metabolism in comparison with the conventional system.

Competing interests
The authors declare that they have no competing interests.

Authors' contributions
BG and CD have contributed for proposing, planning and execution of all the studies whereas RP helped in execution of the confocal microscopy studies and writing the manuscript as well. All authors read and approved the final manuscript.

Acknowledgement
The authors are thankful to Intas Biopharmaceuticals Ltd, India for providing gift sample of Itraconazole and Sigma-Aldrich, USA for providing gift sample of Polycaprolactone. The authors are also thankful to K.C. Patel Research and Development Centre (KRADLE), Charotar University of science and Technology, CHARUSAT Campus, Changa, Gujarat, India, to provide facility for Particle size measurement and to the Director, National Institute for Research in Reproductive Health (NIRRH), Mumbai, India, to provide facility of Confocal Laser Scanning Microscopy.

Author details
[1]Department of Pharmaceutics & Pharmaceutical Technology, Ramanbhai Patel College of Pharmacy, Charotar University of Science and Technology, CHARUSAT Campus, Changa 388 421, Gujarat, India. [2]Department of Pharmaceutics, Indian Institute of Technology, Banaras Hindu University (IIT-BHU), Varanasi 221 005, UP, India.

References

1. R kumar A. Robbins and cotran pathologic basic of disease. 8th ed. New Delhi, India: Elsevier; 2007. p. 320–50.
2. Six K, Daemsa T, Jd H. Clinical study of solid dispersions of itraconazole prepared by hot-stage extrusion. Eur J Pharm Sci. 2005;24:179–86.
3. Kim J-K, Parkb J-S, Kima C-K. Development of a binary lipid nanoparticles formulation of itraconazole for parenteral administration and controlled release. Int J Pharm. 2010;383:209–15.
4. Chen W, Gua B, Wang H. Development and evaluation of novel itraconazole-loaded intravenous nanoparticles. Int J Pharm. 2008;362:133–40.
5. Valencia PM, Basto PA, Zha L. Single-step assembly of homogenous lipid polymeric and lipid quantum dot nanoparticles enabled by microfluidic rapid mixing. Am Chem Soc. 2010;4:1671–9.
6. Clark MA, Jepson MA. Exploiting M cells for drug and vaccine delivery. Adv Drug Deliv Rev. 2001;50:81–106.
7. Lopes MA, Abrahim BA. Intestinal absorption of insulin nanoparticles: contribution of M cells. Nanomedicine. 2014;10:1139–51.
8. Shrestha N, Shahbazi M-A. Chitosan-modified porous silicon microparticles for enhanced permeability of insulin across intestinal cell monolayers. Biomaterials. 2014;35:7172–9.
9. Lee H, Jeong C, Ghafoor K. Oral delivery of insulin using chitosan capsules cross-linked with phytic acid. Biomed Mater Eng. 2011;21:25–36.
10. Li H, Zhao X. Enhancement of gastrointestinal absorption of quercetin by solid lipid nanoparticles. J Control Release. 2009;133:238–44.
11. Zakeri-Milani P, Loveymi BD. The characteristics and improved intestinal permeability of vancomycin PLGA-nanoparticles as colloidal drug delivery system. Colloids Surf B: Biointerfaces. 2013;103:174–81.
12. Mazzaferro S, Bouchemal K. Intestinal permeation enhancement of docetaxel encapsulated into methyl-β-cyclodextrin/poly(isobutylcyanoacrylate) nanoparticles coated with thiolated chitosan. J Control Release. 2012;162:568–74.
13. Liu Y, Di Zang H. In vitro evaluation of mucoadhesion and permeation enhancement of polymeric amphiphilic nanoparticles. Carbohydr Polym. 2012;89:453–60.
14. Kogaa K, Takarada N. Nano-sized water-in-oil-in-water emulsion enhances intestinal absorption of calcein, a high solubility and low permeability compound. Eur J Pharm Biopharm. 2010;74:223–32.
15. Zhang L, Chan JM, Gu FX. Self-assembled lipid polymer hybrid nanoparticles: a robust drug delivery platform. J Am Chem Soc. 2008;2:1696–702.
16. Cheow WS, Hadinoto K. Factors affecting drug encapsulation and stability of lipid–polymer hybrid nanoparticles. Colloids Surf B: Biointerfaces. 2011;85:214–20.
17. Zhang L. Lipid polymer hybrid nanoparticles: synthesis, characterization and applications. World Sci Publishing Company. 2010;1:163–73.
18. Ferreira SL, Bruns RE, Ferreira HS. Box-behnken design: an alternative for the optimization of analytical methods. Anal Chim Acta. 2007;597:179–86.
19. Solanki AB, Parikh JR, Parikh RH. Formulation and optimization of piroxicam proniosomes by 3-factor, 3-level box-behnken design. AAPS PharmSciTech. 2007;8(4):E86.
20. Devarajan PV, Benival DM. Lipomer of doxorubicin hydrochloride for enhanced oral bioavailability. Int J Pharm. 2012;423:554–61.
21. Jain S, Jain AK, Swarnakar NK. The effect of the oral administration of polymeric nanoparticles on the efficacy and toxicity of tamoxifen. Biomaterials. 2011;32:503–15.
22. Ling G, Zhang P, Zhang W. Development of novel self-assembled DS-PLGA hybrid nanoparticles for improving oral bioavailability of vincristine sulfate by P-gp inhibition. J Control Release. 2010;148:241–8.
23. Li Y, Wong HL, Shuhendler AJ. Molecular interactions, internal structure and drug release kinetics of rationally developed polymer–lipid hybrid nanoparticles. J Control Release. 2008;128:60–70.
24. Watanabe ETM, Hayashi M. A possibility to predict the absorbability of poor water-soluble drugs in humans based on the rat intestinal permeability assessed by an in vitro chamber method. Eur J Pharm Biopharm. 2004;58:659–65.
25. Mukherjee S, Ray S, Thakur R. Design and evaluation of itraconazole loaded solid lipid nanoparticulate system for improving the antifungal therapy. Pak J Pharm Sci. 2009;22:131–8.
26. Hillgren KM, Kato A, Borchardt RT. In vitro systems for studying intestinal drug absorption. Med Res Rev. 1995;15:83–109.
27. Wong HL, Bendayan R, Rauth AM. A mechanistic study of enhanced doxorubicin uptake and retention in multidrug resistant breast cancer cells using a polymer-lipid hybrid nanoparticle system. J Pharmacol Exp Ther. 2006;317:1372–81.
28. Belletti D, Rivab G, Tosia G. Novel polymeric/lipidic hybrid systems (PLHs) for effective cidofovir delivery: preparation, characterization and comparative in vitro study with polymeric particles and liposomes. Int J Pharm. 2011;413:220–8.
29. Yang W, Chow KT, Lang B. In vitro characterization and pharmacokinetics in mice following pulmonary delivery of itraconazole as cyclodextrin solubilized solution. Eur J Pharm Sci. 2010;39:336–47.
30. Singhvi G, Singh M. Review: in-vitro drug release characterization models. Int J Pharm Stud Res. 2011;2:77–84.
31. Paulo Costa JML. Modeling and comparison of dissolution profiles. Eur J Pharm Sci. 2001;13:123–33.
32. Wei S, Shirui M, Shi Y. Nanonisation of itraconazole by high pressure homogenisation: stabiliser optimization and effext of particle size on oral absorption. J Pharm Sci. 2011;100:3365–73.
33. Sahoo SK, Panyama J, Prabha S. Residual polyvinyl alcohol associated with poly (D, L-lactide-coglycolide) nanoparticles affects their physical properties and cellular uptake. J Control Release. 2002;82:105–14.
34. Prakobvaitayakit M, Nimmannit U. Optimization of polylactic-co-glycolic acid nanoparticles containing itra-conazole using 23 factorial design. AAPS PharmSciTech. 2003;4:565–73.

The hypoglycemic effect of *Juglans regia* leaves aqueous extract in diabetic patients: A first human trial

Saeed Hosseini[1], Hasan Fallah Huseini[2], Bagher Larijani[1], Kazem Mohammad[3], Alireza Najmizadeh[4], Keramt Nourijelyani[3] and Leila Jamshidi[5]*

Abstract

Background: *Juglans regia* L. (*J. regia*) is one of the medicinal plants traditionally used for treatment of diabetes in Iranian medicine. The effect of this plant has already been investigated on animal models; however, this is the first study conducted on human subjects. The aim of this study is to investigate the hypoglycemic effect of *J. regia* leaves aqueous extract in type 2 diabetes patients. Fifty eight Iranian male and female patients with type 2 diabetes were enrolled. The patients were randomly allocated into two groups. One group (n = 30) received *J. regia* leaves extract while the other group (n = 28) received placebo. Fasting blood samples were collected at the beginning of the study and after two months for determination of HbA1c and blood glucose level as a main outcome and insulin, SGOT, SGPT, and ALP level as secondary outcome.

Results: Our analysis showed that serum fasting HbA1C and blood glucose levels were significantly decreased and the insulin level was increased in patients in the *J. regia* arm.

Conclusions: The results indicate that *J. regia* aqueous extract favorably affects blood levels of glucose, insulin and HbA1C in type 2 diabetic patients.

Keywords: *J. regia*, Insulin, Diabetes mellitus, Glucose, Liver enzymes

Introduction

Diabetes mellitus is a major public health problem in both developed and developing countries. Among the leading causes of death, diabetes mellitus is ranked seventh and when fatal complications are taken into the account, it is ranked third [1]. Recently, there has been increasing interest in the use of medicinal plants. Frequently, however, it is mandatory to provide scientific proof in order to justify the use of a plant or its active components [2]. Several studies confirm the potential therapeutic efficacy of some medicinal plants in treatment of diabetic patients [3]. Since natural products may provide better treatments with fewer side effects than the existing artificial medications, a major focus for suitable anti-hyperglycemic agents has been on plants used in traditional medicine [4]. The probable

efficiency of medicinal plants for treating diabetes and their abundance in most parts of the world facilitate their usage. *J. regia* belongs to the family Juglandaceae. It includes 3 species: *J. nigra*, *J. cinerea*, and *J. regia* although only *J. regia* type is found in Iran [5]. Investigations show that *J. regia* extract contains ellagitannins which contains anti-cancer agent and with anti-inflammatory properties [6]. The key chemical composition of walnut is Juglone (5-hydroxy-1,4-naphthoquinone), the toxic compound which is found only in green and fresh walnuts, but such property disappear in dried leaves [7]. Other several phenolic compounds with antioxidant properties have been identified in *J. regia* leaves [8]. In an experimental study treatment of *J. regia* extracts in experimental animals resulted in a significant decrease in blood glucose, glycosylated hemoglobin, LDL, triglyceride and total cholesterol and a significant increase in insulin and HDL level [9]. In another study the favorable effects of *J. regia* leaves on pancreatic cells in alloxan induced diabetic rat have been

* Correspondence: jamshidi.nutrition@yahoo.com
[5]Department of Nutrition, Tehran University of Medical Sciences, School of Public Health, Tehran, Iran
Full list of author information is available at the end of the article

reported [10]. In addition, Asgary and co-authors showed that fasting blood sugar decreased meaningfully where as insulin level increased and glycosylated hemoglobin decreased significantly in diabetic groups receiving either glibenclamide or *J. regia* extract compared with the diabetic untreated group [11]. In the present study, we evaluated the effect of *J. regia* leaves aqueous extract on type II diabetic patients for the first time.

Methods

Plant material and extraction procedure

J. regia leaves were collected from institute of medicinal plant Farm Karaj Iran. The leaves were washed by distilled water and placed in oven at 37°C to dry. Then, the leaves were completely pulverized using a porcelain mortar and pester. The powder was soaked in distilled water and placed on a magnetic stirrer for 24 hours to resolve completely. The resulting solution was passed through a filter paper and dried under appropriate conditions (in the oven at 37°C).

Participants

Initially, total of 62 patients (37 female and 25 male) with type 2 diabetes were recruited through an announcement made in the Diabetes Clinic of Shariati Hospital. The patients were randomly divided into two equal groups (*J. regia* and placebo). Shortly after the start of the study, 4 patients withdrew for personal reasons and the study continued with the remaining 58 patients (Figure 1) including 35 female and 23 male. The research protocol was approved by the Ethics Committee of the Endocrinology and Metabolism Research Center of Shariati Hospital and written informed consent was obtained of each patient prior to the study. All the patients who participated were aged between 40 and 65 years and had a confirmed diabetes type 2 diagnoses according to ADA criteria [12]. The inclusion criteria were: age 30 to 80, HbA1C > 7% fasting blood glucose less than 250 mg/L and taking maximum dose of two anti- diabetic drug (metformin and glibenclamide). The exclusion criteria were: Immune deficiency, pregnancy and lactation, cardiovascular disease, currently receiving corticosteroids and thiazide, uncontrolled thyroid dysfunction, acute infection, history of diabetic ketoacidosis, Cr > 1.5 for male, Cr > 1.2 for female, acute hepatitis, cirrhosis, proliferative retinopathy and severe weight loss (at least 10% during last 6 months).

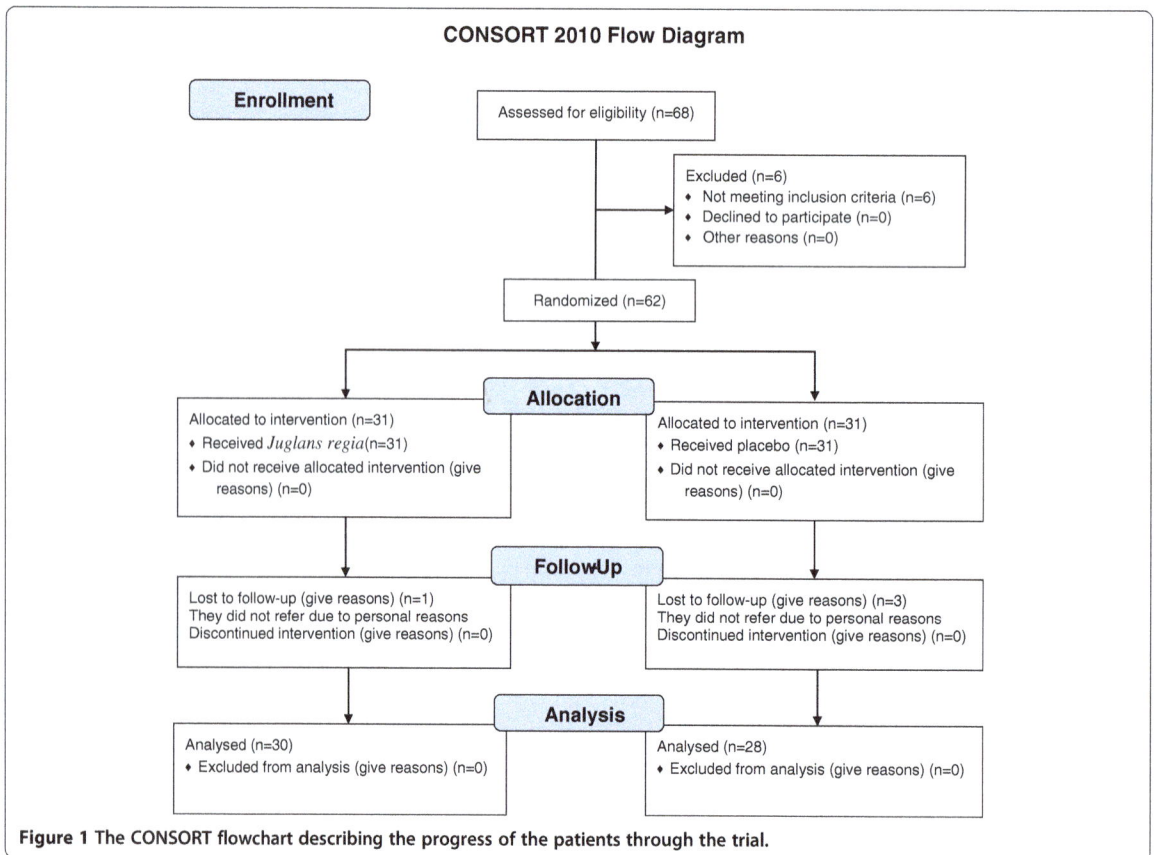

Figure 1 The CONSORT flowchart describing the progress of the patients through the trial.

Protocol

The patients were randomly allocated to two groups using a balanced randomization method. The patients and investigators who carried out clinical and para-clinical assessments were unaware of the treatment groups and the type of medication. *J. regia* (100 mg) and placebo tablets of the same shape were provided by the Institute of Medicinal Plants (Tehran, Iran). The conventional oral hypoglycemic agents (metformin and glibenclamide) continued in both groups. Compliance was assessed indirectly using the pill count method. The first group (32 patients) received one 200 mg *J. regia* tablet two times a day before meal. Also, the control group (29 patients) received a placebo tablet twice a day before meal. The blood levels of HbA1c and fasting blood glucose, insulin, SGOT, SGPT, and ALP were measured at the beginning and after 2 months of the study in both groups. Blood samples were drawn after overnight fasting (12 h). Fasting glucose levels were measured using the gloucose-oxidase method using a Beckman Glucose2 Analyzer immediately after blood sampling at the Endocrine Research Center Laboratory. Glycosylated hemoglobin levels were measured by a D-10 hemoglobin testing system (Bio-Rad Laboratories, Inc.). All other blood sample parameters were measured by an auto analyzer (Hitachi 902) using commercial kits. Patients were visited and examined every month and the efficacy of treatment was checked by measurement of the fasting blood glucose level. Sample size was calculated comparing the main outcome of the study (namely FBS) to detect 10 mg/dl of reduction from the baseline group with 80% of power and 5% sig. level.

Statistical analysis

Paired sample t test was conducted for comparing the pre and post evaluation and independent sample t test was preformed to compare the differences between two groups. Statistical analysis was carried on using R statistical package version3.0.1 (R Core Team 2013. R: A language and environment for statistical computing. R Foundation for Statistical Computing, Vienna, Austria). A p-value less than 0.05 was considered statistically significant (Figure 1).

Results

All 58 patients completed the study with no further dropouts. The patients' demographic characteristics are summarized in Table 1.

The baseline findings of patients in the two groups (*J. regia* and placebo) were compared for FBS, HbA1c, insulin and liver enzymes. The two groups were completely comparable regarding baseline and demographic characteristics (Table 2).

The average fasting blood glucose level in the *J. regia* group was 165 ± 54 mg/dL in the beginning of the study which significantly decreased (p < 0.05) to 144 ± 65 mg/dL

Table 1 The demographic characteristics of patients in placebo and *J. regia* treated groups (mean ± SD)

Groups	*J. regia*	Placebo	p-value
Age (year)	58.1 ± 4.2	56.2 ± 7.3	0.21
Sex (male/female)	11 M/19 F	12 M/16 F	0.69
Duration of disease (year)	5.2 ± 1.6	6.2 ± 1.1	0.006
Weight (kg)	62.3 ± 5.6	60.6 ± 6.1	0.52

after 2 months of treatment with *J. regia*. The average fasting blood glucose level in the placebo group was not significantly changed after 2 months of the study.

The average HbA1c level in the *J. regia* group at the beginning of the study was 8.5 ± 1.6 mg/dL, which decreased significantly (p < 0.05) to 7.6 ± 1.3 mg/dL after 2 months of *J. regia* treatment. The average HbA1c level in the placebo group was 8.3 ± 1.7 mg/dL at the beginning of the study which decreased significantly (p < 0.05) to 7.7 ± 1.5 mg/dL after 2 months of placebo treatment.

The average insulin level in the *J. regia* group was 8.6 ± 4.2 mg/dL in the beginning of the study which increased significantly (p < 0.05) to 10 ± 4.7 mg/dL after 2 months of treatment with *J. regia*. The average insulin level in the placebo group was not significantly changed after 2 months of placebo treatment.

The results of the clinical findings in both groups in the beginning and after 2 months of the study are summarized in Table 3. Finally, No liver functional or other gastrointestinal side effects of the treatment were reported during the study.

Discussion

The results suggest that *J. regia* improves glycemic in the type 2 diabetic patients without any adverse effects on the kidney and hepatic function. The results showed that although there were no significant differences in the main parameters between the two groups of patients at the beginning of the study, *J. regia* extract treatment significantly lowered fasting blood glucose and HbA1c, and increased the insulin level in diabetic patients at the end

Table 2 Para clinical characteristics of the two groups at the beginning of the study (mean ± SD)

	Groups		
	J. regia	Placebo	p-value
FBS (mg/dl)	165 ± 52	168 ± 65	0.82
HbA1c (%)	8.5 ± 1.6	8.3 ± 1.7	0.588
Insulin (ng/ml)	0.9 ± 0.7	0.7 ± 0.4	0.274
SGOT (U/L)	11.7 ± 5.3	12.5 ± 4.2	0.910
SGPT (U/L)	8.7 ± 3.7	9.5 ± 3.1	0.665
ALP (IU/L)	159 ± 34	151 ± 59	0.502

Table 3 The serologic parameters in Placebo and *J. regia* treated groups (mean ± SD)

	J. regia (n = 30)			Placebo (n = 28)			
	Beginning	After 2 month	*p*-value	Beginning	After 2 month	*p*-value	*P*-value Difference of difference
FBS (mg/d L)	165 ± 54	144 ± 65	0.017	169 ± 71	171 ± 61	0.847	0.079
HbA1c (%)	8.5 ± 1.6	7.6 ± 1.3	0.000	8.3 ± 1.7	7.7 ± 1.5	0.042	0.068
Insulin (U/L)	8.6 ± 4.2	10.4 ± 4.7	0.007	8.6 ± 3.6	9.1 ± 3.9	0.413	0.138
SGOT (U/L)	11.6 ± 5.3	12.6 ±5.0	0.293	12.5 ± 4.2	12.2 ± 4.5	0.110	0.879
SGPT (U/L)	8.7 ± 3.7	9.7 ± 2.9	0.849	9.5 ± 3.1	8.5 ± 2.8	0.708	0.692
ALP (IU/L)	159 ± 30	163 ±43	0.469	152 ± 59	152 ± 46	0.228	0.660

HbA1c (%).
8.5% NGSP = 70 mmol/mol IFCC = 198 mg/dL eAG.
7.6% NGSP = 60 mmol/mol IFCC = 171 mg/dL eAG.
8.3% NGSP = 67 mmol/mol IFCC = 191 mg/dL eAG.
7.9% NGSP = 62 mmol/mol IFCC = 179 mg/dL eAG.

of the study. The mechanism underlying the glucose lowering effect of *J. regia* might be due to increase release of insulin from remnant β-cells and/or regenerated β-cells, restore insulin sensitivity [10], interference with the absorption of dietary carbohydrates in the small intestine [13], and facilitate utilization of glucose by peripheral tissues mediated by an insulin dependent glucose transporter [14]. The key compound responsible for antihyperglycemic effect of the plant extract may be phenolic substances, such as gallic acid and caffeoylquinic acid [15]. Phenolic acids and flavonoids are two groups major phenolic compounds existing *J. regia* leaves [8]. Caffeoylquinic acid and acid coumaroylquinic are major phenolic acids in *J. regia* leaves. The main flavonoids in walnut leaves are juglone, quercetin 3-galactoside, quercetin 3-arabinoside, quercetin 3-xyloside, quercetin 3-rhamnoside and quercetin 3-pentoside [16,17]. Histomorphologic studies conducted in animal models of liver sections showed that the diabetic group had moderate inflammation in the portal space, and mild lobular necrosis was also observed where as in diabetic rats treated with the walnut extract, very mild portal inflammation and inflammatory cells were seen without any significant intra-lobular necrosis [18,19]. The same study showed that in diabetic rats treated with walnut leaf extract, serum AST and ALT had a significant decrease when compared to diabetic rats. The decrease in the plasma levels of AST and ALT is due to the decrease in liver cells injury, glucose, cholesterol, triglyceride, hepatic lipid levels and subsequently prevention from the formation of fatty liver. Our findings also indicated that treatment with *J. regia* did not adversely affects SGOT and SGPT levels as indication of its safety. In conclusion, our finding showed that the use of *J. regia* leaves was effective for glycemic control of diabetic patients. Since this study was conducted on human samples for the first time, therefore the lowest dose of the drug was used. Considering the hypoglycemic effect of *J. regia* leaves in present study and to obtain better results, we suggest the efficacy of higher doses investigated in future clinical trials.

Competing interests
The authors declare that they have no competing interests.

Authors' contributions
LJ: Designer and project manager, Sample collection, Article writing. HFH: Sample collection, Doing Statistical Analysis. SH: Designer and project manager. KM: Statistical advisor. BL: Cost of testing. AN: Sample collection. KN: Doing Statistical Analysis. All authors read and approved the final manuscript.

Acknowledgements
This study was supported by a research grant (number: 258/2011) from the Endocrinology and Metabolism Research Center, Tehran University of Medical Sciences, Tehran, Iran. Dr. Ramin Heshmat (Endocrinology & Metabolism Research Center, Tehran University of Medical Sciences) is the guarantor of this work. There is no conflict of interest. The authors wish to thank the Institute of Medical Plants and the medical and nursing staff of the Diabetic Center of Shariati Hospital for their support in providing the necessary facilities for conducting this study.

Author details
[1]Endocrinology and Metabolism Research Center, Endocrinology and Metabolism Clinical Sciences Institute, Tehran University of Medical Sciences, Tehran, Iran. [2]Pharmacology and Applied Medicine Department of Medicinal Plants Research Center, Institute of Medicinal Plants, ACECR, Karaj, Iran. [3]Department of Epidemiology and Biostatistics, Tehran University of Medical Sciences, School of Public Health, Tehran, Iran. [4]Karaj Diabetes Society, Alborz, Karaj, Iran. [5]Department of Nutrition, Tehran University of Medical Sciences, School of Public Health, Tehran, Iran.

References
1. Shaw JE, Sicree RA, Zimmet PZ: Global estimates of the prevalence of diabetes for 2010 and 2030. *Diabetes Res Clin Pract* 2010, 87(1):4–14. PubMed,MedLine, PDF.
2. Shojaii A, Dabaghian FH, Goushegir A, Fard MA: Antidiabetic plants of Iran. *Acta Med Iran* 2011, 49(10):637–642. PubMed,MedLine, PDF.
3. Suksomboon N, Poolsup N, Boonkaew S, Suthisisang CC: Meta-analysis of the effect of herbal supplement on glycemic control in type 2 diabetes. *J Ethnopharmacol* 2011, 137(3):1328–1333.
4. Rahman MA, Mossa JS, Al-Said MS, Al-Yahya MA: Medicinal plant diversity in the flora of Saudi Arabia 1: a report on seven plant families. *Fitoterapia* 2004, 75(2):149–161.
5. Mozafarian V: *Walnut tree. Identification of medicinal and aromatic plants of Iran.* Tehran, Iran: Farhang Moaser press; 2012:473–475.
6. Kaumar S, Harkonen PL, Arora S, Kaur M: Studies on correlation of antimutagenic and antiproliferative activities of *Juglans regia* L. *J Environ Pathol Toxicol Oncol* 2003, 22:59–67. PDF.

7. Amaral JS, Seabra RM, Andrade PB, Valent AOP, Pereira JA, Ferreres F: **Phenolic profile in the quality control of walnut (*Juglans regia* L.) leaves.** *J Food Chem* 2004, **88**:373–379.

8. Pereira JA, Oliveira I, Sousa A, Valenta˜ob P, Andrade PB, Ferreira I, *et al*: **Walnut (*Juglans regia* L.) leaves: phenolic compounds, antibacterial activity and antioxidant potential of different cultivars.** *J Food Chem Tox* 2007, **45**:2287–2295. Pubmed, Medline,Fulltext.

9. Mohammadi J, Sadeqpour K, Delaviz H, Mohammadi B: **Anti-diabetic effects of an alcoholic extract of Juglans regia in an animal model.** *Turk J Med Sci* 2011, **41**:685–691. Pubmed, Medline,PDF.

10. Jelodar G, Mohsen M, Shahram S: **Effect of walnut leaf, coriander and pomegranate on blood glucose and histopathology of pancreas of alloxan induced diabetic rats.** *Afr J Trad CAM* 2007, **43**:299–305. Pubmed, Medline,PDF.

11. Asgary S, Parkhideh S, Solhpour A, Madani H, Mahzouni P, Rahimi P: **Effect of ethanolic extract of *Juglans regia* L. on blood sugar in diabetes-induced rats.** *J Med Food* 2008, **11**:533–538. Pubmed, Medline,PDF.

12. American Diabetes Association: **Screening for type 2 diabetes.** *Diabetes Care* 2003, **26**:21–24. Pubmed, Medline,PDF.

13. Ortiz-Andrade RR, Garcia-Jimenez S, Castillo-Espana P, Ramirez-A G, Villalobos-Molina R, Estrada-Soto S: **α-Glucosidase inhibitory activity of the methanolic extract from Tournefortia hartwegiana: an antihyperglycemic agent.** *J Ethnopharmacol* 2007, **109**:48–53. CrossRef, PubMed, CAS, Web of Science® Times Cited: 28.

14. Del Rio D, Rodriguez-Mateos A, Spencer JP, Tognolini M, Borges G, Crozier A: **Dietary (Poly) phenolics in human health: Structures, bioavailability, and evidence of protective effects against chronic diseases.** *Antioxid Redox Signal* 2013, **18**(14):1818–1892.

15. Pereira JA, Oliveira I, Sousa A, Ferreira I, Bento A, Estevinho L: **Bioactive properties and chemical composition of six walnut (*Juglans regia* L.) cultivars.** *Food ChemToxicol* 2008, **46**:2103–2111. CrossRef, Web of Science®.

16. Savage GP: **Chemical composition of walnuts (*Juglans regia* L.) grown in New Zealand.** *Plant Food Hum Nutr* 2001, **56**:75–82. Pubmed, Medline,PDF.

17. Fukuda T, Ito H, Yoshida T: **Antioxidative polyphenols from walnuts (*Juglans regia* L.).** *Phytochemistry* 2004, **63**:795–801. Pubmed, PDF.

18. Banerji MA, Buckley MC, Chaiken RL, Gordon D, Lebovitz HE, Kral JG: **Liver fat, serum triglycerides and visceral adipose tissue in insulin sensitive and insulin-resistant black men with NIDDM.** *Int J Obes Relat Metab Disord* 1995, **19**:846–850. PubMed, MedLine.

19. Madani H, Rahimi P, Mahzoni P: **Effects of hydroalcoholic extract of *Juglans regia* leaves on activity of AST and ALT enzymes in alloxan-induced diabetic rats.** *Pharmaceut Sci* 2009, **15**(2):213–218. PubMed, MedLine, PDF.

Synthesis and biological evaluation of novel benzyl piperazine derivatives of 5-(5-nitroaryl)-1,3,4-thiadiazoles as Anti-*Helicobacter pylori* agents

Negar Mohammadhosseini[1], Parastoo Saniee[2], Ameneh Ghamaripour[3], Hassan Aryapour[3], Farzaneh Afshar[4], Najmeh Edraki[1], Farideh Siavoshi[2], Alireza Foroumadi[1] and Abbas Shafiee[1*]

Abstract

Background and the purpose of the study: *Helicobacter pylori* is recognized as the main cause of gastritis and gastroduodenal ulcers and classified as class 1 carcinogen pathogen. Different 1,3,4-thiadiazole derivatives bearing 5-nitroaryl moiety have been shown considerable anti- *H. pylori* activity. In attempt to find new and potent derivatives of described scaffold, a new series of 1-(substituted benzyl)-4-(5-(5-nitroaryl-2-yl)-1,3,4-thiadiazol-2-yl) piperazine derivatives were synthesized and evaluated against three metronidazole-resistant isolates of *H. pylori* using paper disk diffusion bioassay test.

Methods: The title compounds were prepared through the reaction of 1-(5-(5-nitroaryl-2-yl)-1,3,4-thiadiazol-2-yl) piperazine **5a-b** and substituted benzyl chloride in DMF. The inhibitory activity of the new derivatives **6a-q** against three metronidazole-resistant isolates of *H. pylori* was evaluated by the disc diffusion method and compared with the commercially available standard drug metronidazole.

Results and discussion: The results of SAR study indicated that the potency and anti-*H. pylori* activity profile of synthesized derivatives is mainly attributed to the substituted nitroaryl moiety at the C-5 position of 1,3,4-thiadiazole ring. Most of 1,3,4-thiadiazole derivatives bearing 5-nitrofuran moiety at C-5 position of central thiadiazole ring, demonstrated more promising anti-*H. pylori* than the 5-nitrothiophen counterpart.

Conclusion: The most potent nitrofuran derivative containing 3-methoxybenzyl piperazine pendant at the C-2 position of 1,3,4-thiadiazole ring (compound **6i**), demonstrated strong anti-*H. pylori* potential at studied concentrations 100-25 μg/disk (IZD > 20 mm) against all studied metronidazole- resistant isolates of *H. pylori*.

Keywords: Anti-*Helicobacter pylori* activity, 1,3,4-Thiadiazole, Nitrofuran, Nitrothiophen

Introduction

Helicobacter pylori, an spiral-shaped Gram-negative bacterium, has been considered as the leading cause of gastritis and gastroduodenal ulcer in developing countries. *H. pylori* is also classified as the class 1 carcinogen pathogen because of its epidemiological relationship to gastric adenocarcinoma and gastric mucosa-associated lymphoid tissue lymphoma [1-3]. Therefore; treatment of *Helicobacter pylori* requires targeted therapeutic strategy.

Different studies show that eradication of *H. pylori* infection resulted to ulcer healing and reduced prevalence of gastric cancer [4]. However, treatment of this infection is complicated and successful eradication of this organism is continuously requiring a combination regime using a minimum of two different antibiotics plus proton pump inhibitor (PPI) agent [3,5,6].

Although several combination therapy regimes using various anti-bacterial agents through different duration of therapy are proposed for eradication of *H. pylori* infection, emergence of resistance strains is a growing global concern. Clinical evaluation of current therapeutic

* Correspondence: ashafiee@ams.ac.ir
[1]Department of Medicinal Chemistry, Faculty of Pharmacy and Pharmaceutical Sciences Research Center, Tehran University of Medical Sciences, Tehran 14176, Iran
Full list of author information is available at the end of the article

agents indicated the incidence of drug-drug interaction, infection relapses and side effects of common drugs [7,8]. These factors have been the rationale for the development of new anti- *Helicobacter pylori* drugs and search for novel therapeutic molecules that offer better protection and decreased relapse towards resistant strains.

Nitrofuran and nitrothiophene heterocyclic derivatives have been extensively studied in therapy against different microbial infections [9-11]. Moreover, the antimicrobial and anti-Helicobacter property of 1,3,4-thiadiazole moiety is well established and attachment of this antimicrobial scaffold with nitro-hetrocyclic moieties would accommodate the bioresponses and antimicrobial activity depending on the type of substituted group and position of attachment [12-14]. In our previous works, we have investigated the anti-Helicobacter potential of different 5-(5-nitroaryl)-1,3,4-thiadiazole scaffold bearing different C-2 attached pendants. Among different nitroheterocycles, 5-nitrofuran, 5-nitrothiophen and 5-nitroimidazole moieties are preferable for substitution at C-5 position of 1,3,4-thiadiazole ring. These nitroheteroaromatic moieties mimic the nitroaromatic part of nitroheterocyclic drugs such as metronidazole and furazolidon (Figure 1) [11,14-17].

In continuation of our research program to find a novel antibacterial agent [18], we have previously demonstrated the considerable antibacterial activity of 5-nitroimidazole-based 1,3,4-thiadiazoles bearing cyclic amine functionality such as pyrrolidine and piperazine derivatives at the C-2 position of thiadiazole ring against resistant strains of *Helicobacter pylori* [15]. In order to find the structural requirement of cyclic amine derivatives of 5-(nitroaryl)-1,3,4-thiadiazole as anti-*H. pylori* agents, herein, we describe the synthesis and anti-*Helicobacter* evaluation of a new series of 5-(nitrothienyl) and 5-(nitrofuryl)-1,3,4-thiadiazoles containing different piperazine side chain at 2-position of 1,3,4-thiadiazole ring system (Figure 1).

Material and methods
Chemistry
A Kofler hot stage apparatus was used for the measurement of reported melting. The IR spectra were recorded on a Nicollet FT-IR Magna 550 spectrometer. The ^{1}H NMR spectra were recorded on a Varian FT-400 MHz or Bruker FT-500 MHz spectrometer and chemical shifts (δ) are reported in ppm relative to internal tetramethylsilane. The

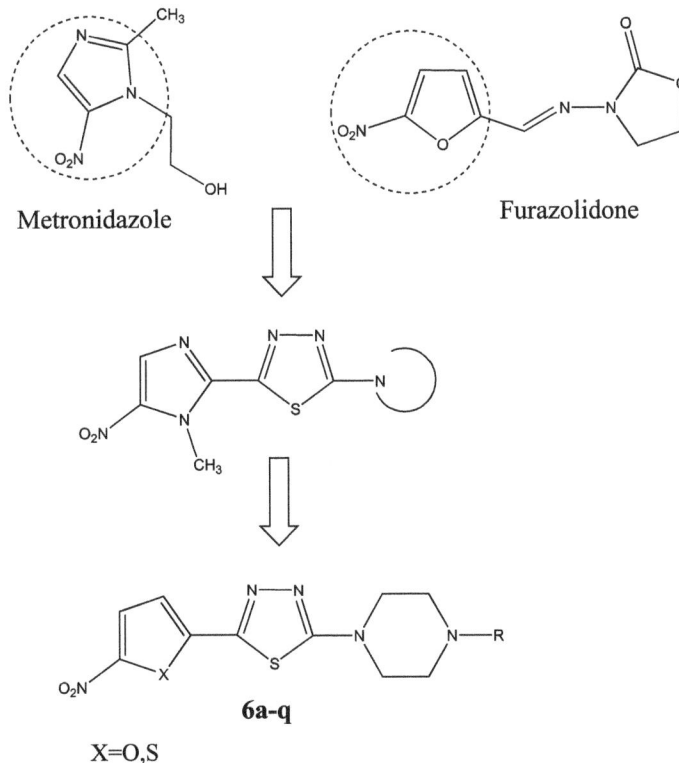

Figure 1 Chemical structure of current nitroheterocyclic drugs (Metronidazole and Furazolidone) used in the treatment of *H.pylori* infection and designed 5-(nitroaryl)-1,3,4-thiadiazoles bearing piperazine derivatives 6a-q.

mass spectra were run on a Agilent 1100/Bruker Daltonic (Ion trap) VL instrument. at 70 eV. Fross- Heraeus CHN-O rapid analyzer was used for elemental analysis of synthesized compounds and the results are within ± 0.4% of the theoretical values. Analytical thin-layar chromatography (TLC) on Merck silicagel 60 F254 plates using various mobile phases of different polarities was performed in order to confirm the purity of final products.

General method for the synthesis of 1-substitutedbenzyl-4-(5-(5-nitroaryl-2-yl)-1,3,4-thiadiazol-2-yl)piperazine 6a-q

To a mixture of 1-(5-(5-nitroaryl-2-yl)-1,3,4-thiadiazol-2-yl)piperazine **5a-b** (1.0 mmol) and different benzyl chloride derivatives (1.0 mmol) in DMF (15 mL), NaHCO$_3$ (0.21 mmol) was added and the resulted mixture was stirred at room temperature overnight. After completion of the reaction, water was added, and the resulted precipitate was filtered off, washed with water, and crystallized from ethanol.

1-(2-nitrobenzyl)-4-(5-(5-nitrothiophen-2-yl)-1,3,4-thiadiazol-2-yl)piperazine (6a)

Yield 40%; m.p. 219-221°C; IR(KBr): 1343, 1527 cm^{-1} (NO$_2$); ^{1}H-NMR(CDCl$_3$) δ: 2.48-2.64 (m, 4H, piperazine), 3.48-3.63 (m, 2H, CH$_2$), 3.48-3.63 (m, 4H, piperazine), 7.16 (bs, 1H, thiophene), 7.45 (bs, 1H, phenyl), 7.52-7.60 (m, 2H, phenyl), 7.80-7.92 (m, 2H, phenyl-thiophene); MS: m/z (%) 432 (M$^+$, 1), 415 (21), 241 (15), 191 (81), 172 (15), 136 (100), 120 (33), 91 (34), 69 (93), 42 (25). Anal. Calcd. For C$_{17}$H$_{16}$N$_6$O$_4$S$_2$: C, 47.21; H, 3.73; N, 19.43; Found: C, 47.03; H, 3.51; N, 19.67.

1-(3-nitrobenzyl)-4-(5-(5-nitrothiophen-2-yl)-1,3,4-thiadiazol-2-yl)piperazine (6b)

Yield 33%; m.p. 205-206°C; IR(KBr): 1344, 1528 cm^{-1} (NO$_2$); ^{1}H-NMR(CDCl$_3$) δ: 2.26-2.69 (m, 4H, piperazine), 3.60-3.72 (m, 4H, piperazine and 2H, CH$_2$), 7.16 (bs, 1H, thiophene), 7.58 (t, 1H, phenyl, J = 7.5Hz), 7.68 (bs, 1H, phenyl), 7.86 (bs, 1H, thiophene), 8.15 (bs, 1H, phenyl), 8.24 (s, 1H, phenyl); MS: m/z (%) 432 (M$^+$, 2), 241 (14), 191 (88), 172 (14), 155 (16), 136 (100), 111 (16), 90 (60), 73 (18), 56 (47). Anal. Calcd. For C$_{17}$H$_{16}$N$_6$O$_4$S$_2$: C, 47.21; H, 3.73; N, 19.43; Found: C, 47.54; H, 3.61; N, 19.83.

1-(4-nitrobenzyl)-4-(5-(5-nitrothiophen-2-yl)-1,3,4-thiadiazol-2-yl)piperazine (6c)

Yield 60%; m.p. 232-234°C; IR(KBr): 1340, 1509 cm^{-1} (NO$_2$); ^{1}H-NMR(CDCl$_3$) δ: 2.35-2.50 (m, 4H, piperazine), 3.40-3.60 (m, 4H, piperazine and 2H, CH$_2$), 7.02 (s, 1H, thiophene), 7.37 (d, 2H, phenyl, J = 7.6Hz), 7.70 (s, 1H, thiophene), 8.02 (d, 2H, phenyl, J = 7.6 Hz); MS: m/z (%)432 (M$^+$, 16), 415 (16), 395 (46), 368 (11), 313 (11), 296 (14), 241 (32), 191 (100), 172 (33), 155 (12),

136 (77), 106 (31), 78 (37), 56 (30). Anal. Calcd. For C$_{17}$H$_{16}$N$_6$O$_4$S$_2$ C, 47.21; H, 3.73; N, 19.43; Found: C, 47.56; H, 3.99; N, 19.07.

1-(2,6-difluorobenzyl)-4-(5-(5-nitrothiophen-2-yl)-1,3,4-thiadiazol-2-yl)piperazine (6d)

Yield 31%; m.p. 198-199°C; IR(KBr): 1343, 1503 cm^{-1} (NO$_2$); ^{1}H-NMR(CDCl$_3$) δ: 2.64-2.76 (m, 4H, piperazine), 3.60-3.71 (m, 4H, piperazine), 3.79 (s, 2H, CH$_2$), 6.92 (t, 3H, phenyl, J = 7.6Hz), 7.14 (d, 1H, thiophene, J = 3.6Hz), 7.85 (d, 1H, thiophene, J = 3.6Hz); MS: m/z (%) 423 (M$^+$, 2), 182 (100), 166 (30), 127 (100), 111 (15), 83 (21), 57 (31), 41 (23). Anal. Calcd. For C$_{17}$H$_{15}$F$_2$N$_5$O$_2$S$_2$: C, 48.22; H, 3.57; N, 16.54; Found: C, 48.49; H, 3.34; N, 16.16.

1-(2,4,5-trifluorobenzyl)-4-(5-(5-nitrothiophen-2-yl)-1,3,4-thiadiazol-2-yl)piperazine (6e)

Yield 33%; m.p. 213-215°C; IR(KBr): 1342, 1513 cm^{-1} (NO$_2$); ^{1}H-NMR(CDCl$_3$) δ: 2.64 (bs, 4H, piperazine), 3.59 (s, 2H, CH$_2$), 3.65 (bs, 4H, piperazine), 6.90-7.00 (m, 1H, phenyl), 7.12 (bs, 1H, thiophene), 7.20-7.38 (m, 1H, phenyl), 7.87 (bs, 1H, thiophene); MS: m/z (%) 441 (M$^+$, 5), 241 (13), 200 (86), 182 (19), 145 (100), 128 (11), 69 (11), 42 (14). Anal. Calcd. For C$_{17}$H$_{14}$F$_3$N$_5$O$_2$S$_2$: C, 46.25; H, 3.20; N, 15.86; Found: C, 45.88; H, 3.44; N, 16.03.

1-(2,5-diChlorobenzyl)-4-(5-(5-nitrothiophen-2-yl)-1,3,4-thiadiazol-2-yl)piperazine (6f)

Yield 93%; m.p. 210-211°C; IR(KBr): 1344, 1504 cm^{-1} (NO$_2$); ^{1}H-NMR(CDCl$_3$) δ: 2.65-2.74 (m, 4H, piperazine), 3.60-3.74 (m, 2H, CH$_2$ and 4H, piperazine), 7.13-7.32 (m, 3H, phenyl-thiophene), 7.50 (s, 1H, phenyl), 7.86 (d, 1H, thiophene, J = 3.6 Hz); MS: m/z (%) 459 (M$^+$+4, 0.4), 457 (M$^+$+2, 3), 455 (M$^+$, 4), 214 (93), 192 (18), 159 (100), 123 (18). Anal. Calcd. For C$_{17}$H$_{15}$Cl$_2$N$_5$O$_2$S$_2$: C, 44.74; H, 3.31; N, 15.35; Found: C, 44.51; H, 3.70; N, 15.67.

1-(3,4-dichlorobenzyl)-4-(5-(5-nitrothiophen-2-yl)-1,3,4-thiadiazol-2-yl)piperazine (6g)

Yield 36%; m.p. 183-185°C; IR(KBr): 1343, 1508 cm^{-1} (NO$_2$); ^{1}H-NMR(CDCl$_3$) δ: 2.51-2.63 (m, 4H, piperazine), 3.52 (s, 2H, CH$_2$), 3.60-3.68 (m, 4H, piperazine), 7.13-7.24 (m, 2H, phenyl-thiophene), 7.40 (dd, 2H, phenyl), 7.85 (s, 1H, thiophene); MS: m/z (%) 459 (M$^+$+4, 0.5), 457 (M$^+$+2, 3), 455 (M$^+$, 5), 241 (18), 214 (81), 159 (100), 124 (16), 89 (12), 56 (19). Anal. Calcd. For C$_{17}$H$_{15}$Cl$_2$N$_5$O$_2$S$_2$: C, 44.74; H, 3.31; N, 15.35; Found: C, 44.46; H, 3.62; N, 15.14.

1-(4-bromobenzyl)-4-(5-(5-nitrothiophen-2-yl)-1,3,4-thiadiazol-2-yl)piperazine (6h)

Yield 50%; m.p. 207-208°C; IR(KBr): 1343, 1509 cm^{-1} (NO$_2$); ^{1}H-NMR(CDCl$_3$) δ: 2.53-2.68 (m, 4H, piperazine), 3.52 (s, 2H, CH$_2$), 3.60-3.69 (m, 4H, piperazine),

7.14-7.20 (m, 3H, phenyl-thiophene), 7.44-7.50 (m, 2H, phenyl), 7.85 (s, 1H, thiophene); MS: m/z (%) 467 (M$^+$+2, 13), 465 (M$^+$, 14), 296 (16), 280 (14), 265 (10), 254 (41), 239 (100). Anal. Calcd. For $C_{17}H_{16}BrN_5O_2S_2$: C, 43.78; H, 3.46; N, 15.02; Found: C, 43.94; H, 3.74; N, 14.78.

1-(3-methoxybenzyl)-4-(5-(5-nitrofuran-2-yl)-1,3,4-thiadiazol-2-yl)piperazine (6i)

Yield 54%; m.p. 126-127°C; IR(KBr): 1355, 1536 cm^{-1} (NO$_2$); ^{1}H-NMR(CDCl$_3$) δ: 2.63 (t, 4H, piperazine, J = 5.1 Hz), 3.57 (s, 2H, CH$_2$), 3.67 (t, 4H, piperazine, J = 5.1Hz), 3.83 (s, 3H, OCH$_3$), 6.84-6.87 (m, 1H, phenyl), 6.92-6.95 (m, 2H, phenyl), 7.17 (d, 1H, furan, J = 3.7 Hz), 7.21-7.23 (m, 1H, phenyl), 7.44 (d, 1H, furan, J = 3.7 Hz); MS: m/z (%) 401 (M$^+$, 7), 176 (86), 147 (13), 121 (100), 91 (24), 57 (18), 40 (14). Anal. Calcd. For $C_{18}H_{19}N_5O_4S$: C, 53.85; H, 4.77; N, 17.45; Found: C, 53.97; H, 4.54; N, 17.79.

1-(2-nitrobenzyl)-4-(5-(5-nitrofuran-2-yl)-1,3,4-thiadiazol-2-yl)piperazine (6j)

Yield 43%; m.p. 197-199°C; IR(KBr): 1353,1529 cm^{-1} (NO$_2$); ^{1}H-NMR(CDCl$_3$) δ: 2.62 (t, 4H, piperazine, J = 5.1 Hz), 3.62 (t, 4H, piperazine, J = 5.1 Hz), 3.89 (s, 2H, CH$_2$), 7.17 (d, 1H, furan, J = 3.8 Hz), 7.44 (d, 1H, furan, J = 3.8 Hz),7.45-7.48 (m, 1H, phenyl), 7.56-7.59 (m, 2H, phenyl), 7.85 (d, 1H, phenyl, J = 7.8 Hz); MS: m/z (%) 416 (M$^+$, 2), 399 (46), 381 (13), 225 (18), 191 (86), 166 (14), 136 (100), 105 (12), 78 (44), 56 (19). Anal. Calcd. For $C_{17}H_{16}N_6O_5S$:C, 49.03; H, 3.87; N, 20.18; Found: C, 49.28; H, 3.64; N, 20.42.

1-(3-nitrobenzyl)-4-(5-(5-nitrofuran-2-yl)-1,3,4-thiadiazol-2-yl)piperazine (6k)

Yield 50%; m.p. 144-146°C; IR(KBr): 1353, 1529 cm^{-1} (NO$_2$); ^{1}H-NMR(CDCl$_3$) δ: 2.66 (t, 4H, piperazine, J = 5.0 Hz), 3.69 (t, 4H, piperazine, J = 5.0 Hz), 3.71 (s, 2H, CH$_2$), 7.18 (d, 1H, furan, J = 3.9 Hz), 7.44 (d, 1H, furan, J = 3.9 Hz), 7.54 (t, 1H, phenyl, J = 7.9 Hz), 7.71 (d, 1H, phenyl, J = 7.9 Hz), 8.17 (d, 1H, phenyl, J = 7.9 Hz), 8.26 (bs, 1H, phenyl); MS: m/z (%) 416 (M$^+$, 7), 399 (12), 225 (19), 191 (100), 166 (20), 136 (86), 90 (37), 57 (21), 40 (18). Anal. Calcd. For $C_{17}H_{16}N_6O_5S$: C, 49.03; H, 3.87; N, 20.18; Found: C, 48.88; H, 3.56; N, 20.44.

1-(4-nitrobenzyl)-4-(5-(5-nitrofuran-2-yl)-1,3,4-thiadiazol-2-yl)piperazine (6l)

Yield 50%; m.p. 212-213°C; IR(KBr): 1348, 1505 cm^{-1} (NO$_2$); ^{1}H-NMR(CDCl$_3$) δ: 2.65 (t, 4H, piperazine, J = 5.1 Hz), 3.69(s, 2H, CH$_2$), 3.70 (t, 4H, piperazine, J = 5.1 Hz), 7.18 (d, 1H, furan, J = 3.9 Hz), 7.44 (d, 1H, furan, J = 3.9 Hz), 7.56 (d, 2H, phenyl, J = 8.6 Hz), 8.23 (d, 2H, phenyl, J = 8.6 Hz); MS: m/z (%) 416 (M$^+$, 9), 399 (13), 225 (21), 191 (100), 166 (12), 136 (87), 106 (36), 78 (49), 60 (11), 42 (40). Anal. Calcd. For $C_{17}H_{16}N_6O_5S$: C, 49.03; H, 3.87; N, 20.18; Found: C, 49.31; H, 3.58; N, 20.36.

1-(2,6-difluorobenzyl)-4-(5-(5-nitrofuran-2-yl)-1,3,4-thiadiazol-2-yl)piperazine (6m)

Yield 50%; m.p. 176-179°C; IR (KBr): 1353, 1540 cm^{-1} (NO$_2$); ^{1}H-NMR(CDCl$_3$) δ: 2.69 (t, 4H, piperazine, J = 4.6 Hz), 3.67 (t, 4H, piperazine, J = 4.6 Hz), 3.79 (s, 2H, CH$_2$), 6.93 (t, 2H, phenyl, J = 7.4 Hz), 7.16 (d, 1H, furan, J = 3.8 Hz), 7.28-7.38 (m, 1H, phenyl), 7.43 (d, 1H, furan, J = 3.8 Hz); MS: m/z (%) 407 (M$^+$, 5), 182 (85), 149 (11), 127 (100), 69 (11), 42 (11). Anal. Calcd. For $C_{17}H_{15}F_2N_5O_3S$:C, 50.12; H, 3.71;N, 17.19; Found: C, 50.35; H, 3.45; N, 17.54.

1-(2,4,5-trifluorobenzyl)-4-(5-(5-nitrofuran-2-yl)-1,3,4-thiadiazol-2-yl)piperazine (6n)

Yield 41%; m.p. 174-175°C; IR(KBr): 1355, 1517 cm^{-1} (NO$_2$); ^{1}H-NMR(CDCl$_3$) δ: 2.65 (t, 4H, piperazine, J = 5.2 Hz), 3.60 (s, 2H, CH$_2$), 3.68 (t, 4H, piperazine, J = 5.2 Hz), 6.84-6.86 (m, 1H, phenyl), 7.18 (d, 1H, furan, J = 3.8 Hz), 7.25-7.26 (m, 1H, phenyl), 7.74 (d, 1H, furan, J = 3.8 Hz); MS: m/z (%) 425 (M$^+$, 6), 225 (13), 200 (94), 166 (11), 145 (100), 82 (12). Anal. Calcd. For $C_{17}H_{14}F_3N_5O_3S$: C, 48.00; H, 3.32; N, 16.46; Found: C, 48.35; H, 3.44; N, 16.18.

1-(2,5-dichlorobenzyl)-4-(5-(5-nitrofuran-2-yl)-1,3,4-thiadiazol-2-yl)piperazine (6o)

Yield 92%; m.p. 165-167°C; IR(KBr): 1353, 1549 cm^{-1} (NO$_2$); ^{1}H-NMR(CDCl$_3$) δ: 2.71 (t, 4H, piperazine, J = 4.6 Hz), 3.67 (s, 2H, CH$_2$), 3.68 (t, 4H, piperazine, J = 4.6 Hz), 7.17 (d, 1H, furan, J = 3.6 Hz), 7.22 (dd, 1H, phenyl, J = 8.5 Hz, J = 2.0 Hz), 7.32 (d, 1H, phenyl, J = 8.5 Hz, J = 2.0 Hz), 7.45 (d, 1H, furan, J = 3.6 Hz), 7.51 (d, 1H, phenyl, J = 2.0 Hz); MS: m/z (%) 443 (M$^+$+4, 0.4), 441 (M$^+$+2, 3), 439 (M$^+$, 6), 313 (12), 236 (16), 214 (95), 192 (16), 159 (100), 123 (16), 99 (13), 82 (16), 57 (20), 40 (16). Anal. Calcd. For $C_{17}H_{15}Cl_2N_5O_3S$: C, 46.37; H, 3.43; N, 15.91; Found: C, 46.65; H, 3.67; N, 15.69.

1-(3,4-dichlorobenzyl)-4-(5-(5-nitrofuran-2-yl)-1,3,4-thiadiazol-2-yl)piperazine (6p)

Yield 62%; m.p. 161-162°C; IR(KBr): 1353, 1503 cm^{-1} (NO$_2$); ^{1}H-NMR(CDCl$_3$) δ: 2.62 (t, 4H, piperazine, J = 5.0 Hz), 3.53 (s, 2H, CH$_2$), 3.67 (t, 4H, piperazine, J = 5.0 Hz), 7.17 (d, 1H, furan, J = 3.8 Hz), 7.19 (dd, 1H, phenyl, J = 8.3 Hz, J = 2.0 Hz), 7.41-7.45(m, 2H, phenyl), 7.47 (d, 1H, furan, J = 3.8 Hz); MS: m/z (%) 443 (M$^+$+4, 0.5), 441 (M$^+$+2, 3), 439 (M$^+$, 5), 273 (12), 238 (11), 214 (93), 159 (100), 123 (16), 100 (7), 82 (13), 56 (15). Anal. Calcd. For $C_{17}H_{15}Cl_2N_5O_3S$: C, 46.37; H, 3.43; N, 15.91; Found: C, 46.68; H, 3.16; N, 16.09.

1-(4-bromobenzyl)-4-(5-(5-nitrofuran-2-yl)-1,3,4-thiadiazol-2-yl)piperazine (6q)

Yield 28%; m.p. 192-193°C; IR(KBr): 1353, 1508 cm^{-1} (NO_2); ^{1}H-NMR(CDCl$_3$) δ: 2.61 (t, 4H, piperazine, $J = 5.0$ Hz), 3.54 (s, 2H, CH_2), 3.66 (t, 4H, piperazine, $J = 5.0$ Hz), 7.17 (d, 1H, furan, $J = 3.9$ Hz), 7.23 (d, 2H, phenyl, $J = 8.3$Hz), 7.44 (d, 1H, furan, $J = 3.9$ Hz), 8.25 (d, 2H, phenyl, $J = 8.3$ Hz); MS: m/z (%) 451 (M$^+$+2, 1), 449 (M$^+$, 2), 210 (20), 169 (100), 90 (44), 56 (22), 40 (21). Anal. Calcd. For $C_{17}H_{16}BrN_5O_3S$: C, 45.34; H, 3.58; N, 15.55; Found: C, 45.59; H, 3.92; N, 15.27.

Biological activity

Patients and bacterial strains

Different isolates of *H. pylori* were obtained from 160 dyspeptic patients consisted of 78 men and 82 women whose mean ages were 48 and 43 years, respectively. Based on the endoscopic diagnosis, the patients were classified into three groups: gastritis (124, 77.5%), ulcers (32, 20%) and cancer.

Antral biopsies demonstrating positive urease tests were transported to the microbiology lab in semisolid (0.1% agar) normal saline. The biopsies were cultured using selective medium containing brucella agar (Merck), 7% defibrinated sheep blood, vancomycin (5 mg/L), trimethoprim (5 mg/L), polymyxin B (50 mg/L), and amphotericin B (4 mg/L). Incubation of cultured isolates was performed at 37°C under microaerobic conditions (CO_2 incubator; Heraeus, Germany). After 3–5 days, all cultures were examined for observation of pinpoint (1–2 mm) glistening colonies. Identification of *H. pylori* isolates was carried out according to the spiral microscopic appearance, Gram negative stain and some biochemical examinations such as urease, oxidase and catalase positive test and negative activities of nitrate and H_2S.

The protocol of this research was approved by Pharmaceutical Sciences Research Center ethics committee (number 90-3-29: 1-1).

Consent

Written informed consent was obtained from the patient for the publication of this report.

Antimicrobial susceptibility test

Antimicrobial susceptibility test was performed using disk diffusion method (DDM). Recruited antibiotics included metronidazole, tetracycline. In the first step of the susceptibility evaluation, one hundred and ten strains were recruited. As a result of remarkable resistance of different studied bacterial isolates to recruited antibiotics and in attempt to increase the accuracy of the metronidazole resistant rates, in the second step of our study, an additional fifty strains of *H. Pylori* isolates were recruited for susceptibility testing with metronidazole (32, 16, 8, and 4 µg/mL)

and with 2, 1, and 0.5 µg/mL of tetracycline. The susceptibility tests were repeated twice for the resistant strains. Bacterial suspensions were prepared in normal saline with the turbidity of Mac-Farland standard No.2 (equivalent to 6×108cell/mL). 100 µl of each bacterial suspension were inoculated in the surface of non- selective blood agar plates and the culture plates were allowed to dry at room temperature (10 min). Sterile blank disks were deposited on the surface of inoculated plates. 10 µL of each antibiotic dilution was poured into a blank disk. Moreover, control plates with growth positive bacterial culture were prepared using the introduction of 10 µl of the antibiotic solvent into the blank disks.

Plates were incubated at described condition and the inhibition zone diameters (IZD) were examined after 3–5 days. Susceptible and resistant isolates of *H.pylori* demonstrated IZDs ≥ 20 mm and ≤ 10 mm for metronidazole, respectively. The antibacterial activities of target compounds were evaluated against three metronidazole-resistant isolates of *H. pylori*. All experiments were performed in triplicate and the mean of IZDs produced by test compounds in four concentrations (100, 50, 25 and 12.5 µg/mL) was considered as antibacterial activity.

Anti-Helicobacter pylori activity assay

As mentioned earlier, the growth inhibitory potential of test compounds was evaluated against three metronidazole resistant isolates of *H. pylori* by the filter paper disk diffusion method at 37°C, under microqerophilic condition on selective Brucella agar with 7% defibrinated horse blood. Four concentrations of titled compounds in dimethylsulfoxide (DMSO) were used for evaluation of anti *Helicobacter* activity assay. Blank standard disks (6 mm in diameter) were deposited on the surface of test plates and impregnated with $10\,\mu L$ of different concentrations of target compounds. Test plates were incubated at 37°C for 3–5 days and the inhibition zone around each disk (average diameter) was measured. The control disks were impregnated with $10\,\mu L$ of DMSO. All antibacterial activity experiments were performed in triplicate and the antibacterial activity was expressed as the mean of IZDs (mm) produced by the test compounds at each evaluated concentration.

Result and discussion

Chemistry

The synthetic pathway for the target compounds **6a-q** is depicted in the Scheme 1. A mixture of 5-nitroaryl-2-carboxaldehyde diacetate **1a-b** with thiosemicarbazide was refluxed in ethanol to afford thiosemicarbazone **2a-b**. Amino-1,3,4-thiadiazoles **3a-b,** were synthesized through the oxidative cyclization of **2a-b** in presence of ammonium ferric sulfate. In the next step, diazotization of **3a-b** in hydrochloric acid and in the presence of copper powder

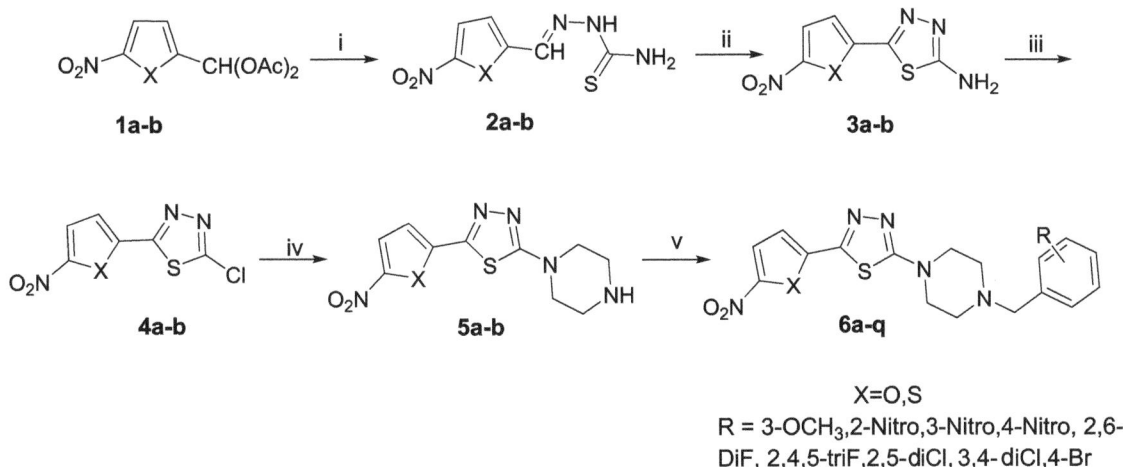

Scheme 1 Reagents and conditions: (i) thiosemicarbazide, EtOH, HCl, reflux, 1.5 h; (ii) $NH_4Fe(SO_4)_2$, $12H_2O$, H_2O reflux, 25 h; (iii) $NaNO_2$, HCl, Cu, °C→ rt, 3 h; (iv) Piperazine hydrate, EtOH, $NaHCO_3$ 1 h; (v) DMF, Substituted benzyl chloride, 4 h.

yielded chloro-1,3,4-thiadiazole **4a-b**. 1-(5-(5-nitroaryl-2-yl)-1,3,4-thiadiazol-2-yl)piperazine **5a-b** were prepared through the reaction of chloro-1,3,4-thiadiazole derivatives **4a-b** with piperazine hydrate in stirred ethanol.

The prepared key intermediates **5a-b** were further reacted with different substituted benzyl chlorides in refluxing DMF to give the corresponding 1-substituted-benzyl-4-(5-(5-nitroaryl-2-yl)-1,3,4-thiadiazol-2-yl)piperazine **6a-q**. The structures of compounds **6a-q** were determined using spectroscopic methods including mass spectrometry,^{1}H NMR, IR, and elemental analysis. The chemical structure of target compounds are shown in Figure 2.

Anti-*Helicobacter pylori* activity and structure-activity relationship study

The *in vitro* anti-Helicobacter activity of synthesized derivatives was determined by paper disk diffusion bioassay against three metronidazole resistant *H. pylori* isolates. The average of inhibition zone diameters (IZD) of compounds against three isolates at four different concentrations (100, 50, 25 and 12.5 µg/ disk) is summarized in Figure 2. The anti-*H. pylori* activity of target derivatives could be simply categorized as follows: strong response, zones range diameter >20 mm; moderate response, zone diameter 16–20 mm; weak response, zone diameter 11–15 mm; and little or no response, zone diameter <10 mm [15].

Investigation of the IZD of studied compounds revealed that the target derivatives demonstrated a wide

spectrum of anti-*H. pylori* activity varied from little (IZD <10 mm) to strong (IZD >20 mm) response at concentration of 100 µg/disk against metronidazole resistant strains. In view of the obtained data, the following structure-activity relationship might be developed:

Assessment of nitroheterocyclic moiety

Based on the substituted nitroaromatic group, the studied 1,3,4-thiadiazole derivatives could be classified into two groups: Nitrothiophen **6a-h** and nitrofuran **6i-q** derivatives. The results of anti-*H. pylori* activity indicated that the inhibitory responses of test compounds is mainly attributed to the substituted nitroaryl moiety at the C-5 position of 1,3,4-thiadiazole ring. While all of nitrothiophene derivatives **6a-h** demonstrated weak (IZD = 11–15 mm) to little (IZD <10 mm) inhibitory response at concentration of 100 µg/disk against three metronidazole resistant isolates, most of nitrofurane derivatives **6i-q** showed strong (IZD > 20 mm) to moderate (IZD = 16–20) growth inhibitory potential at the same concentration.

It could be concluded that nitrofuran **6i-q** derivatives of 1,3,4-thiadiazole scaffold, are more potent than the nitrothiophen **6a-h** counterpart.

Investigation of substituted group into the benzyl piperazine pendant

In order to find the structural requirement of substituted moiety at C-2 position of 1,3,4-thiadiazole scaffold,

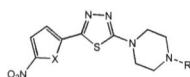

Compound	X	R	Average of Inhibition Zone Diameters (range, mm)[a]			
			100 µg/disk	50 µg/disk	25 µg/disk	12.5 µg/disk
6a	S	(2-NO₂ benzyl)	14.7 (11-16)	10 (9-10)	6	6
6b	S	(3-NO₂ benzyl)	12 (10-14)	6	6	6
6c	S	(4-NO₂ benzyl)	15 (11-18)	11 (9-11)	6	6
6d	S	(2,6-F₂ benzyl)	13 (10-15)	6	6	6
6e	S	(F₃ benzyl)	13.5 (10-15)	6	6	6
6f	S	(Cl₂ benzyl)	14 (12-16)	6	6	6
6g	S	(Cl₂ benzyl)	13.5 (15-14)	6	6	6
6h	S	(4-Br benzyl)	14 (11-16)	6	6	6
6i	O	(3-OCH₃ benzyl)	28 (25-30)	24 (21-28)	21.5 (16-24)	20 (15-22)
6j	O	(2-NO₂ benzyl)	16 (12-20)	8 (6-13)	3.6 (6-11)	6
6k	O	(3-NO₂ benzyl)	22 (19-25)	19.5 (18-20)	17 (15-20)	16 (14-18)
6l	O	(4-NO₂ benzyl)	11 (10-11)	6	6	6
6m	O	(2,6-F₂ benzyl)	20 (17-22)	19 (17-21)	17 (15-20)	14.5 (12-18)
6n	O	(F₃ benzyl)	23 (22-24)	21 (20-22)	19 (15-21)	17 (13-20)
6o	O	(Cl₂ benzyl)	12 (12-17)	5 (6-15)	4 (6-12)	3.6 (6-11)
6p	O	(Cl₂ benzyl)	16 (12-19)	11.5 (11-12)	4 (6-11)	3.3 (6-10)
6q	O	(4-Br benzyl)	18 (11-25)	13 (6-22)	12 (6-20)	10.5 (6-18)

[a] The anti-Helicobacter pylori activity was determined by the paper disk diffusion bioassay. All tests were performed in triplicate and the antibacterial activity was expressed as the mean of inhibition zone diameters (mm) produced by title compounds.

Figure 2 Average of inhibition zone diameters of compounds 6a-q at four different concentrations against three metronidazole resistant *H. pylori* isolates.

different benzyl piperazine derivatives were substituted at the described position. Among the nitrofuran derivatives **6i-q**, 3-methoxybenzyl piperazine derivative **6i**, demonstrated strong anti-*H. pylori* potential at studied concentrations 100–25 µg/disk (IZD > 20 mm) against studied isolates. Investigation of the growth inhibitory potential of the nitrofuran series **6i-q** revealed that substitution of nitro group at the *meta* position of the benzyl piperazine side chain, resulted in compound with strong (IZD = 20 mm) to moderate (IZD = 16–20 mm) growth inhibitory potential at 100 and 50–12.5 µg/disk, respectively. However, introduction of nitro substitute at *ortho* or *para* position of the benzyl piperazine pendant, resulted in compound with diminished inhibitory potential against resistant strains of *H. pylori* isolates (compounds **6j** (IZD = 16 mm, moderate response) and **6l** (IZD = 11 mm, weak response) respectively. Moreover, substitution of fluorine groups at different positions of benzyl pieperzine side chain influenced the growth inhibitory potential of compounds which is mainly dependent on the position and number of substituted fluorine groups; compound **6n** containing 2,4,5-triflouro benzyl piperazine pendant at C-2 position of 5-nitrofuran-1,3,4-thiadiazole scaffold, produced strong inhibitory response at 100 and 50 µg/disk (IZD =23 and 21 mm, respectively); while the anti-*H. pylori* potential of 2,5-difluoro benzyl piperazine counterpart was diminished to weak (IZD = 12 mm) to no response (IZD = 5 mm) at 100 and 50 µg/disk, respectively.

Conclusion

A novel series of 5-(5-nitroaryl)-1,3,4-thiadiazole derivatives containing various benzyl piperazine moiety at C-2 position of 1,3,4-thiadiazole ring were synthesized and evaluated against three metronidazole-resistant isolates of *H.pylori* using paper disk diffusion bioassay test. Structure-activity relationship study of these derivatives indicated that 1,3,4-thiadiazole derivatives bearing 5-nitrofuran moiety at C-5 position of central thiadiazole ring, demonstrated more promising anti-*H. pylori* than the 5-nitrothiophen counterpart. The most potent nitrofuran derivative had 3-methoxybenzyl piperazine pendant at the C-2 position of 1,3,4-thiadiazole ring. The results indicated that the anti-*H. pylori* potential of the nitrofurane derivatives of 1,3,4-thiadiazole scaffold is mainly attributed to the type and position of the substituted group at the benzyl piperazine pendant. Future studies may be aimed at designing more potent derivatives of these series in order to investigate the structure-activity relationship of cyclic amine derivatives of 5-(nitroaryl)-1,3,4-thiadiazole derivatives as Anti-*H. pylori* agents.

Competing interests
The authors declare that they have no competing interests.

Authors' contributions

NM: Synthesis of some target compounds. PS: Evaluation of the antibacterial activities (10%). AG: Evaluation of the antibacterial activities. HA: Evaluation of the antibacterial activities (10%). FA: Synthesis of the intermediates and some target compounds. NE: Collaboration in identifying of the structures of target compounds. FS: Evaluation of the antibacterial activities. AF: Collaboration in design and identifying of the structures of target compounds, manuscript preparation. AS: Design of target compounds and management of the synthetic and pharmacological parts. All authors read and approved the final manuscript.

Acknowledgements

This work was financially supported by grants from Research Council of Tehran University of Medical Sciences grant No.90/d/425/236 and Iran National Science Foundation (INSF).

Author details

[1]Department of Medicinal Chemistry, Faculty of Pharmacy and Pharmaceutical Sciences Research Center, Tehran University of Medical Sciences, Tehran 14176, Iran. [2]Department of Microbiology, Faculty of Sciences, University of Tehran, P.O. Box: 14155–6455, Tehran, Iran. [3]Department of Biology, Faculty of Science, Golestan University, Gorgan, Iran. [4]Department of Chemistry, Science and Research Branch, Islamic Azad University, Arak, Iran.

References

1. Marshall BJ, Warren JR: Unidentified curved bacilli in the stomach of patients with gastritis and peptic ulceration. *Lancet* 1984, 1(8390):1311–1315.
2. Bardhan PK: Epidemiological features of *H. pylori* infection in developing countries. *Clin Infect Dis* 1997, 25:973–978.
3. Gisbert JP, Pajares JM: Treatment of *H. pylori* infection: the past and the future. *Eur J Intern Med* 2010, 21:357–359.
4. Sepulveda AR, Coelho LG: *H. pylori* and gastric malignancies. *Helicobacter* 2002, 7:37–42.
5. Egan BJ, Katicic M, O'Connor HJ, O'Morain CA: Treatment of *H. pylori*. *Helicobacter* 2007, 12:31–37.
6. Petersen AM, Krogfelt KA: *H. pylori*: an invading microorganism? A review. *FEMS Immunol Med Microbiol* 2003, 36:117–126.
7. Gisbert JP: Review: second-line rescue therapy of *H. pylori* infection. *Therap Adv Gastroenterol* 2009, 2:331–356.
8. Kivi M, Tindberg Y, Sörberg M, Casswall TH, Befrits R, Hellström PM, Bengtsson C, Engstrand L, Granström M: Concordance of *H. pylori* strains within families. *J Clin Microbiol* 2003, 41:5604–5608.
9. Nair MD, Nagarajan K: Nitroimidazoles as chemotherapeutic agents. *Prog Drug Res* 1983, 27:163–252.
10. Foroumadi A, Pournourmohammadi S, Soltani F, Asgharian-Rezaee M, Dabiri S, Kharazmi A, Shafiee A: Synthesis and in vitro leishmanicidal activity of 2-(5-nitro-2-furyl) and 2-(5-nitro-2-thienyl)-5-substituted-1,3,4-thiadiazoles. *Bioorg Med Chem Lett* 2005, 15:1983–1985.
11. Foroumadi A, Emami S, Pournourmohammadi S, Kharazmi A, Shafiee A: Synthesis and in vitro leishmanicidal activity of 2-(1-methyl-5-nitro-1H-imidazol-2-yl)-5-substituted-1,3,4-thiadiazole derivatives. *Eur J Med Chem* 2005, 40:1346–1350.
12. Tahghighi A, Razmi S, Mahdavi M, Foroumadi P, Ardestani SK, Emami S, Kobarfard F, Dastmalchi S, Shafiee A, Foroumadi A: Synthesis and anti-leishmanial activity of 5-(5-nitrofuran-2-yl)-1,3,4-thiadiazol-2-amines containing N-[(1-benzyl-1H-1,2,3-triazol-4-yl)methyl] moieties. *Eur J Med Chem* 2012, 50:124–128.
13. Poorrajab F, Ardestani SK, Emami S, Behrouzi-Fardmoghadam M, Shafiee A, Foroumadi A: Nitroimidazolyl-1,3,4-thiadiazole-based anti-leishmanial agents: synthesis and in vitro biological evaluation. *Eur J Med Chem* 2009, 44:1758–1762.
14. Foroumadi A, Sorkhi M, Moshafi MH, Safavi M, Rineh A, Siavoshi F, Shafiee A, Emami S: 2-Substituted-5-nitroheterocycles: in vitro anti- *H. pylori* activity and structure-activity relationship study. *Med Chem* 2009, 5:529–534.
15. Moshafi MH, Sorkhi M, Emami S, Nakhjiri M, Yahya-Meymandi A, Negahbani AS, Siavoshi F, Omrani M, Alipour E, Vosooghi M, Shafiee A, Foroumadi A:
5-Nitroimidazole-based 1,3,4-thiadiazoles: heterocyclic analogs of metronidazole as anti- *H. pylori* agents. *Arch Pharm* 2011, 344:178–183.
16. Mirzaei J, Siavoshi F, Emami S, Safari F, Khoshayand MR, Shafiee A, Foroumadi A: Synthesis and in vitro anti- *H. pylori* activity of N-[5-(5-nitro-2-heteroaryl)-1,3,4-thiadiazol-2-yl]thiomorpholines and related compounds. *Eur J Med Chem* 2008, 43:1575–1580.
17. Foroumadi A, Rineh A, Emami S, Siavoshi F, Massarrat S, Safari F, Rajabalian S, Falahati M, Lotfali E, Shafiee A: Synthesis and anti- *H. pylori* activity of 5-(nitroaryl)-1,3,4-thiadiazoles with certain sulfur containing alkyl side chain. *Bioorg Med Chem Lett* 2008, 18:3315–3320.
18. Mohammadhosseini N, Alipanahi Z, Alipour E, Emami S, Faramarzi M, Samadi N, Khoshnevis N, Shafiee A, Foroumadi A: Synthesis and antibacterial activity of novel levofloxacin derivatives containing a substituted thienylethyl moiety. *DARU* 2012, 20:16.

Silymarin effect on amyloid-β plaque accumulation and gene expression of APP in an Alzheimer's disease rat model

Parichehreh Yaghmaei[1*], Katia Azarfar[1], Mehrooz Dezfulian[2] and Azadeh Ebrahim-Habibi[3,4*]

Abstract

Background: The deposition of amyloid peptides is associated with Alzheimer's disease (AD). These amyloid peptides are derived from the amyloid protein precursor (APP). Silymarin, a standardized extract of milk thistle, which is currently used in liver diseases, may be effective in the inhibition of amyloid formation. However, its effect has not been assessed on APP expression.

Results: In this study, first, the effect of silymarin was examined on the passive avoidance learning in a rat model of AD. This model was induced by the intracerebroventricular injection of Aβ peptide ($A\beta_{1-42}$) in Wistar rats. Rats were treated with 70 and 140 mg/kgof the extract, once a day, for 4 weeks. Memory function that was evaluated in a shuttle-cage test, showed improvement upon administration of this extract. Brain amyloid plaques had also decreased upon administration of the extract. Furthermore, APP gene expression was compared in treated and untreated groups. The result showed that silymarin was able to suppress APP expression.

Conclusion: Our results are in accordance with the *in vitro* tests concerning the positive antiamyloidogenic property of the main component of silymarin, namely silibinin. We suggest that the beneficial effect of sylimarin in the AD model is related to its capacity to disaggregate amyloid plaques and to suppress APP expression. Considering the limited side effects of silymarin, this compound could be of use in AD therapy.

Keywords: Silymarin, RT-PCR, Passive avoidance learning, Alzheimer's disease, Beta amyloid

Background

Alzheimer's disease (AD) is a progressive neurodegenerative disorder which has been characterized by the existence of extraneuronal aggregates of amyloid β (Aβ) peptide as well as intraneuronal deposits of hyperphosphorylated tau [1]. It is usually assumed that Aβ (abeta) aggregation in the brain is the starting trigger of a pathological cascade which ultimately leads to synaptic dysfunction and loss, neuronal death, and eventually cognitive dysfunction [2]; the process includes also oxidative stress and inflammatory response, which play their roles in neuronal dysfunction [3,4]. It is suggested that the reactive microglia and astrocytes that surround the Aβ plaques in the AD brain may release reactive oxygen species and proinflammatory molecules [5].

Various isoforms of Aβ peptide with lengths varying from 14 to 42 aminoacids have been characterized which are derivated from "APP", the amyloid precursor protein (APP) [6,7]. However, it is generally accepted that the main dominant forms of Aβ (40 and 42 aminoacids) are the toxic species involved in AD pathophysiology, as for example, it has been shown that the presence of Aβ 42 in cerebrospinal fluid could be a reliable predictor of AD progression [8].

The intracerebroventricular administration of Aβ peptide into rodent brain has been used as a mean to simulate AD disease, since this injection could induce histological and biochemical changes as well as oxidative damage and inflammatory responses which result into memory deficits [9,10]. With this animal model, *in vivo* studies could be performed to test potential new candidates for AD therapy.

* Correspondence: yaghmaei_p@srbiau.ac.ir; aehabibi@sina.tums.ac.ir
[1]Department of Biology, Science and Research Branch, Islamic Azad University, Tehran, Iran
[3]Biosensor Research Center, Endocrinology and Metabolism Molecular-Cellular Sciences Institute, Tehran University of Medical Sciences, Tehran, Iran
Full list of author information is available at the end of the article

The flavonoid silibinin (or sylibin) [(2R,3R)-3,5,7-tri-hydroxy-2-[(2R,3R)-3-(4-hydroxy-3-methoxyphenyl)-2-(hydroxy-methyl)-2,3-dihydrobenzo[b][1,4]doxin-6-yl] chroman-4-one] is the main compound of the herb milk thistle (*Silybum marianum*) extract (silymarin) [11]. This compound possess anti-inflammatory and antioxidative effects [12]. It has also been reported that silymarin has protective effects against ethanol-induced brain injury [13], and neurotoxicity induced by lipopolysaccharide (LPS) [14]. In this study, we investigated the effect of silymarin on the memory impairment induced by Aβ1-42 injection in rats. We also examined its effect on changes in APP gene expression in the rats' brain.

Materials and methods

Animals

Male Wistar rats weighing 250 ±300 g were housed at six per cage (42 × 26 cm), 23 ± 0.5°C, under a 12/12-h light/dark cycle (lights on from 8:00 AM to 8:00 PM). Animals had free access to standard pellet food and water. Behavioral experiments were carried out in a sound-attenuated room, to which the rats were habituated for at least 1 hour. All experiments were performed in accordance with to the international guidelines set out in the *Guide for the Care and Use of Laboratory Animals* (Institute of Laboratory Animal Resources, 1996) and approved by the Research and Ethics Committee of Science and Research Branch, Azad University.

Inducing Alzheimer's disease in animals and used compound

Aβ1-42 (Sigma, St Louis, MO, USA), was dissolved in PBS and incubated at 37°C for 7 days, after which bilateral surgery and injection of Aβ1-42 peptide was done in rats hippocampus with the help of a stereotaxic apparatus (SR-6 N Narishig, Japan) [15]. Ketamine and xylazin (Alfasan,Woerden-Holland) were used to anesthetize the rats. Injection was performed slowly into the CA1 region of the hippocampus at both sides of the brain as mentioned in the Paxinos atlas [16].

Silymarin tablets, containing ethyl acetate extracted Silymarin, were purchased from Goldaru Pharmaceutical Laboratory, (Isfahan, Iran) and suspended in a distilled water solution. Treatment group was administered two different dosages of the compound (70 and 140 mg/kg/day P.O.) for 4 weeks after the injection with A*β1–42*. A volume of 0.1 ml/10 g body weight was used.

Animals were divided into four groups with n = 6: the control group did not undergo surgery, the sham group underwent surgery (AD inducing) and ws given distilled water 7 days after surgery, the experimental groups Exp1 and Exp2 received 70 and 140 mg/kg/day of the compound respectively (7 days after surgery).

Testing the treatment efficacy

a. Passive avoidance test

A shuttle-cage consisting of two compartments of equal size (26 × 26 cm) separated by a sliding door (8 × 8 cm) was used. The shock compartment was dark in contrast to the starting compartment. Each experiment started with a pre-training trial, where the rat was placed in the starting compartment for 5 seconds, after which the sliding door was raised, and the rat was allowed to stay in the dark compartment for 10 seconds. The rat was then put back in its cage and stayed there for 30 minutes after which it was again put into the shuttle box, and this time, after entering the dark compartment, a footshock (50 Hz, 1 mA, and 5 s) was delivered. The rat was then put back into cage and stayed there for 120 seconds. When put back in the shuttle box, if a latency (in the order of 120 seconds) is observed before entering the dark compartment, successful acquisition of passive avoidance is recorded. A similar procedure was used 24 hours after training sessions to make a retention test for evaluating long-term memory. Higher or lower latencies are taken as indicative of increase or decrease in memory retention [17].

b. Histological studies of brain tissue

At the end of experiment animals were decapitated under anesthesia and their brain removed for histological assessments. First, the brains were fixed in 10% formalin and later processed for embedding with paraffin, after which serial sections in 6 mm of thickness were prepared. For staining of hippocampus cells, Thioflavin-S method which is detected by fluorescent microscopy was used [18].

c. Assessing amyloid precursor protein (APP) expression

Semi-quantitative RT-PCR was performed to assess APP expression. RNA was extracted from the homogenized brain tissue of the rats by use of RNX plus kit (CinnaGen, Iran). Isolated RNA was reverse-transcribed using the following gene-specific primers: 5'-GGA TGC GGA GTT CGG ACA TG –3' (forward) and 5'-GTT CTG CAT CTG CTC AAA G –3'(reverse). GAPDH was used as housekeeping gene as a control [5'- GACATGCCGCCTGGAGAAAC –3 ' (forward) and 5'- AGCCCAGGATGCCCTTTAGT –3' (reverse)]. The difference in threshold cycles between APP gene and GAPDH gives the standardized expression level. PCR were performed using the One-Step SYBR PrimeScript RT-PCR kit (Cinagen,Tehran-Iran). The reaction profile consisted of a first round at 95°C for 3 min and then 40 cycles of denaturation at 95°C for 30 s, annealing at 57°C for 30 s, and extension at 72°C for30 s, with a final extension reaction carried out at

72°C for 10 min. The RT-PCR products were loaded onto agarose gels and the resulting bands from electrophoresis were photographed with a UV transillumnator.

Statistical analyses

The results are expressed as the mean ± S.E.M. Statistical significance was determined with the one-way ANOVA followed by Tukey's multiple comparisons test. A Pearson correlation analysis was performed to elucidate the relationships. $p < 0.05$ was taken as a significant level of difference.

Results

Passive avoidance test

Both experimental groups showed significantly longer step-through latency compared to control group ($p < 0.05$) both in the training (Figure 1A) and test (Figure 1B) days.

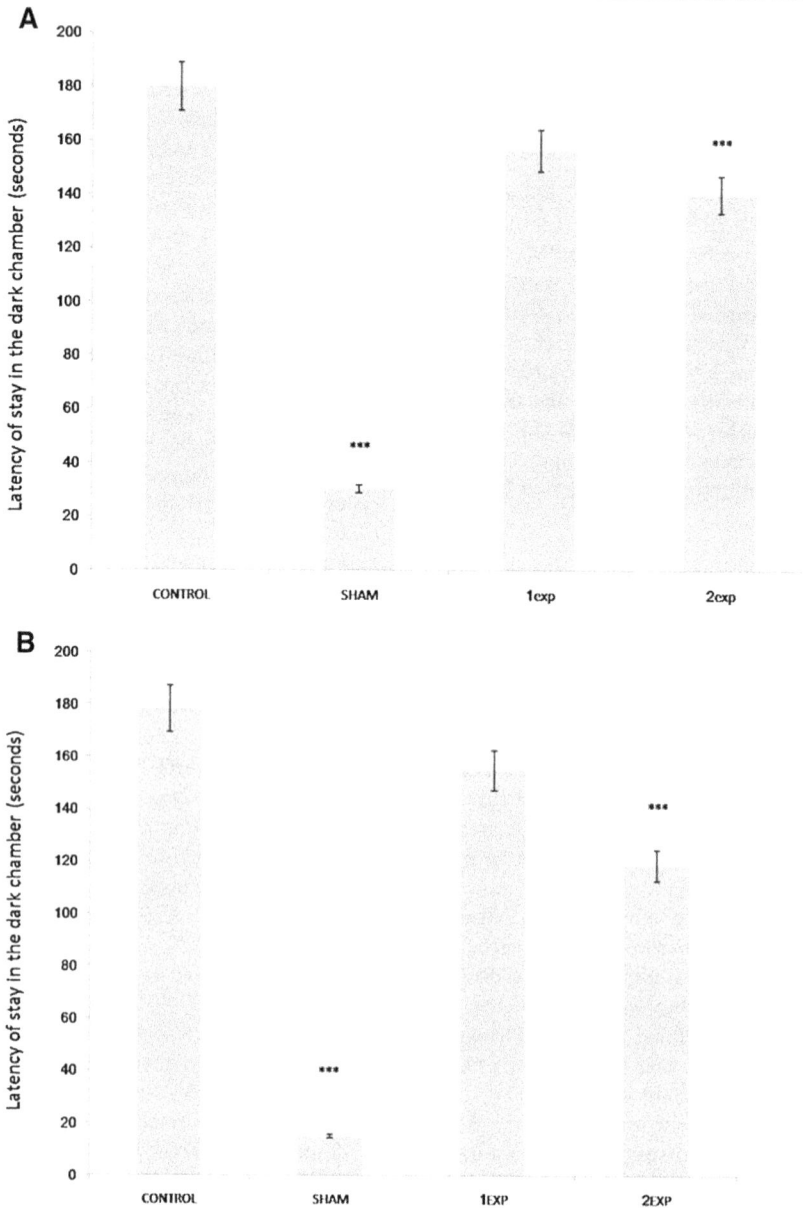

Figure 1 The mean latency to enter the dark chamber on the training (A) and test day (B). *** is indicative of ($P < 0.001$). 1Exp group was treated with 70 mg/kg Silymarinan and 2Exp group had received 140mg/kg Silymarin.

However, it is interesting to note that the 2Exp group, which had received a higher dose of silymarin showed slightly lower results in comparison with the 1Exp group. The 1Exp group has no significant difference in the step-through latency compared with the control group.

Histological studies of brain tissue

ThT staining was used to show the formation of plaques in the abeta-treated brain tissues. Usually, amyloid plaques could be detected in different areas of the brain, including the hippocampus and cortex (for an example of whole brain sections showing plaques distribution see Figure three A,B in reference # [19]). In the present study, both these areas were observed separately with regard to plaques concentration. The normal hippocampus and cortex tissues are showed in Figure 2A. Upon injection of abeta, plaques are formed in both tissues and observed as lighter areas (Figure 2B and C showing the cortex and hippocampus respectively). Treatment with silymarin is effective in diminishing the plaques amount, but here too, administration of 70 mg/Kg of the compound (Figure 2D and E) has a better effect than the higher used dose of 140 mg/Kg (Figure 2F and G).

Amyloid precursor protein (APP) expression

Results of electrophoresis are shown in Figure 3. When the housekeeping gene GAPDH is seen in all samples,

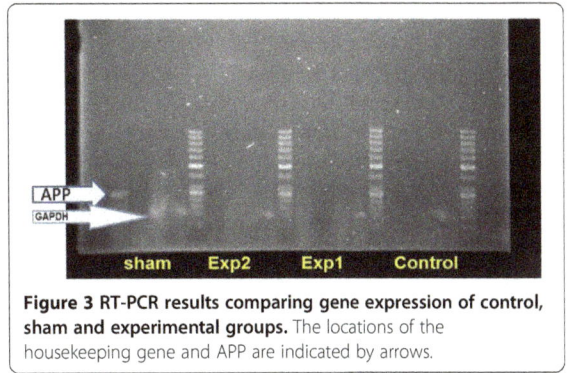

Figure 3 RT-PCR results comparing gene expression of control, sham and experimental groups. The locations of the housekeeping gene and APP are indicated by arrows.

APP expression is detected in the sham group, which had only received the compound solvent, and is absent in both experimental groups.

Discussion

From the different theories that try to explain AD pathology, two have been more focused on: the cholinergic theory, which points to the decrease of acetyl choline as the main cause of the disease [20,21] and the amyloid hypothesis, which considers the aggregation of different derivatives of APP as having an important role in the pathophysiology of AD [22]. Therapeutic approaches may

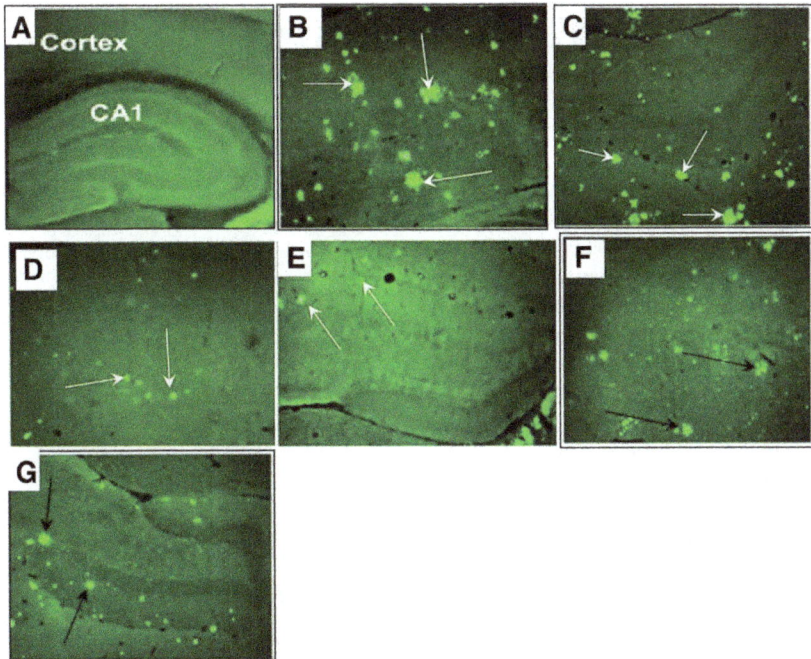

Figure 2 Brain slices from the frontal cortex &hippocampus with a magnification of 40. (A), control group, **(B,C)**, sham group: arrows indicate positions where abeta plaques accumulation has occured, **(D,E)** 1Ex group which was treated with 70 mg/kg silymarin and **(F,G)** 2Ex group which was treated with 140mg/kg silymarin. **B,D,** and **E** correspond to the cortex whereas **C,E,** and **G** correspond to the hippocampus.

include the design of acetyl cholinesterase inhibitors [23] as well as efforts toward finding Aβ aggregation blockers [24], or compounds that would inhibit secretases, i.e. enzymes which cleave APP to Aβ peptides of various length [25]. Some researchers have also tried to employ two or more therapeutic approaches simultaneously, or to find molecules that could affect more than one therapeutic target [26].

Abeta deposits are directly associated with AD. Various isoforms of abeta are derived from the precursor APP, including Aβ25–35 which is one of the most toxic species detected in the brain of AD patients [27,28]. At any rate, administration of abeta variants has led to cognitive impairment [9,29,30] which has also been observed in the present study. The hippocampus is known to be the part of the brain which is first affected by AD [31] and the result of this damage shows itself by cognitive impairment [32] that has been assessed here by the shuttle-box test.

Silymarin, the extract of *Silybum marianum* that contains flavonolignans, has been shown to possess multiple therapeutic properties, including protective effect against nerve damage and brain aging [33,34]. This extract may act via its antioxidant which could protect cells from oxidative stress damage [33], as it has been shown that silymarin effect against oxidative stress may be the result of an increase in reduced glutathione, ascorbic acid and superoxide dismutase levels [35]. Silymarin had also a neuroprotective effect in diabetic mice brains [36], and in mice treated with the brain damaging drug metamphetamine [37]. Previous studies have also reported the beneficial effect of silymarin on Aβ plaques formation, and the effect was suggested to be related to microglial inflammation reduction and direct effect on Aβ accumulation by blocking its aggregation in an Alzheimer's disease model of transgenic mice [19].

As a matter of fact, silibinin has the ability to inhibit the amyloid structure formation of various model or pathogenic proteins *in vitro*, including Aβ$_{1-42}$ [38] human islet amyloid polypeptide [39], and human insulin and albumin [40]. This may be suggestive of a generic anti-amyloidogenic effect for this compound, as it has been suggested/observed for various other aromatic/polyphenolic molecules [41,42]. It should be pointed out that in the present study, what has been observed is a disaggregative effect of silymarin on Aβ plaques, since the decrease of plaques was observed *after* they had been formed. This is an important fact, which is directly suggestive of a potential therapeutic effect for the compounds that are able to act on existing fibrils. The current view in the search for AD therapeutic compounds is preferably directed toward compounds that could preserve the native conformation of peptides that may form amyloid structure [43] or to focus on compounds that inhibit the formation

of intermediate structures in the course of amyloid formation [44,45]. However, it could make sense to include the compounds that have destabilizing effect on pre-formed fibrils into the spectra of potential AD therapies.

Flavonoids are able to cross the blood brain barrier [46], a fact that should also be true about silymarin, given its established neuroprotective effect [47]. Furthermore, this extract presents few side effects and drug interactions [48] which makes it a quite interesting potential drug for AD. Silymarin is already used as adjuvant therapy in liver insufficiency [49], which is another positive point for a potential drug candidate.

The beneficial effect of silymarin on the short term memory of rats is thus related with less abeta plaques, but also, as demonstrated in the present study, with a negative regulatory effect on the APP gene expression. Increased expression of APP has been detected in the ageing brain [50], and specifically related to AD pathophysiology [51]. Furthermore, the overexpression of APP that is present in the established transgenic mouse model of AD is definitely linked to the pathological characteristics of the model [52].

As far as we know, this should be a first report about the extract effect on APP, which is expanding our knowledge about the mechanism of action of silibinin in attenuating AD symptoms.

Competing interests
The authors declare that they have no competing interest.

Authors' contributions
PY has designed and supervised the project, analyzed the data and advised on writing the paper. This report is part of the results of KA MSc thesis project who performed experiments and wrote the first draft of the manuscript. MD has been an advisor to the thesis, supervised studies and analyzed data. A.E-H. advised on the project, analyzed data, and finalized the manuscript. All authors read and approved the final manuscript.

Author details
[1]Department of Biology, Science and Research Branch, Islamic Azad University, Tehran, Iran. [2]Department of Microbiology, College of Science, Islamic Azad University, Karaj Branch, Karaj, Iran. [3]Biosensor Research Center, Endocrinology and Metabolism Molecular-Cellular Sciences Institute, Tehran University of Medical Sciences, Tehran, Iran. [4]Endocrinology and Metabolism Research Center, Endocrinology and Metabolism Clinical Sciences Institute, Tehran University of Medical Sciences, North Kargar Avenue, 1411413137 Tehran, Iran.

References
1.   Blennow K, de Leon MJ, Zetterberg H: Alzheimer's disease. *Lancet* 2006, 368(9533):387–403.
2.   Walsh DM, Selkoe DJ: Deciphering the molecular basis of memory failure in Alzheimer's disease. *Neuron* 2004, 44(1):181–193.
3.   Butterfield DA, Reed T, Newman SF, Sultana R: Roles of amyloid beta-peptide-associated oxidative stress and brain protein modifications in the pathogenesis of Alzheimer's disease and mild cognitive impairment. *Free Radic Biol Med* 2007, 43(5):658–677.
4.   Farfara D, Lifshitz V, Frenkel D: Neuroprotective and neurotoxic properties of glial cells in the pathogenesis of Alzheimer's disease. *J Cell Mol Med* 2008, 12(3):762–780.

5. Combs CK, Karlo JC, Kao S-C, Landreth GE: **Beta-amyloid stimulation of microglia and monocytes results in TNF alpha dependent expression of inducible nitric oxide synthase and neuronal apoptosis.** *J Neurosci* 2001, 21(4):1179–1188.

6. Portelius E, Brinkmalm G, Tran AJ, Zetterberg H, Westman-Brinkmalm A, Blennow K: **Identification of novel APP/Abeta isoforms in human cerebrospinal fluid.** *Neurodegener Dis* 2009, 6(3):87–94.

7. Portelius E, Mattsson N, Andreasson U, Blennow K, Zetterberg H: **Novel a isoforms in Alzheimers disease-their role in diagnosis and treatment.** *Curr Pharm Des* 2011, 17(25):2594–2602.

8. van Harten AC, Visser PJ, Pijnenburg YA, Teunissen CE, Blankenstein MA, Scheltens P, van der Flier WM: **Cerebrospinal fluid Abeta42 is the best predictor of clinical progression in patients with subjective complaints.** *Alzheimers Dement* 2013, 9(5):481–487.

9. Frautschy SA, Baird A, Cole GM: **Effects of injected Alzheimer beta-amyloid cores in rat brain.** *Proc Natl Acad Sci U S A* 1991, 88(19):8362–8366.

10. Maurice T, Lockhart BP, Privat A: **Amnesia induced in mice by centrally administered beta-amyloid peptides involves cholinergic dysfunction.** *Brain Res* 1996, 706(2):181–193.

11. Kvasnicka F, Biba B, Sevcik R, Voldrich M, Kratka J: **Analysis of the active components of silymarin.** *J Chromatogr A* 2003, 990(1–2):239–245.

12. Kren V, Walterova D: **Silybin and silymarin–new effects and applications.** *Biomed Pap Med Fac Univ Palacky Olomouc Czech Repub* 2005, 149(1):29–41.

13. la Grange L, Wang M, Watkins R, Ortiz D, Sanchez ME, Konst J, Lee C, Reyes E: **Protective effects of the flavonoid mixture, silymarin, on fetal rat brain and liver.** *J Ethnopharmacol* 1999, 65(1):53–61.

14. Lu P, Mamiya T, Lu LL, Mouri A, Zou LB, Nagai T, Hiramatsu M, Ikejima T, Nabeshima T: **Silibinin prevents amyloid β peptide-induced memory impairment and oxidative stress in mice.** *Br J Pharmacol* 2009, 157(7):1270–1277.

15. Cetin F, Dincer S: **The effect of intrahippocampal beta amyloid (1–42) peptide injection on oxidant and antioxidant status in rat brain.** *Ann N Y Acad Sci* 2007, 1100:510–517.

16. Paxinos G, Watson C: *The rat brain in stereotaxic coordinates: hard cover edition.* The Netherlands: Academic Press, Elsevier; 2006.

17. Guaza C, Borrell J: **Prolonged ethanol consumption influences shuttle box and passive avoidance performance in rats.** *Physiol Behav* 1985, 34(2):163–165.

18. Gandy S: **The role of cerebral amyloid beta accumulation in common forms of Alzheimer disease.** *J Clin Invest* 2005, 115(5):1121–1129.

19. Murata N, Murakami K, Ozawa Y, Kinoshita N, Irie K, Shirasawa T, Shimizu T: **Silymarin attenuated the amyloid beta plaque burden and improved behavioral abnormalities in an Alzheimer's disease mouse model.** *Biosci Biotechnol Biochem* 2010, 74(11):2299–2306.

20. Boller F, Forette F: **Alzheimer's disease and THA: a review of the cholinergic theory and of preliminary results.** *Biomed Pharmacother* 1989, 43(7):487–491.

21. Robbins T, McAlonan G, Muir J, Everitt B: **Cognitive enhancers in theory and practice: studies of the cholinergic hypothesis of cognitive deficits in Alzheimer's disease.** *Behav Brain Res* 1997, 83(1):15–23.

22. Selkoe DJ: **Toward a comprehensive theory for Alzheimer's disease. Hypothesis: Alzheimer's disease is caused by the cerebral accumulation and cytotoxicity of amyloid beta protein.** *Ann N Y Acad Sci* 2000, 924(1):17–25.

23. Wilkinson DG, Francis PT, Schwam E, Payne-Parrish J: **Cholinesterase inhibitors used in the treatment of Alzheimer's disease.** *Drugs Aging* 2004, 21(7):453–478.

24. Cheng B, Gong H, Xiao H, Petersen RB, Zheng L, Huang K: **Inhibiting toxic aggregation of amyloidogenic proteins: a therapeutic strategy for protein misfolding diseases.** *Biochimica et Biophysica Acta (BBA)-General Subjects* 2013, 1830(10):4860–4871.

25. Citron M: **Beta-Secretase inhibition for the treatment of Alzheimer's disease-promise and challenge.** *Trends Pharmacol Sci* 2004, 25(2):92–97.

26. Bajda M, Guzior N, Ignasik M, Malawska B: **Multi-Target-Directed ligands in Alzheimer's disease treatment.** *Curr Med Chem* 2011, 18(32):4949–4975.

27. Pike CJ, Walencewicz-Wasserman AJ, Kosmoski J, Cribbs DH, Glabe CG, Cotman CW: **Structure-activity analyses of beta-amyloid peptides: contributions of the beta 25–35 region to aggregation and neurotoxicity.** *J Neurochem* 1995, 64(1):253–265.

28. Kubo T, Nishimura S, Kumagae Y, Kaneko I: **In vivo conversion of racemized beta-amyloid ([D-Ser 26]A beta 1–40) to truncated and toxic fragments ([D-Ser 26]A beta 25-35/40) and fragment presence in the brains of Alzheimer's patients.** *J Neurosci Res* 2002, 70(3):474–483.

29. Alkam T, Nitta A, Mizoguchi H, Itoh A, Nabeshima T: **A natural scavenger of peroxynitrites, rosmarinic acid, protects against impairment of memory induced by Abeta(25–35).** *Behav Brain Res* 2007, 180(2):139–145.

30. Tsunekawa H, Noda Y, Mouri A, Yoneda F, Nabeshima T: **Synergistic effects of selegiline and donepezil on cognitive impairment induced by amyloid beta (25–35).** *Behav Brain Res* 2008, 190(2):224–232.

31. Busche MA, Chen X, Henning HA, Reichwald J, Staufenbiel M, Sakmann B, Konnerth A: **Critical role of soluble amyloid beta for early hippocampal hyperactivity in a mouse model of Alzheimer's disease.** *Proc Natl Acad Sci* 2012, 109(22):8740–8745.

32. Sabuncu MR, Desikan RS, Sepulcre J, Yeo BTT, Liu H, Schmansky NJ, Reuter M, Weiner MW, Buckner RL, Sperling RA: **The dynamics of cortical and hippocampal atrophy in Alzheimer disease.** *Arch Neurol* 2011, 68(8):1040.

33. Raza SS, Khan MM, Ashafaq M, Ahmad A, Khuwaja G, Khan A, Siddiqui MS, Safhi MM, Islam F: **Silymarin protects neurons from oxidative stress associated damages in focal cerebral ischemia: a behavioral, biochemical and immunohistological study in Wistar rats.** *J Neurol Sci* 2011, 309(1):45–54.

34. Galhardi F, Mesquita K, Monserrat JM, Barros DM: **Effect of silymarin on biochemical parameters of oxidative stress in aged and young rat brain.** *Food Chem Toxicol* 2009, 47(10):2655–2660.

35. Nencini C, Giorgi G, Micheli L: **Protective effect of silymarin on oxidative stress in rat brain.** *Phytomedicine* 2007, 14(2):129–135.

36. Marrazzo G, Bosco P, la Delia F, Scapagnini G, di Giacomo C, Malaguarnera M, Galvano F, Nicolosi A, Li Volti G: **Neuroprotective effect of silibinin in diabetic mice.** *Neurosci Lett* 2011, 504(3):252–256.

37. Lu P, Mamiya T, Lu L, Mouri A, Niwa M, Kim HC, Zou LB, Nagai T, Yamada K, Ikejima T, et al: **Silibinin attenuates cognitive deficits and decreases of dopamine and serotonin induced by repeated methamphetamine treatment.** *Behav Brain Res* 2010, 207(2):387–393.

38. Yin F, Liu J, Ji X, Wang Y, Zidichouski J, Zhang J: **Silibinin: a novel inhibitor of Abeta aggregation.** *Neurochem Int* 2011, 58(3):399–403.

39. Cheng B, Gong H, Li X, Sun Y, Zhang X, Chen H, Liu X, Zheng L, Huang K: **Silibinin inhibits the toxic aggregation of human islet amyloid polypeptide.** *Biochem Biophys Res Commun* 2012, 419(3):495–499.

40. Chinisaz M, Ghasemi A, Larijani B, Ebrahim-Habibi A: **Amyloid formation and inhibition of an all-beta protein: a study on fungal polygalacturonase.** *J Mol Struct* 2014, 1059:94–100.

41. Ono K, Yoshiike Y, Takashima A, Hasegawa K, Naiki H, Yamada M: **Potent anti-amyloidogenic and fibril-destabilizing effects of polyphenols in vitro: implications for the prevention and therapeutics of Alzheimer's disease.** *J Neurochem* 2003, 87(1):172–181.

42. Choi Y-T, Jung C-H, Lee S-R, Bae J-H, Baek W-K, Suh M-H, Park J, Park C-W, Suh S-I: **The green tea polyphenol (–)-epigallocatechin gallate attenuates β-amyloid-induced neurotoxicity in cultured hippocampal neurons.** *Life Sci* 2001, 70(5):603–614.

43. Johnson SM, Petrassi HM, Palaninathan SK, Mohamedmohaideen NN, Purkey HE, Nichols C, Chiang KP, Walkup T, Sacchettini JC, Sharpless KB: **Bisaryloxime ethers as potent inhibitors of transthyretin amyloid fibril formation.** *J Med Chem* 2005, 48(5):1576–1587.

44. Hafner-Bratkovič I, Gašperšič J, Šmid LM, Bresjanac M, Jerala R: **Curcumin binds to the α-helical intermediate and to the amyloid form of prion protein–a new mechanism for the inhibition of PrPSc accumulation.** *J Neurochem* 2008, 104(6):1553–1564.

45. Liu D, Xu Y, Feng Y, Liu H, Shen X, Chen K, Ma J, Jiang H: **Inhibitor discovery targeting the intermediate structure of β-amyloid peptide on the conformational transition pathway: implications in the aggregation mechanism of β-amyloid peptide.** *Biochemistry* 2006, 45(36):10963–10972.

46. Youdim KA, Shukitt-Hale B, Joseph JA: **Flavonoids and the brain: interactions at the blood–brain barrier and their physiological effects on the central nervous system.** *Free Radic Biol Med* 2004, 37(11):1683–1693.

47. Baluchnejadmojarada T, Roghanib M, Mafakheria M: **Neuroprotective effect of silymarin in 6-hydroxydopamine hemi-parkinsonian rat: involvement of estrogen receptors and oxidative stress.** *Neurosci Lett* 2010, 480(3):206–210.

48. Jacobs BP, Dennehy C, Ramirez G, Sapp J, Lawrence VA: **Milk thistle for the treatment of liver disease: a systematic review and meta-analysis.** *Am J Med* 2002, 113(6):506–515.

49. Feher J, Lengyel G: **Silymarin in the prevention and treatment of liver diseases and primary liver cancer.** *Curr Pharm Biotechnol* 2012, 13(1):210–217.

50. Lukiw WJ: **Gene expression profiling in fetal, aged, and alzheimer hippocampus: a continuum of stress-related signaling.** *Neurochem Res* 2004, 29(6):1287–1297.

51. Theuns J, Brouwers N, Engelborghs S, Sleegers K, Bogaerts V, Corsmit E, de Pooter T, van Duijn CM, de Deyn PP, van Broeckhoven C: **Promoter mutations that increase amyloid precursor-protein expression are associated with Alzheimer disease.** *Am J Hum Genet* 2006, **78**(6):936–946.
52. Howlett DR, Richardson JC: **The pathology of APP transgenic mice: a model of Alzheimer's disease or simply overexpression of APP?** *Histol Histopathol* 2009, **24**(1):83–100.

16

Introduction of a mathematical model for optimizing the drug release in the patient's body

Mohammad Reza Nabatchian[1*], Hamid Shahriari[1] and Mona Shahriari[2]

Abstract

Background: Drug release in a patient's body is of particular interest to the pharmaceutical industry. One of the most essential types of drug release is the gradual release based on a behavior, which is called a profile or modified release. The investigation of the time-oriented quality characteristic is one of the newest topics in the area of product design. There are already several approaches addressing this issue. In this paper, a mathematical model is proposed to find the suitable values of the controllable factors in a drug to achieve the profile of the drug release in the patient's body.

Results: The proposed method has several advantages over the existing methods.

Conclusion: The authors feel that by adjusting the control factors during the production process the drug release profile become closer to the reference profile.

Keywords: Drug release, Time-oriented quality characteristic, Parameter design, Desirability function, Release profile

Introduction

The amount of time it takes a drug to release in a patient's body as well as the time it takes to exert its effects on the target organ are very important factors used to measure the effectiveness of a drug. If this releasing manner is not based on a pre-defined profile, it may cause a reduction of curative properties of the drug and can even have some negative effects on the patient's body. Similarly, in the area of quality engineering, the time-oriented quality characteristics are also assessed. The time-oriented profile of the quality characteristic is specified and the aim of the designer is to find the pre-defined profile with minimum deviation from the target. The quality characteristics are then monitored using the defined profile. In this study, we aim to establish a logical relationship between these two areas and to apply a mathematical modeling approach to investigate the drug release problem in pharmaceutics. In this paper some basic definitions of drug release and quality engineering are presented and then we introduce the four existing approaches for these types of problems and

their deficiencies. The proposed method is presented in the next section. Several examples are provided to evaluate the suggested model and in the final section, the conclusions are made.

Definitions

In this section some of the basic terms included in the paper are defined to familiarize the reader with the concepts of the discussion.

Drug release

Drug release is an important stage in the drug life cycle. When the drug is released based on a pre-defined profile, it is more effective on the patient's body. One of the most applicable approaches for measuring the amount of released drugs is to measure the plasma concentration of the drug. The drug is considered effective when the plasma concentration is somewhere between minimum effective concentration (MEC) and minimal toxic concentration (MTC) as is shown in Figure 1 [1-3].

Drugs are usually classified based on the drug release mechanism as follows:

* Correspondence: mrnabatchian@dena.kntu.ac.ir
[1]Department of Industrial Engineering, K.N. Toosi University of Technology, No 7, Pardis St., Mollasadra Ave., Tehran, Iran
Full list of author information is available at the end of the article

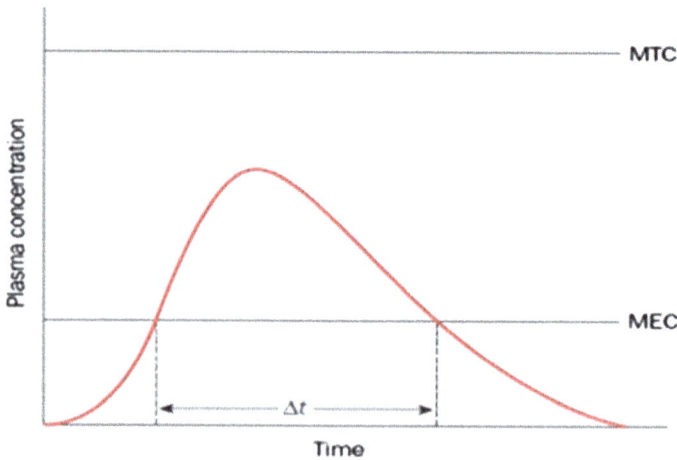

Figure 1 Plasma concentration versus time profile [1].

Immediate release drugs: In this group, the drug is quickly released in the body. This is particularly suitable for drugs that need to take affect rapidly such as painkillers [1,4].

Modified drug release: In this case by using the pharmaceutical techniques, the time, the amount and the target organ for the drug release is determined. The delayed release and extended release are the methods being used. In the delayed release the drug is released after a pre-determined delay. Figure 2 shows the plasma concentration for this modified release method [1,4].

In the extended release technique, the drug is released gradually over a longer period of time. It is classified into two categories: sustained release and controlled release. In sustained release, the drug is released continuously with a constant rate. In controlled release, the drug is released intelligently so that the concentration

remains almost constant in the body. Figure 3 shows the plasma concentration when using this method of drug release [1,5].

Time-oriented quality characteristics

There are several definitions of the quality characteristics in the quality management literature. The most comprehensive of them is the degree of adaptability of the quality characteristic by the user's requirements [6]. Furthermore, the design phase is the principal stage of a product life cycle, because the quality is formed in this stage and control actions at the end of the production process cannot improve the quality of a product with poor quality of design [7].

The Taguchi robust design is a famous design procedure. It is an engineering method for optimizing the product or process condition to minimize the product

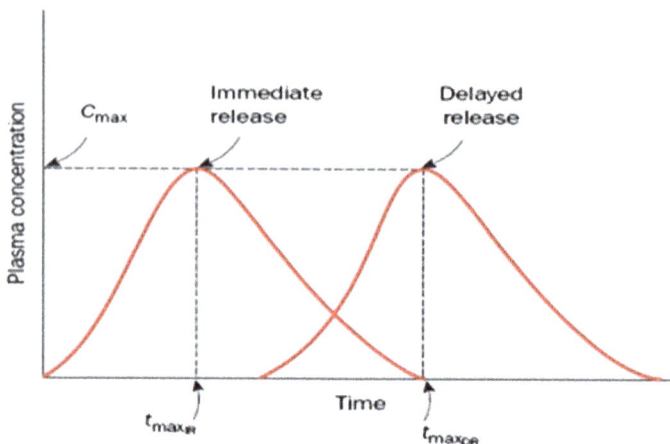

Figure 2 Plasma concentration versus time profile for an immediate release drug and a delayed release drug [1].

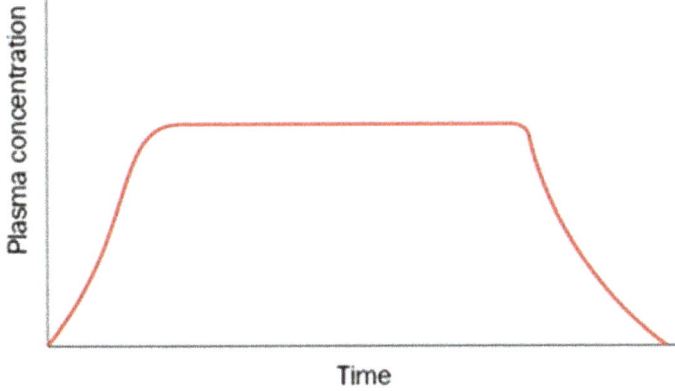

Figure 3 Plasma concentration versus time profile for a controlled release formulation [1].

sensitivity to the noise factors in the environment, such as: ambient temperature, humidity, air pressure and direct sunlight [8]. So, a product with high quality and low cost is being produced. One property of this approach is to investigate the quality characteristics numerically. In this approach the quality characteristics are grouped into three classes as: nominal the best (NTB), larger the better (LTB) and smaller the better (STB). Each of these quality characteristics could be constant or variable over time [9].

The target value and the specification limits for the time-oriented quality characteristics are being changed over time. So, for the design of a product with these quality characteristics, the parameters are designed such that the quality characteristics are being as close to their pre-specified target values as possible.

In this regard, three basic topics need to be introduced.

Design of experiments (DOE)
A collection of statistical methods that are used to find the influenced factors on a quality characteristic and to optimize its conditions. There are several types of DOE techniques including factorial experiments and fractional factorial experiments [10,11].

Response surface methodology (RSM)
A statistical and mathematical method for modeling, analyzing and optimizing the problems with response variables which are directly related to some other independent variables [12].

Desirability function
Is one of the common methods to simultaneously optimize multi response problems. The most applicable method of this type is the Derringer and Suich's which is defined for several types of quality characteristics as follows [13]:

NTB quality characteristic:

$$DF(y) = \begin{cases} \left[\dfrac{y-LSL}{T-LSL}\right]^r &, \quad LSL < y < T \\ \left[\dfrac{y-USL}{T-USL}\right]^s &, \quad T < y < USL \\ 0 &, \quad y < LSL; y > USL \end{cases} \quad (1)$$

LTB quality characteristic:

$$DF(y) = \begin{cases} 1 &, \quad y > y_i^* \\ \left[\dfrac{y-y_{i_*}}{y_i^*-y_{i_*}}\right]^r &, \quad y_{i_*} < y < y_i^* \\ 0 &, \quad y < y_{i_*} \end{cases} \quad (2)$$

STB quality characteristic

$$DF(y) = \begin{cases} 1 &, \quad y < y_{i_*} \\ \left[\dfrac{y_i^*-y}{y_i^*-y_{i_*}}\right]^r &, \quad y_{i_*} < y < y_i^* \\ 0 &, \quad y > y_i^* \end{cases} \quad (3)$$

In the above equations:

y: value observed for the quality characteristic

T: The target value for quality characteristic applicable for NTB quality characteristic.

USL: Upper specification Limit of NTB quality characteristic

LSL: Lower specification Limit of NTB quality characteristic

y_i^*: optimum point for LTB quality characteristic and highest acceptable value for STB quality characteristic

y_i*: Optimum point for STB quality characteristic and lowest acceptable value for LTB quality characteristic

r, s: Weight values, positive constants.

Problem definition

The drugs have a pre-determined profile for release based on the drug's controlled-release mechanism. The aim in any drug laboratory is to find optimum adjustment of the controllable factors, such as material, production machine settings and so on to produce drugs that achieve the pre-determined profile as much as possible. Four methods already exist for parameter design of a drug to achieve its pre-determined profile:

Contour overlay method

This method is applied by Gohel and Amin [14] to find the optimal values to the Diclofenac Sodium formulation. The aim is to determine the suitable values for the three main controllable factors: stirring speed, concentration of $CaCl_2$ and percentage of liquid paraffin, all of which influence the drug efficacy. The pre-determined profile of release is defined in advance. Then, the regression function of the drug release as a response variable and the above-mentioned control factors as independent variables is obtained by the least square method. For each point of time, the response is computed and compared to the pre-specified value. In this method, one variable is kept fixed and a two dimensional plot is used to find the optimal values.

The disadvantage of this method is that when the number of control factors increases, the efficiency of the method to introduce optimal values decreases.

Profile selection

In situations where the profile properties are hard to identify, selection of the best profile is done by using the pre-defined indices. Two of these indices are f_1 and f_2 defined as:

$$f_1 = \frac{\sum_{t=1}^{n}|R_t - T_t|}{\sum_{t=1}^{n} R_t} * 100 \tag{4}$$

$$f_2 = 50 * Log\left\{\left[1 + \frac{1}{n}\sum_{t=1}^{n}(R_t - T_t)^2\right]^{-0.5} * 100\right\} \tag{5}$$

Where:

R_t: Percentage of drug release obtained from the reference formulation

T_t: Percentage of drug release obtained from the test formulation

n: number of observations

The first index, f_1 is defined as the dissimilarity index. As long as its value is small; the profile is close to the

reference profile. The second index, f_2 is defined as similarity index and when its value is large; the profile is near to the reference profile [15,16].

MSE minimizing method

This method is applied in three articles. Truong et al. [17] used this method to determine the optimum values for control factors of a regenerative drug based on a profile of seven points.

Park et al. [18] used this method to investigate two quality characteristics separately for six and seven point profiles. Shin et al. [19] used this method to assess two quality characteristics separately for eight and eleven point profiles.

The first step in this method is to gather data and to calculate the basic statistics such as the mean and the variance. Then the RSM for these statistics are computed at each point of time. The optimal values for the control factors are obtained such that the following objective function is minimized.

$$Minimize \sum_{q=1}^{w}\left(\hat{M}(x, t_q) - T_q\right)^2 + \sum_{q=1}^{w}\hat{v}(x, t_q), \ S.t: x \in \Omega \tag{6}$$

Where:

$\hat{M}(x, t_q)$: The mean of the responses at time t_q.

$\hat{v}(x, t_q)$: The variance of the responses at time t_q.

T_q: The pre-specified target value for the response variable for the time q.

w: The number of points in time under study.

Method of minimizing the total cost

This method is used by Goethals and Cho [20] and also the experiment of Gohel and Amin [14] on the Diclufenac Sodium is reassessed. The logic behind this method is to find the optimal values for control factors that minimize the following objective function:

$$Minimize \ E[TC] = \sum_{q=1}^{w}\left[\int_{LSL_q}^{USL_q} L[Y(q)].f[Y(q)].dY(q)\right.$$
$$+ \int_{-\infty}^{LSL_q} NC_{q1}.f[y(q)]dY(q)$$
$$\left. + \int_{USL_q}^{+\infty} NC_{q2}.f[Y(q)]dY(q)\right] \tag{7}$$

Where:

LSL_q and USL_q: are the lower and the upper specification limits for the quality characteristic, respectively.

$f(y(q))$: is the probability distribution function for response variable at time q.

NC_{q1} and NC_{q2}: are the costs corresponding to being greater than USL and smaller than LSL, respectively.

$L(y\,(q))$: is the quality loss function for the quality characteristic within the acceptable region, but not on the target.

w: is the number of time points under study.

The proposed method

The proposed method is a systematic and straightforward technique for determining the optimum values for the control factors for a drug. So that in a specified time interval, the drug release follows its premeditated profile. This method requires the following steps:

1. Determination of the drug release profile: Considering the kind of drug and its mechanism of release, the pharmaceutics design of the release profile of a drug by consulting the specialist physicians. To facilitate the comparison between the standard profile and the drug profile function, some points on time are considered and the experiments are run in these points. At each time point, the target value and the upper and the lower specification limits are determined. Selection of the number of points under study is based on the type of the drug and its life cycle in the patient's body.

2. Determination of the experiment templates: In this stage, many controllable factors such as raw material and production factors for the drug under study are determined. Several combinations of these controllable factors are being tested by running the experiments. One important logic of the DOE is to find as much as information possible from the minimum number of experiments. For each combination of the factor levels at each time point some data is collected. Then, the data are organized based on the Table 1. The primary statistics such as the mean, the variance and the coefficient of variation for each time point and the covariance between observations in different time points are calculated. The computational formulas used to compute these statistics are as follows:

$$\bar{y}_{qr} = \frac{\sum_{w=1}^{m} y_{qrw}}{m} \tag{8}$$

$$s_{qr}^2 = \frac{\sum_{w=1}^{m}\left(y_{qrw}-\bar{y}_{qr}\right)^2}{m-1} \tag{9}$$

$$\left(\frac{s}{m}\right)_{qr} = \frac{s_{qr}}{\bar{y}_{qr}} \tag{10}$$

$$s_{i,j} = \frac{\sum_{r=1}^{m}\left(y_{ipr}-\bar{y}_{ip}\right)\left(y_{jpr}-\bar{y}_{jp}\right)}{m-1} \tag{11}$$

3. Determination of the relationships among the statistics and the control factors: By using RSM technique, the relationships are defined. For the sake of simplicity and prevention of using data with several scales, the control factors are coded by linear relationships.

$$\hat{\mu}_q(x) = x\hat{\beta}_{\mu q}\ ,\quad \hat{\beta}_{\mu q} = \left(x'x\right)^{-1}x'\bar{y}_q\ ,\quad x = \begin{bmatrix} 1 & \cdots & x_{1,k-1} \\ \vdots & \ddots & \vdots \\ 1 & \cdots & x_{n,k-1} \end{bmatrix}$$

$$\bar{y}_q = \left[\bar{y}_{q1},\bar{y}_{q2},\dots,\bar{y}_{qn}\right]' \tag{12}$$

$$\hat{s}_q^2(x) = x\hat{\beta}_{s^2 q}\ ,\quad \hat{\beta}_{s^2 q} = \left(x'x\right)^{-1}x's_q^2\ ,\quad x = \begin{bmatrix} 1 & \cdots & x_{1,k-1} \\ \vdots & \ddots & \vdots \\ 1 & \cdots & x_{n,k-1} \end{bmatrix}$$

$$s_q^2 = \left[s_{q1}^2,s_{q2}^2,\dots,s_{qn}^2\right]' \tag{13}$$

$$\left(\left(\frac{\hat{s}}{m}\right)\right)_q (x) = x\hat{\beta}_{(s/m)}q\ ,\quad \hat{\beta}_{(s/m)}q = \left(x'x\right)^{(-1)}x'(s/m)_q,$$

$$x = \begin{bmatrix} 1 & \cdots & x_{1,k-1} \\ \vdots & \ddots & \vdots \\ 1 & \cdots & x_{n,k-1} \end{bmatrix} \tag{14}$$

$$\left(\frac{s}{m}\right)_q = \left[\left(\frac{s}{m}\right)_{q1},\left(\frac{s}{m}\right)_{q2},\dots,\left(\frac{s}{m}\right)_{qn}\right]'$$

Table 1 Experimental format [20]

Run	x	Y(1)	$\bar{y}_1$	s_1^2	...	Y(w)	$\bar{y}_w$	s_w^2
1	Control factor settings	$y_{111}\dots y_{11m}$	$\bar{y}_{11}$	s_{11}^2	...	$y_{w11}\dots y_{w1m}$	$\bar{y}_{w1}$	s_{w1}^2
2		$y_{121}\dots y_{12m}$	$\bar{y}_{12}$	s_{12}^2	...	$y_{w21}\dots y_{w2m}$	$\bar{y}_{w2}$	s_{w2}^2
.		...	...	...	...	...	...	...
r		$y_{1r1}\dots y_{1rm}$	$\bar{y}_{1r}$	s_{1r}^2	...	$y_{wr1}\dots y_{wrm}$	$\bar{y}_{wr}$	s_{wr}^2
.		...	...	...	...	...	...	...
n		$y_{1n1}\dots y_{1nm}$	$\bar{y}_{1n}$	s_{1n}^2	...	$y_{wn1}\dots y_{wnm}$	$\bar{y}_{wn}$	s_{wn}^2

$$\hat{s}_{i,j}(x) = x\hat{\beta}_{s_{i,j}}, \hat{\beta}_{s_{i,j}} = (x'x)^{-1}x's_{i,j}, x = \begin{bmatrix} 1 & \cdots & x_{1,k-1} \\ \vdots & \ddots & \vdots \\ 1 & \cdots & x_{n,k-1} \end{bmatrix}$$

$$s_{i,j} = [s_{i,j,1}, s_{i,j,2}, ..., s_{i,j,n}]'$$

$$(15)$$

In the interest of time and cost, the number of control factors is reduced before running the experiments by using any technique such as screening experiments, as well as the forward, backward and stepwise regression.

4 Model optimization: Using the desirability function method, the optimal values for control factors are determined based on the type of quality characteristics and their specification limits such that their values come as close to the target values as possible. The desirability function of interest is:

$$MaximizeD_{total} = \left\{ \left[\prod_{i=1}^{n} D(\mu_i)^{w_i} \right] \cdot \left[\prod_{i=1}^{n} D(s_i^2)^{w_i'} \right] \cdot \left[\prod_{i=1}^{n} D\left(\frac{s_i}{m_i}\right)^{w_i''} \right] \cdot \left[\prod_{i=1}^{n} D(s_{i,j})^{w_i'''} \right] \right\}$$

$$\times \left(\frac{1}{\sum_{i=1}^{n} (w_i + w_i' + w_i'') + \sum_{i=1}^{n} w_i'''} \right)$$

$$(16)$$

The results are robust as long as the covariances between the observations for each pair of points are close to zero. So, when there is a deviation in some time intervals, they would not be transmitted to the other points.

The other advantage of the proposed method is its ability to be used for any part of the desirability function. For instance when we don't have access to the entire data and only the mean and the variance of the observations are available, the covariance part of the model may be eliminated. Or if the mean of the observations at each point of time for different combinations is in hand, only the mean part of the model is being used. Also, by using the desirability function and its weighted values, one may use any indices in some points under study. For the sake of simplicity, in the examples provided in Section 5, equal weights are assigned to all statistical indices in all time periods.

Numerical examples

To illustrate the applications of the proposed method, seven examples for different drugs are presented in this section adapted from credible pharmaceutical papers.

These examples are solved by the proposed method to find the optimum values for the control factors of the drugs. The required material, the methods of pharmaceutical experiments and the data for each example are presented in the stated indicated references.

Example 1
Diclufenac Sodium
The release profile of this drug is investigated by Gohel [14] and Goethals [20]. The contour overlay and the minimization of quality loss function methods are introduced in their papers, respectively. This drug has three main control factors given in Table 2.

The first step is to code the control factors using the following relationships:

$$x_{1(new)} = \frac{x_1 - 1000}{500}, x_{2(new)} = \frac{x_2 - 10}{5}, x_{3(new)} = \frac{x_3 - 25}{25}$$

In this research, three points of time for the drug release profile are being investigated with properties shown in Table 3.

The response surface relationships for the mean, the variance, the coefficient of variation and the covariance between each pair of points under study are presented in the Appendix 1. Optimum values are shown in Table 4.

Example 2
Terazosin HCl dehydrate
The release profile for this drug is investigated by Shin [19] and the problem is solved by the MSE minimization method. This experiment has ten control factors as shown in Table 5.

Noticing the large number of control factors in this example, five control factors x_1, x_3, x_7, x_8 and x_{10} are identified as significant control factors by using the stepwise regression method. The control factors are coded by the following relationships:

$$x_{i-new} = \begin{cases} \frac{x_i - 93.71}{7.03}, i = 1 \\ \frac{x_i}{7.03}, i = 2, 3, ..., 10 \end{cases}$$

In this research, 11 points of time of drug release profile are being investigated as presented in Table 6.

Table 2 Main control factors influencing Diclufenac Sodium release

Variable	Control factor	Level 1	Level 2	Level 3
x_1	Stirring speed (RPM)	500	1000	1500
x_2	Concentration of calcium chloride	5%	10%	15%
x_3	Percentage of liquid paraffin	0%	25%	50%

Table 3 The target values and lower and upper values for example 1

Response	Delay after usage	LSL	Target	USL
y_1	1 hour	20%	30%	40%
y_2	6 hour	50%	60%	70%
y_3	8 hour	65%	72.5%	80%

The response surface relationships for the mean and the variance of the underlying data are presented in Appendix 2. Optimum values for this example are shown in Table 7.

Example 3
Verapamil HCl
The release profile of this drug is investigated by Siva [21]. The three main control factors for this drug are presented in Table 8.

The control factors are coded by the following relationships:

$$x_{1(new)} = \frac{x_1 - 11}{3}, x_{2(new)} = \frac{x_2 - 36}{12}, x_{3(new)} = \frac{x_3 - 90}{30}$$

In this research, five points of time are investigated from release profile as shown in Table 9.

The RSM relationships for the mean, the variance and the coefficient of variation for the points in Table 8 are presented in Appendix 3. By using the desirability function method the optimum values obtained for control factors are shown in Table 10.

Example 4
Metformin
The release profile for this drug is investigated by Nagrava [22]. The three main control factors are defined for this drug release as shown in Table 11.

The values of the control factors are coded using the following relationships:

$$x_{1(new)} = \frac{x_1 - 1.758}{1.25}, x_{2(new)} = \frac{x_2 - 0.25}{0.25}, x_{3(new)} = \frac{x_3 - 3.75}{1.25}$$

The three points of time for the release profile are investigated in this research have the properties provided in Table 12.

The RSM relationships for the mean, the variance and the coefficient of variation for the data are presented in

Table 4 Optimum values for example 1

Variable	Control factor	Coded value	Uncoded value
x_1	Stirring speed (RPM)	−0.7576	621.2 rpm
x_2	Concentration of calcium chloride	−0.3939	8.0305%
x_3	Percentage of liquid paraffin	1	50%

Table 5 Control factors influencing Terazosin HCl dehydrate release

Variable	Control factor	Level 1	Level 2	Level 3	Level 4	Level 5
x_1	PEO	93.71	100.77	107.77	171.04	234.31
x_2	LH-11	0	7.03	14.06	77.33	140.6
x_3	Syloid	0	7.03	14.06	77.33	140.6
x_4	Ac-Di-Sol	0	7.03	14.06	77.33	140.6
x_5	Na-CMC	0	7.03	14.06	77.33	140.6
x_6	HEC	0	7.03	14.06	77.33	140.6
x_7	NaH_2PO_4	0	7.03	14.06	77.33	140.6
x_8	Citric acid	0	7.03	14.06	77.33	140.6
x_9	Pharma coat 603	0	7.03	14.06	77.33	140.6
x_{10}	Polyox N10	0	7.03	14.06	77.33	140.6

Appendix 4. By using the desirability function method the optimum values obtained for control factors are shown in Table 13.

Example 5
Rhinetedin
The release profile of this drug is investigated by Patel [23]. The two main control factors for this drug are presented in Table 14.

The control factors are coded by the following relationships:

$$x_{1(new)} = \frac{x_1 - 672}{168}, x_{2(new)} = \frac{x_2 - 168}{84}$$

In this research three time points are investigated from release profile are shown in Table 15.

In this example, the index f_2 is the measure of similarity between the drug release profile and the target profile. The RSM relationships are presented in Appendix 5 and the optimum values are shown in Table 16.

Example 6
Metoprolol
The release profile for this drug is investigated by Gohel [24]. The two main control factors defined for this drug are shown in Table 17.

The control factor values are coded by using the following relationships:

$$x_{1(new)} = \frac{x_1 - 30}{10}, x_{2(new)} = \frac{x_2 - 20}{10}$$

The three points of time for the drug release profile are presented in Table 18.

In the study of this drug, f_2, t_{50} (the time required for 50% of drug to be released) and mean dissolution time (MDT) are the measures of the similarity factor between

Table 6 The target values and lower and upper values for example 2

	y_1	y_2	y_3	y_4	y_5	y_6	y_7	y_8	y_9	y_{10}	y_{11}
Time	0.5 h	1 h	1.5 h	2 h	3 h	4 h	6 h	8 h	10 h	12 h	24 h
LSL	4.8	8.8	10.24	12.88	18.08	23.84	34.8	41.12	48.24	54.8	65.84
Target	6	11	12.8	16.1	22.6	29.8	43.5	51.4	60.3	68.5	82.3
USL	7.2	13.2	15.36	19.32	27.12	35.76	52.2	61.68	72.36	82.2	98.76

release profile and the predefined profile, the time required to dissolve half of the drug and the mean dissolution time, respectively. The RSM relationships for the means and these measures are presented in Appendix 6. By using the proposed method, the optimum values are obtained as shown in Table 19.

Comparison of the proposed method and the existing ones

The disadvantages of the existing methods are:

Contour overlay method:

This method has a limited application and when the number of variables exceeds from two, the model may not be optimized unless the additional variables are being fixed at a constant level.

Profile selection method:

In this method, the number of test profiles is adjusted based on the experimenter point of view and the best profile is selected among the existing ones. It is possible that the optimum values for the control factors may not be included in these profiles.

MSE minimizing method:

In this method, there is no attention paid to the specification limits, while in the real world, passing these limits has substantial penalties.

Minimizing the total cost method:

In this method all deviations from the target values are evaluated by means of money terms, while in human problems, e.g. pharmaceutical studies, adverse events may have human fallout which cannot be measured by money terms.

The proposed method overcomes all the above disadvantages.

Conclusions

Investigation of the pharmaceutics problems in an industrial engineering framework is very constructive. The key point here is the problem presentation by the engineering terms. In this research, the drug release problem which is an important subject of pharmaceutics is being studied. In this area, applying the complex formulas is avoided. So, the experts with minimum knowledge of mathematics and statistics may apply this approach to solve the pharmaceutics problems. The results of the examples show the ability of the proposed model for solving the controlled release problems and to assure that the intended drug is resolved as its predefined profile. The simultaneous optimization of drugs with multi time-oriented quality characteristics is a topic for the future research.

Appendix 1

$$\mu_{1(1h)} = 39.929 + 2.365x_1 - 2.206x_2 - 1.959x_3 \\ + 0.202x_1^2 + 1.971x_2^2 - 0.912x_3^2 - 1.389x_1x_2 \\ + 0.797x_1x_3 + 0.079x_2x_3$$

$$\mu_{2(6h)} = 73.368 + 4.388x_1 - 5.031x_2 - 2.379x_3 \\ + 0.399x_1^2 + 0.579x_2^2 - 0.127x_3^2 - 1.525x_1x_2 \\ - 0.062x_1x_3 - 0.359x_2x_3$$

$$\mu_{3(8h)} = 83.203 + 4.165x_1 - 4.562x_2 - 2.498x_3 \\ - 0.624x_1^2 - 0.907x_2^2 + 1.176x_3^2 - 2.37x_1x_2 \\ + 0.151x_1x_3 - 1.632x_2x_3$$

$$V_{1(1h)} = 7.31 - 0.642x_1 + 0.032x_2 + 2.799x_3 \\ + 1.698x_1^2 + 5.377x_2^2 + 4.895x_3^2 + 5.543x_1x_2 \\ + 1.893x_1x_3 - 0.686x_2x_3$$

$$V_{2(6h)} = 5.74 - 1.195x_1 + 1.609x_2 - 5.458x_3 \\ + 7.112x_1^2 + 0.037x_2^2 + 9.608x_3^2 + 11.9x_1x_2 \\ - 4.042x_1x_3 + 0.98x_2x_3$$

$$V_{3(8h)} = 11.548 - 6.216x_1 + 3.632x_2 - 0.354x_3 \\ + 2.053x_1^2 + 2.293x_2^2 + 2.581x_3^2 - 5.282x_1x_2 \\ + 2.575x_1x_3 - 5.902x_2x_3$$

Table 7 Optimum values for control factors for example 2

Variable	Control factor	Coded value	Uncoded value
x_1	PEO	15.556	203.069
x_3	Syloid	0.691	4.858
x_7	NaH_2PO_4	14.748	103.675
X_8	Citric acid	0	0
X_{10}	Polyox N10	20	140.6

Table 8 Main control factors influencing Verapamil HCl release

Variable	Control factor	Level 1	Level 2	Level 3
x_1	Coating weigh gain	8%	11%	14%
x_2	Duration of coating	24 h	36 h	48 h
x_3	Amount of plasticizer	60%	90%	120%

Table 9 The target values and lower and upper values for example 3

	y_1	y_2	y_3	y_4	y_5
Time	2 h	4 h	6 h	9 h	12 h
LSL	13.36%	26.64%	40%	50%	80%
Target	16.7%	33.3%	50%	75%	100%
USL	20.04%	39.96%	60%	90%	120%

Table 11 Main control factors for example 3

Variable	Control factor	Level 1	Level 2	Level 3
x_1	Concentration of sodium alginate	1.25%	1.75%	2.25%
x_2	Concentration of gellan gum	0%	0.25%	0.5%
x_3	Concentration of metformin	2.5%	3.75%	5%

$$\left(\frac{s}{m}\right)_{1(1h)} = 0.063 - 0.005x_1 - 0.001x_2 + 0.012x_3 \\ + 0.007x_1^2 + 0.008x_2^2 + 0.014x_3^2 \\ + 0.021x_1x_2 + 0.008x_1x_3 - 0.003x_2x_3$$

$$\left(\frac{s}{m}\right)_{2(6h)} = 0.04 - 0.002x_1 + 0.007x_2 - 0.003x_3 \\ + 0.006x_1^2 - 0.004x_2^2 + 0.009x_3^2 \\ + 0.013x_1x_2 - 0.008x_1x_3 + 0.004x_2x_3$$

$$\left(\frac{s}{m}\right)_{3(8h)} = 0.039 - 0.009x_1 + 0.008x_2 + 0.002x_3 \\ - 0.0002x_1^2 + 0.004x_2^2 + 0.006x_3^2 - 0.007x_1x_2 \\ + 0.002x_1x_3 - 0.006x_2x_3$$

$$(s_{12})_{(1h-6h)} = 1.89 + 2.507x_1 - 0.799x_2 + 0.299x_3 \\ + 0.677x_1^2 - 2.227x_2^2 - 4.571x_3^2 - 2.594x_1x_2 \\ - 0.655x_1x_3 - 2.289x_2x_3$$

$$(s_{13})_{(1h-8h)} = 1.091 + 1.603x_1 1.572x_2 + 3.023x_3 \\ - 3.872x_1^2 - 3.299x_2^2 + 3.353x_3^2 - 1.879x_1x_2 \\ + 0.966x_1x_3 + 2.559x_2x_3$$

$$(s_{23})_{(6h-8h)} = -2.945 - 1.711x_1 - 1.729x_2 - 3.296x_3 \\ + 2.541x_1^2 + 2.411x_2^2 - 2.738x_3^2 - 0.22x_1x_2 \\ + 3.237x_1x_3 + 3.732x_2x_3$$

Appendix 2

$$\mu_{1(0.5h)} = 4.844 - 0.039x_1 + 0.023x_3 - 0.006x_7 - 0.005x_8 \\ - 0.001x_{10} + 0.0001x_1^2 - 0.00007x_3^2 + 0.00006x_7^2 \\ + 0.00002x_8^2 + 0.00003x_{10}^2 + 0.0006x_1x_3$$

$$V_{1(0.5h)} = 0.71 - 0.008x_1 + 0.0001x_3 - 0.00078x_7 \\ + 0.006x_8 - 0.006x_{10} + 0.00003x_1^2 \\ + 0.000006x_3^2 + 0.00003x_7^2 - 0.00002x_8^2 \\ + 0.00004x_{10}^2 - 0.00003x_1x_3$$

$$\mu_{2(1h)} = 7.644 - 0.027x_1 + 0.015x_3 - 0.01x_7 + 0.017x_8 \\ - 0.014x_{10} + 0.0001x_1^2 + 0.000001x_3^2 + 0.0001x_7^2 \\ + 0.0002x_8^2 + 0.0001x_{10}^2 + 0.0004x_1x_3$$

$$V_{2(1h)} = 1.103 - 0.041x_1 - 0.027x_3 - 0.002x_7 \\ + 0.021x_8 + 0.006x_{10} + 0.0001x_1^2 \\ + 0.00008x_3^2 + 0.00002x_7^2 - 0.00007x_8^2 \\ - 0.00002x_{10}^2 + 0.0009x_1x_3$$

$$\mu_{3(1.5h)} = 7.228 + 0.109x_1 + 0.018x_3 - 0.029x_7 + 0.033x_8 \\ - 0.035x_{10} - 0.0003x_1^2 - 0.0005x_3^2 + 0.0003x_7^2 \\ + 0.0003x_8^2 + 0.0002x_{10}^2 - 0.0044x_1x_3$$

$$V_{3(1.5h)} = 0.292 + 0.021x_1 + 0.035x_3 - 0.031x_7 \\ + 0.033x_8 - 0.004x_{10} - 0.00005x_1^2 - 0.000009x_3^2 \\ + 0.0002x_7^2 - 0.0001x_8^2 + 0.00003x_{10}^2 - 0.0009x_1x_3$$

$$\mu_{4(2h)} = 8.611 + 0.165x_1 + 0.248x_3 - 0.074x_7 \\ + 0.074x_8 - 0.05x_{10} - 0.0005x_1^2 - 0.0007x_3^2 \\ + 0.0006x_7^2 + 0.0002x_8^2 + 0.0003x_{10}^2 - 0.006x_1x_3$$

$$V_{4(2h)} = 1.582 - 0.082x_1 - 0.05x_3 - 0.033x_7 + 0.058x_8 \\ + 0.027x_{10} + 0.0003x_1^2 + 0.0002x_3^2 \\ + 0.0002x_7^2 - 0.0002x_8^2 - 0.0001x_{10}^2 + 0.002x_1x_3$$

$$\mu_{5(3h)} = 12.428 + 0.207x_1 + 0.309x_3 - 0.09x_7 \\ + 0.089x_8 - 0.049x_{10} - 0.0006x_1^2 - 0.0008x_3^2 \\ + 0.0007x_7^2 + 0.0003x_8^2 + 0.0004x_{10}^2 - 0.008x_1x_3$$

$$V_{5(3h)} = 1.69 - 0.078x_1 - 0.033x_3 - 0.021x_7 + 0.052x_8 \\ + 0.033x_{10} + 0.0003x_1^2 + 0.0001x_3^2 \\ + 0.0001x_7^2 - 0.0002x_8^2 - 0.0001x_{10}^2 + 0.001x_1x_3$$

$$\mu_{6(4h)} = 16.417 + 0.287x_1 + 0.388x_3 - 0.11x_7 \\ + 0.126x_8 - 0.07x_{10} - 0.0008x_1^2 - 0.001x_3^2 \\ + 0.0009x_7^2 + 0.0003x_8^2 + 0.0005x_{10}^2 - 0.011x_1x_3$$

Table 10 Optimum values for control factors for example 3

Variable	Control factor	Coded value	Uncoded value
x_1	Coating weigh gain	−0.6566	9.0302
x_2	Duration of coating	0.5152	29.8176
x_3	Amount of plasticizer	1	120

Table 12 The target values and lower and upper values for example 4

Response	Delay after usage	LSL	Target	USL
y_1	0.5 hour	21%	23.5%	26%
y_2	3.5 hours	62%	63.5%	65%
y_3	8 hours	91%	92.5%	94%

Table 13 Optimum values of control factors for example 4

Variable	Control factor	Coded value	Uncoded value
x_1	Concentration of sodium alginate	1	2.25%
x_2	Concentration of gellan gum	−0.9192	0.0202%
x_3	Concentration of metformin	−1	2.5%

Table 15 The target values and lower and upper specifications for example 5

Response	Delay after usage	LSL	Target	USL
y_1	1 hour	26%	32.5%	39%
y_2	5 hours	54%	67.5%	81%
y_3	10 hours	68%	85%	102%

$$V_{6(4h)} = 3.123 - 0.134x_1 - 0.074x_3 - 0.035x_7 + 0.061x_8 + 0.053x_{10} + 0.0005x_1^2 + 0.0002x_3^2 + 0.0002x_7^2 - 0.0002x_8^2 - 0.0002x_{10}^2 + 0.003x_1x_3$$

$$\mu_{7(6h)} = 21.874 + 0.563x_1 + 0.691x_3 - 0.174x_7 + 0.109x_8 - 0.084x_{10} - 0.002x_1^2 - 0.002x_3^2 + 0.001x_7^2 + 0.0006x_8^2 + 0.0007x_{10}^2 - 0.02x_1x_3$$

$$V_{7(6h)} = 4.719 - 0.22x_1 - 0.104x_3 - 0.056x_7 + 0.073x_8 + 0.105x_{10} + 0.0008x_1^2 + 0.0003x_3^2 + 0.0003x_7^2 - 0.0002x_8^2 - 0.0004x_{10}^2 + 0.005x_1x_3$$

$$\mu_{8(8h)} = 28.588 + 0.811x_1 + 0.963x_3 - 0.221x_7 + 0.073x_8 - 0.11x_{10} - 0.002x_1^2 - 0.003x_3^2 + 0.001x_7^2 + 0.0007x_8^2 + 0.001x_{10}^2 - 0.03x_1x_3$$

$$V_{8(8h)} = 5.417 - 0.226x_1 - 0.064x_3 - 0.072x_7 + 0.061x_8 + 0.158x_{10} + 0.0008x_1^2 + 0.0001x_3^2 + 0.0004x_7^2 - 0.0002x_8^2 - 0.0006x_{10}^2 + 0.004x_1x_3$$

$$\mu_{9(10h)} = 37.1 + 0.886x_1 + 1.086x_3 - 0.249x_7 + 0.058x_8 - 0.094x_{10} - 0.003x_1^2 - 0.003x_3^2 + 0.002x_7^2 + 0.001x_8^2 + 0.001x_{10}^2 - 0.032x_1x_3$$

$$V_{9(10h)} = 7.351 - 0.28x_1 - 0.085x_3 - 0.088x_7 + 0.046x_8 + 0.201x_{10} + 0.001x_1^2 + 0.0002x_3^2 + 0.0005x_7^2 - 0.0002x_8^2 - 0.0008x_{10}^2 + 0.005x_1x_3$$

$$\mu_{10(12h)} = 44.362 + 1.017x_1 + 1.237x_3 - 0.229x_7 + 0.055x_8 - 0.144x_{10} - 0.003x_1^2 - 0.004x_3^2 + 0.001x_7^2 + 0.0006x_8^2 + 0.001x_{10}^2 - 0.036x_1x_3$$

$$V_{10(12h)} = 7.482 - 0.267x_1 - 0.049x_3 - 0.095x_7 + 0.055x_8 + 0.217x_{10} + 0.001x_1^2 + 0.00001x_3^2 + 0.0005x_7^2 - 0.0002x_8^2 - 0.001x_{10}^2 + 0.004x_1x_3$$

$$\mu_{11(24h)} = 82.688 + 0.577x_1 + 0.705x_3 - 0.056x_7 + 0.06x_8 + 0.044x_{10} - 0.002x_1^2 - 0.002x_3^2 + 0.004x_7^2 - 0.00004x_8^2 + 0.0001x_{10}^2 - 0.02x_1x_3$$

$$V_{11(24h)} = 7.503 - 0.104x_1 - 0.025x_3 - 0.097x_7 - 0.005x_8 - 0.004x_{10} + 0.0005x_1^2 + 0.00004x_3^2 + 0.0006x_7^2 - 0.0001x_8^2 - 0.0001x_{10}^2 + 0.001x_1x_3$$

Appendix 3

$$\mu_{1(2h)} = 12.986 - 2.16x_1 - x_2 + 0.68x_3 + 0.121x_1^2 - 0.279x_2^2 + 0.221x_3^2 + 0.038x_1x_2 + 0.038x_1x_3 + 0.163x_2x_3$$

$$v_{1(2h)} = 1.274 + 0.057x_1 + 0.33x_2 - 0.235x_3 - 0.064x_1^2 + 0.056x_2^2 - 0.298x_3^2 - 0.002x_1x_2 + 0.426x_1x_3 + 0.292x_2x_3$$

$$\left(\frac{s}{m}\right)_{1(2h)} = 0.082 + 0.013x_1 + 0.017x_2 - 0.015x_3 - 0.006x_1^2 + 0.011x_2^2 - 0.016x_3^2 + 0.002x_1x_2 + 0.014x_1x_3 + 0.015x_2x_3$$

$$\mu_{2(4h)} = 25.121 - 5.2x_1 - 2x_2 + 1.43x_3 + 0.47x_1^2 - 0.331x_2^2 + 0.619x_3^2 + 0.163x_1x_2 + 0.063x_1x_3 + 0.338x_2x_3$$

$$v_{2(4h)} = 1.747 + 0.112x_1 + 0.004x_2 - 0.564x_3 - 1.017x_1^2 + 1.813x_2^2 - 0.732x_3^2 - 0.442x_1x_2 + 0.185x_1x_3 - 0.185x_2x_3$$

$$\left(\frac{s}{m}\right)_{2(4h)} = 0.046 + 0.01x_1 + 0.002x_2 - 0.011x_3 - 0.013x_1^2 + 0.025x_2^2 - 0.009x_3^2 - 0.004x_1x_2 + 0.0004x_1x_3 - 0.004x_2x_3$$

$$\mu_{3(6h)} = 42.938 - 7.27x_1 - 2.87x_2 + 2.31x_3 - 0.257x_1^2 - 0.257x_2^2 - 0.057x_3^2 + 0.913x_1x_2 + 0.463x_1x_3 - 0.688x_2x_3$$

$$v_{3(6h)} = 3.412 + 0.072x_1 + 0.965x_2 + 0.052x_3 + 3.869x_1^2 - 1.106x_2^2 - 1.351x_3^2 - 1.126x_1x_2 + 0.936x_1x_3 - 0.049x_2x_3$$

$$\left(\frac{s}{m}\right)_{3(6h)} = 0.042 + 0.009x_1 + 0.008x_2 - 0.002x_3 - 0.023x_1^2 - 0.005x_2^2 - 0.007x_3^2 - 0.006x_1x_2 + 0.004x_1x_3 + 0.001x_2x_3$$

Table 14 Main control factors for example 5

Variable	Control factor	Level 1	Level 2	Level 3
x_1	Amount of gelucire 43/01	504	672	840
x_2	Amount of ethylcellulose	84	168	252

Table 16 Optimum values for example 5

Variable	Control factor	Coded value	Uncoded value
x_1	Amount of gelucire 43/01	−0.909	657.7288
x_2	Amount of ethylcellulose	1	252

Table 17 Main control factors for example 7

Variable	Control factor	Level 1	Level 2	Level 3
x_1	% of xanthan gum	20%	30%	40%
x_2	% of Methocel	10%	20%	30%

Table 19 Optimum values for example 7

Variable	Control factor	Coded value	Uncoded value
x_1	% of xanthan gum	0.0458	30.458
x_2	% of Methocel	0.6726	26.726

$$\mu_{4(9h)} = 67.278 - 11.37x_1 - 3.02x_2 + 3.27x_3 - 2.541x_1^2 \\ + 3.709x_2^2 - 3.841x_3^2 + 0.125x_1x_2 + 0.825x_1x_3 \\ + 0.05x_2x_3$$

$$v_{4(9h)} = 3.563 + 0.311x_1 - 0.064x_2 + 0.085x_3 - 0.895x_1^2 \\ + 0.32x_2^2 + 0.425x_3^2 + 0.523x_1x_2 - 0.208x_1x_3 \\ - 0.09x_2x_3$$

$$\left(\frac{s}{m}\right)_{4(9h)} = 0.027 + 0.007x_1 + 0.002x_2 - 0.002x_3 - 0.001x_1^2 \\ + 0.001x_2^2 + 0.003x_3^2 + 0.003x_1x_2 \\ - 0.002x_1x_3 - 0.001x_2x_3$$

$$\mu_{5(12h)} = 82.395 - 12.84x_1 - 5.25x_2 + 3.8x_3 - 0.567x_1^2 \\ - 0.417x_2^2 + 0.333x_3^2 - 0.675x_1x_2 + 0.625x_1x_3 \\ + 0.125x_2x_3$$

$$v_{5(12h)} = 3.944 - 0.428x_1 + 0.038x_2 - 0.142x_3 + 1.018x_1^2 \\ - 1.592x_2^2 - 0.662x_3^2 + 0.705x_1x_2 - 0.065x_1x_3 \\ + 0.643x_2x_3$$

$$\left(\frac{s}{m}\right)_{5(12h)} = 0.024 + 0.002x_1 + 0.002x_2 - 0.002x_3 \\ + 0.004x_1^2 - 0.006x_2^2 - 0.002x_3^2 + 0.003x_1x_2 \\ - 0.001x_1x_3 + 0.003x_2x_3$$

$$\mu_{2(3.5h)} = 64.474 - 6.603x_1 - 4.648x_2 + 3.1x_3 - 0.977x_1^2 \\ + 4.658x_2^2 + 1.287x_3^2 - 1.168x_1x_2 - 0.65x_1x_3 \\ - 0.705x_2x_3$$

$$v_{2(3.5h)} = 0.841 - 0.063x_1 + 0.215x_2 + 0.12x_3 - 0.173x_1^2 \\ + 0.765x_2^2 + 0.048x_3^2 - 0.084x_1x_2 - 0.56x_1x_3 \\ - 0.371x_2x_3$$

$$\left(\frac{s}{m}\right)_{2(3.5h)} = 0.011 + 0.001x_1 + 0.003x_2 - 0.001x_3 \\ - 0.001x_1^2 + 0.007x_2^2 - 0.0003x_3^2 - 0.00003x_1x_2 \\ - 0.004x_1x_3 - 0.002x_2x_3$$

$$\mu_{3(8h)} = 92.466 - 4.383x_1 - 2.878x_2 + 1.811x_3 - 1.242x_1^2 \\ + 2.206x_2^2 - 0.987x_3^2 - 1.1x_1x_2 + 0.168x_1x_3 \\ + 2.018x_2x_3$$

$$v_{3(8h)} = 0.895 - 0.192x_1 + 0.213x_2 - 0.302x_3 \\ + 0.029x_1^2 - 0.564x_2^2 + 0.786x_3^2 - 0.135x_1x_2 \\ + 0.088x_1x_3 - 0.284x_2x_3$$

$$\left(\frac{s}{m}\right)_{3(8h)} = 0.01 - 0.001x_1 + 0.001x_2 - 0.001x_3 \\ + 0.0001x_1^2 - 0.004x_2^2 + 0.004x_3^2 - 0.001x_1x_2 \\ + 0.001x_1x_3 - 0.001x_2x_3$$

Appendix 4

$$\mu_{1(0.5h)} = 31.153 - 3.546x_1 - 3.884x_2 + 3.243x_3 \\ + 0.667x_1^2 + 1.874x_2^2 - 3.391x_3^2 \\ + 2.897x_1x_2 - 0.767x_1x_3 + 1.175x_2x_3$$

$$v_{1(0.5h)} = 0.669 - 0.456x_1 - 0.45x_2 - 0.839x_3 + 1.542x_1^2 \\ - 1.429x_2^2 + 2.026x_3^2 - 1.309x_1x_2 - 1.167x_1x_3 \\ + 0.649x_2x_3$$

$$\left(\frac{s}{m}\right)_{1(0.5h)} = 0.028 + 0.002x_1 + 0.0004x_2 - 0.016x_3 \\ + 0.01x_1^2 - 0.01x_2^2 + 0.022x_3^2 - 0.016x_1x_2 \\ - 0.01x_1x_3 + 0.002x_2x_3$$

Table 18 The target values and lower and upper specification limits for example 7

Response	Delay after usage	LSL	Target	USL
y_1	1 hour	15%	17.5%	20%
y_2	4 hours	20%	30%	40%
y_3	12 hours	60%	65%	70%
t_{50}	-	6 h	7 h	8 h
MDT	-	8 h	9 h	10 h

Appendix 5

$$\mu_{1(1h)} = 37.191 - 7.918x_1 - 3.955x_2 + 1.148x_1^2 - 1.432x_2^2 \\ - 0.558x_1x_2$$

$$v_{1(1h)} = 1.957 + 0.862x_1 - 0.693x_2 - 0.105x_1^2 - 0.04x_2^2 \\ - 1.32x_1x_2$$

$$\left(\frac{s}{m}\right)_{1(1h)} = 0.038 + 0.015x_1 - 0.003x_2 - 0.002x_1^2 - 0.001x_2^2 \\ - 0.012x_1x_2$$

$$\mu_{2(5h)} = 75.29 - 6.358x_1 - 8.795x_2 + 1.035x_1^2 - 1.345x_2^2 \\ + 0.745x_1x_2$$

$$v_{2(5h)} = 5.129 + 0.25x_1 + 0.915x_2 - 2.223x_1^2 - 0.583x_2^2 \\ - 1.18x_1x_2$$

$$\left(\frac{s}{m}\right)_{2(5h)} = 0.031 + 0.003x_1 + 0.006x_2 - 0.009x_1^2 \\ - 0.002x_2^2 - 0.005x_1x_2$$

$$\mu_{3(10h)} = 89.216 - 8.49x_1 - 7.528x_2 + 3.797x_1^2 - 1.728x_2^2 \\ - 3.195x_1x_2$$

$$v_{3(10h)} = 3.026 - 0.145x_1 - 1.292x_2 + 2.372x_1^2 - 1.968x_2^2 \\ + 0.75x_1x_2$$

$$\left(\frac{s}{m}\right)_{3(10h)} = 0.017 + 0.002x_1 - 0.003x_2 + 0.007x_1^2 \\ -0.004x_2^2 - 0.003x_1x_2$$

$$f_2value = 50.157 + 7.52x_1 + 9.473x_2 - 5.26x_1^2 - 1.49x_2^2 \\ -0.66x_1x_2$$

Appendix 6

$$\mu_{1(1h)} = 20.778 - 3.317x_1 - 4.017x_2 + 0.183x_1^2 - 0.917x_2^2 \\ -0.325x_1x_2$$

$$\mu_{2(4h)} = 38.678 - 4.5x_1 - 5.7x_2 + 1.583x_1^2 - 1.467x_2^2 \\ -1.425x_1x_2$$

$$\mu_{3(12h)} = 68.822 - 5.483x_1 - 5.5x_2 + 2.317x_1^2 - 1.333x_2^2 \\ + 0.15x_1x_2$$

$$\mu_{4(t_{50})} = 6.222 + x_1 + 1.167x_2 - 0.333x_1^2 + 0.167x_2^2$$

$$\mu_{5(MDT)} = 8.222 + 0.767x_1 + 0.933x_2 - 0.333x_1^2 \\ + 0.267x_2^2 - 0.1x_1x_2$$

$$\mu_{6(f2)} = 68.556 + 11.183x_1 + 11.45x_2 - 2.483x_1^2 \\ -3.583x_2^2 - 1.525x_1x_2$$

Abbreviations

MEC: Minimum effective concentration; MTC: Minimal toxic concentration; NTB: Nominal the best; LTB: Larger the better; STB: Smaller the best; DOE: Design of experiments; RSM: Response surface methodology; LSL: Lower specification limit; USL: Upper specification limit; MDT: Mean dissolution time.

Competing interests

The authors declare that they have no competing interests.

Authors' contributions

Authors contributed to the manuscript according to their responsibility. MRN designed and carried out the study. HS was the dissertation supervisor. MS validated the findings and proofread the final version. All authors read and approved the final manuscript.

Acknowledgements

This research was part of Mohammad Reza Nabatchian PhD Dissertation.

Author details

[1]Department of Industrial Engineering, K.N. Toosi University of Technology, No 7, Pardis St., Mollasadra Ave., Tehran, Iran. [2]Department of Dermatology, University of Connecticut Health Center, Farmington, CT, USA.

References

1. Perrie Y, Rades T: *Pharmaceutics-drug delivery and targeting*. UK: Pharmaceutical press; 2012:7–14.
2. Hillery A, Loyd A, Swarbrick J: *Drug delivery and targeting*. USA: Taylor and Francis; 2005:20–42.
3. Li X, Jasti B: *Design of controlled release drug delivery systems*. USA: McGraw-Hill; 2006:10–35.
4. Wen H, Park K: *Oral Controlled Release formulation design and drug delivery*. USA: John Wiley & Sons; 2010:21–46.
5. Rathbone M, Hadgraft J: *Modified-release drug delivery technology*. USA: Marcel Dekker, Inc; 2003:1–20.
6. Juran J, Godrey A: *Juran's quality handbook*. 5th edition. USA: McGraw-Hill; 1999:5–20.
7. Taguchi G, Chowdhury S, Taguchi S: *Taguchi's quality engineering handbook*. USA: John Wiley & Sons; 2005:20–60.
8. Phadke M: *Quality engineering using robust design*. USA: Prentice-hall international; 1989:5–40.
9. Park S, Antony J: *Robust design for quality engineering and six sigma*. USA: World Scientific; 2008:25–60.
10. Montgomery DC: *Design and analysis of experiments*. 5th edition. USA: John Wiley & Sons; 2001:21–60.
11. Dean A, Lewis S: *Screening: methods for experimentation in industry, drug discovery and genetics*. USA: Springer; 2006:1–45.
12. Myers R, Montgomery DC: *Response surface methodology*. 2nd edition. USA: John Wiley & Sons; 2002:20–50.
13. Derringer G, Suich R: Simultaneous optimization of several response variables. *J Qual Technol* 1980, **12**(4):214–219.
14. Gohel A, Amin A: Formulation optimization if controlled release diclofenac sodium microspheres using factorial design. *J Control Release* 1998, **51**:115–122.
15. Moore J, Flanner H: Mathematical comparison of curves with an emphasis on in-vitro dissolution profiles. *J Pharm Technol* 1996, **20**(6):67–74.
16. Freitag G: Guidelines on dissolution profile comparison. *Drug Inf J* 2001, **35**:865–874.
17. Truong N, Shin S, Choi Y, Jeong S, Cho B: Robust design with time-oriented responses for regenerative medicine industry. In *Proceeding of the 3rd International Conference on the Development of biomedical engineering: 11-14 January 2010*. Edited by Toi V, Khoa T. Vietnam: Springer; 2010:67–70.
18. Park J, Shin J, Truong N, Shin S, Choi Y, Lee J, Yoon J, Jeong S: A pharma robust design method to investigate the effect of PEGand PEO on matrix tablets. *Int J Pharm* 2010, **393**:79–87.
19. Shin S, Choi D, Truong N, Kim N, Chu K, Jeong S: Time-oriented experimental design method to optimize hydrophilic matrix formulations with gelatin kinetics and drug release profiles. *Int J Pharm* 2011, **407**:53–62.
20. Goethals P, Cho B: The development of a robust design methodology for time-oriented dynamic quality characteristics with a target profile. *Qual Reliability Eng Int* 2011, **27**:403–414.
21. Vaithiyalingam S, Khan M: Optimization and characterization of controlled release multi-particulate beads formulated with a customized cellulose acetate butyrate dispersion. *Int J Pharm* 2002, **234**:179–193.
22. Nagarwal R, Srinatha A, Pandit J: In situ forming formulation: development, evaluation, and optimization using 3^3 factorial design. *AAPS pharm sci tech* 2009, **10**(3):977–983.
23. Patel D, Patel N, Patel V, Bhatt D: Floating granules of ranitidine hydrochloride-gelucire 43/01: formulation optimization using factorial design. *AAPS pharm sci tech* 2007, **8**(2):1–7.
24. Gohel M, Parikh R, Nagori S, Jena D: Fabrication of modified release tablet formulation of metoprolol succinate using hydroxypropyl methylcellulose and xanthan gum. *AAPS pharm sci tech* 2009, **10**(1):62–68.

17

Factors affecting viability of *Bifidobacterium bifidum* during spray drying

Zahra Shokri[1], Mohammad Reza Fazeli[2*], Mehdi Ardjmand[1], Seyyed Mohammad Mousavi[3] and Kambiz Gilani[4]

Abstract

Background: There is substantial clinical data supporting the role of *Bifidobacterium bifidum* in human health particularly in benefiting the immune system and suppressing intestinal infections. Compared to the traditional lyophilization, spray-drying is an economical process for preparing large quantities of viable microorganisms. The technique offers high production rates and low operating costs but is not usually used for drying of substances prone to high temperature. The aim of this study was to establish the optimized environmental factors in spray drying of cultured bifidobacteria to obtain a viable and stable powder.

Methods: The experiments were designed to test variables such as inlet air temperature, air pressure and also maltodextrin content. The combined effect of these variables on survival rateand moisture content of bacterial powder was studied using a central composite design (CCD). Sub-lethal heat-adaptation of a *B. bifidum* strain which was previously adapted to acid-bile-NaCl led to much more resistance to high outlet temperature during spray drying. The resistant *B. bifidum* was supplemented with cost friendly permeate, sucrose, yeast extract and different amount of maltodextrin before it was fed into a Buchi B-191 mini spray-dryer.

Results: Second-order polynomials were established to identify the relationship between the responses andthe three variables. Results of verification experiments and predicted values from fitted correlations were in close agreement at 95% confidence interval. The optimal values of the variables for maximum survival and minimum moisture content of *B. bifidum* powder were as follows: inlet air temperature of 111.15°C, air pressure of 4.5 bar and maltodextrin concentration of 6%. Under optimum conditions, the maximum survival of 28.38% was achieved while moisture was maintained at 4.05%.

Conclusion: Viable and cost effective spray drying of *Bifidobacterium bifidum* could be achieved by cultivating heat and acid adapted strain into the culture media containing nutritional protective agents.

Keywords: Spray drying, *Bifidobacterium bifidum*, Viability, Moisture, Response surface methodology

Introduction

Probiotics are live microbial feed supplements that beneficially affect hosts by improving its intestinal microbial balance [1]. Bacterial strains selected as probiotics are predominantly from the genera *Bifidobacteria* and *Lactobacilli*, which are indigenous to the human gastrointestinal tract [2]. These strains possess unique ability to establish in the human intestine and are associated with restoration of normal intestinal flora by outcompeting harmful flora and human pathogens [3]. They are also believed to have detoxifying ability against mycotoxins [4]. Because of their positive effect on host's health, production and consumption of live probiotic supplements and food products enriched with friendly microorganisms have been of focus [5]. Both freeze-dying and spray-drying which are currently used to dry probiotic cultures expose the culture to extreme environmental conditions [6]. Spray drying is however more economic and efficient because of its continuous high production rate behavior, but viability of bacteria is usually affected due to use of extreme heat [7].

During spray drying bacteria are exposed to multiple stresses, i.e. heat (both wet and dry), oxidation, dehydration-related stresses (osmotic, acidic and thermal

* Correspondence: morfazeli@yahoo.com
[2]Probiotic Research Laboratory, Department of Drug and Food Control, Pharmaceutical Sciences Research Center, Faculty of Pharmacy, Tehran University of Medical Sciences, Tehran, Iran
Full list of author information is available at the end of the article

shock, accumulation of toxic compounds, etc.) which potentially could lead to cell death. Loss of viability appears to be principally caused by cell membrane damage [8]; moreover, the cell wall, ribosome and DNA are also affected at higher temperatures [9].

Thermal shock is the most influential factor in this field. Compared to the untreated bacteria, those which are pre-treated in water bath are usually more resistant to dry heat of outlet air temperature during spray drying [10]. High temperatures could lead to heat or stress proteins. The induction of heat shock on bacterial has led to the production of heat shock protein (HSP) or stress proteins. The role of protective proteins is to prevent malicious connections between intracellular amino acids. These proteins are produced by the genes present in all living cells. In 2005, Joana Silva and colleagues showed that the growth of the bacteria in non-controlled pH conditions results in induction of heat shock proteins and results in more bacteria to survive during spray drying and storage [11]. Also water drainage which contributes to the stability of biological molecules and probiotic strains, may cause irreversible changes in the structural and functional integrity of bacterial membranes and proteins. Preservation of these essential functions and structure is crucial for the survival of bacteria and the retention of their functionality.

The residual moisture content should be low enough to prevent damage to the product during storage. Too low moisture content of probiotic powders can also be injurious [8]. Humidity below 2% is also harmful because it can increase the risk of oxidation of unsaturated fatty acids in the cell membrane of bacteria and it can destroy the units of hydration around these fatty acids [12]. Based on the measurements of glass transition temperature (T_g), critical water content 4-7% (w/v) is necessary and appropriate for the storage of culture powders at room temperature of 25°C [13,14].

As data on optimized spray drying of B. bifidum is trace we have tried to investigate the optimum spray drying conditions for preparation of viable B. bifidum powder with suitable moisture content.

Materials and methods

Microorganism and cultivation conditions

The bacterial strain of Bifidobacterium bifidum PTCC 1644 (Persian Type Culture Collection- Iran) was previously adapted to gastrointestinal conditions such as acid, bile and NaCl [15].

Heat adaptation of bacterial cultures

Bacteria underwent heat adaptation according to Jewell and Kashket [16]. Test tubes containing aliquots of 20 ml of 30 hours fresh bacterial culture (37°C and 5% CO_2) in MRS broth (Merck GmbH, Germany) were treated at 60°C for 15 minutes. The survived and heat adapted strains were collected after further incubation of viable strains on MRS agar medium and after 48 hours incubation (temperature, 37°C and 5% CO_2). The experiments were repeated at higher temperatures of 65°C and 75°C and the adapted strains were stored at -80°C for subsequent use in the spray drying. Strains subcultured on MRS broth were enriched with 0.05% L-cysteine (Merck GmbH, Germany), at 37°C for 30 hours [15]. Following incubation under 5% CO_2 cells were harvested by centrifugation at 2000 rpm for 15 min, and were further resuspended in sterile PBS-glycerol (20% v/v) solution and finally stored in 1mlcryotubes at -80°C.

Preparation of spray drying feed suspensions

All feed solutions contained 10% permeate powder (Shirpooyan Yazd Co., Iran), 2.5% saccharose, 2.5% yeast extract as well as 2-6% maltodextrin (Merck GmbH, Germany) and were autoclaved at 121°C for 15 min before use.

A cryo-tube containing 1ml of the adapted Bifidobacterium bifidumwas inoculated into the feed and was further incubated anaerobically (H2/CO2/N2; 10:5:85, Anoxomat WS8000, Mart_ Microbiology, Lichtenvoorde, Netherlands) at 37°C for 30 hours. The harvested feed contained 10^8-10^9cfu/ml prior to spray drying.

Spray drying condition

A mini spray-dryer Buchi B-191 (Buchi, Flawil, Switzerland) and the adopted protocol of Johnson and Etzel [17] was used. The feed solution was transformed from a fluid state into a dried form by spraying it into a hot drying air. The process involved atomization of a liquid feedstock into a spray of droplets. Independent variables for optimized method of spray drying process design included:

- atomizing air pressure (bar)
- inlet air temperature (°C)
- outlet air temperature (°C)
- flow rate of fees suspension ($\frac{ml}{min}$)
- flow rate of drying air (aspiration ($\frac{m^3}{h}$))

The aspiration was set on 80% in all runs. The outlet temperature measured between drying chamber and cyclone was regarded as the drying temperature. Adjustment of outlet temperature was performed by holding flow rate of the feed suspension at a constant value (25% pump capacity ~ 5 ml min^{-1}) for all outlet temperatures. The inlet temperature was varied, as shown in Table 1.

Design of experiments and statistical modeling

Response surface methodology is a combination of mathematical and statistical techniques used for developing, improving and optimizing the processes. It is used to

Table 1 The level of variables in central composite design (CCD)

Factor	Low axial (- $\alpha = -1.68$)	Low factorial (-1)	Center (0)	High factorial (+1)	High axial (+ $\alpha = +1.68$)
A: Inlet temperature (°C)	79.77	90	105	120	130.23
B: Air pressure (bar)	3.32	4	5	6	6.68
C: Maltodextrin ($\frac{gr}{ml}$)	0.64	2	4	6	7.36

evaluate the relative significance of several affecting factors, even in the presence of complex interactions [18,19]. The most popular response surface methodology is the central composite design (CCD) [20], which was used to design the experiment. CCD has three set of experimental runs: (1) fractional factorial runs in which factors are studied at +1 and -1 levels; (2) center points that all factors are at their center levels, which aids with determining the curvature and replication, helps to estimate pure error; and (3) axial points, which are similar to center point, but one factor takes the values above and below the median of the two factorial levels, typically both outside their range. Axial points make the design rotatable [21]. Empirical models describing the experimental results were developed using data collected from the designed experiments and were generated using the least-squares method. Model parameters were estimated using a second-order model of the form (Eq. (1)) [22]:

$$Y = \beta_0 + \sum_{i=1}^{k}\beta_i X_i + \sum_{i=1}^{k}\sum_{j=1}^{k}\beta_{ij}X_i X_j \quad (1)$$

Where Y is the expected value of the response variables, β_0, β_i, β_j are the model parameters, X_i and X_j are the coded factors evaluated, and k is the number of factors being studied. In this study, inlet air temperature, air pressure and maltodextrin concentration were selected as main factors. As shown in Table 1, each factor was examined in five levels, whereas the other parameters were kept constant. Accordingly, 20 experiments were conducted with 14 experiments organized in a factorial design and the 6 remaining experiments were involved in the replication of the central point to get good estimate of experimental error. The statistical software package, Design-Expert 7.0.0 (Stat-Ease, Inc., Minneapolis, MN, USA), was used for both the regression analysis of the experimental data, and the plot of the response contours and surface graphs. DX−7 is the windows-compatible software which provides efficient design of experiments (DOEs) for identification of vital factors that affect the process and uses RSM to determine optimal conditions [23,24]. The optimization module in DX−7 searches for a combination of factor levels that simultaneously satisfy the requirements placed on each of several responses [25,26].

Enumeration of *Bifidobacterium bifidum*

Colony forming units (CFU) of the individual runs of bifidobacterial cultures before and after spray drying were determined by serial dilution of feed suspension and powders, followed by pour plating into MRS agar. Plates were incubated at 37°C, for 48 hours, under anaerobic condition. Survival rates were calculated as follows: Survival (%) = $N/N0 \times 100$, where $N0$ and N represent the number of bacteria before and after drying respectively.

Determination of moisture content in spray dried powders

Moisture content of spray dried powder which is defined as the ratio of dried water to initial powder weight, was determined by oven-drying at 102° [27]. This involved determination of the difference in weight before and after oven-drying. Moisture content was then expressed as a percentage of initial powder weight.

Results and discussion

Twenty experiments were designed using CCD. The design matrix and the corresponding results of CCD experiments to determine the effects of the three independent variables are shown in Table 2.

Quadratic model was found to be adequate for the prediction of the response variables.

$$Y_1 = +28.82-9.15A-2.74B-0.62C-3.93AB + 0.98AC + 0.52BC-4.72A^2-0.51B^2 + 2.52C^2 \quad (2)$$

$$Y_2 = +4.39-1.10A-0.032B-0.24C-0.095AB -0.33AC-0.18BC + 0.16A^2 + 0.16B^2 + 0.29C^2 \quad (3)$$

Where Y_1 and Y_2, predicted Survival rate (%) and Moisture content (%) respectively; A is Inlet air temperature level; B is air pressure level; and C is maltodextrin concentration level. The statistical significance of the model equations (Eqs. (2)–(3)) and the model terms were evaluated by the F-test for analysis of variance (ANOVA), which indicated that the regressions were statistically significant. The results of analysis of variance (ANOVA) of the developed models are shown in Table 3.

Table 2 Experimental plan and results of spray drying of *B. bifidum*

Run	Factors			Responses	
	A (°C)	B (bar)	C ($\frac{gr}{ml}$)	S (%)	Moisture (%)
1	105.00	5.00	4.00	29.80	4.40
2	90.00	4.00	6.00	30.25	6.19
3	105.00	5.00	4.00	28.52	4.10
4	120.00	4.00	2.00	24.80	4.10
5	130.23	5.00	4.00	3.12	2.98
6	105.00	3.32	4.00	35.30	5.34
7	105.00	5.00	4.00	28.30	4.46
8	120.00	6.00	6.00	9.72	3.30
9	120.00	6.00	2.00	6.83	4.29
10	105.00	5.00	0.64	36.78	6.37
11	105.00	5.00	7.36	41.18	4.56
12	105.00	5.00	4.00	28.40	4.49
13	79.77	5.00	4.00	33.90	7.19
14	90.00	6.00	6.00	30.06	6.04
15	120.00	4.00	6.00	17.91	3.66
16	105.00	6.68	4.00	25.50	4.83
17	105.00	5.00	4.00	28.35	4.40
18	90.00	6.00	2.00	38.78	5.89
19	105.00	5,00	4,00	28,50	4.40
20	90.00	4.00	2.00	33.33	5.15

It illustrates that the two fitted models are significant with 95% confidence intervals (p-value < 0.05).

Figure 1 represents predicted against actual values for survival and moisture content of *B. bifidum*, respectively. Actual values are the measured response data for a particular run, and the predicted values are evaluated using the approximating functions generated for the models (Eqs. (2)–(3)).

The fit quality of the second-order polynomial models equations (Eqs. (2)–(3)) were expressed by the coefficient of determination (R^2). The value of R^2 indicates that the quadratic equation is capable of representing the system under the given experimental domain. The coefficients of determination (R^2) of the models were 0.92 for Y_1 and 0.91 for Y_2, which further indicates that the models (Eqs. (1)–(2)) were suitable for adequate representation of the real relationships among the variables. Since R^2 and adjusted- R^2 differ insignificantly, there is a good chance that the models include the important terms. Adequate precision is a measure of the range in predicted response relative to its associated error which provides a measure of the "signalto-noise ratio". Its desired value is 4 or more [24]. In the present study, adequate precision was 13.24 for survival and 11.87 for moisture. Simultaneously, low values of the coefficient of variation (CV) (14.82 for survival and 9.16 for moisture)

indicated good precision and reliability of the experiments. The CV as the ratio of the standard error of estimate to the mean-value of the observed response (as a percentage) was used as a measure of reproducibility of the model. All results showed that this model can be used to navigate the space defined by the CCD.

The p-value was used as a tool to check the significance of each coefficient. Low p-values indicate that the factor has a significant effect on results. A model term with a p-value < 0.05 is considered to be significant [28]. According to the p-values of the model terms (Table 3), A (Inlet air temperature), B (air pressure), interaction variable AB (Inlet air temperature × air pressure) and quadratic variable A^2 are significant terms in the Survival of *B. bifidum* model. Furthermore, the only significant factor in moisture content of *B. bifidum* model is A (Inlet air temperature).

A negative sign for the coefficients of factors in the fitted models for Y_1 and Y_2 (Eq. 2 and 3) indicated that the level of the Survival of *B. bifidum* and the moisture content of *B. bifidum* increased with decreasing levels of factors. Also, the greatest coefficients of factor A (Inlet air temperature) revealed the high sensitivities of the both responses to this factor. Additionally the survival rate of *B. bifidum* was inversely proportional to air pressure and maltodextrin conc., but it seems that air pressure was

Table 3 Analysis of variance for response surface models

Responses		Sum of square	DOF	Mean square	F-value	P-value
	Model	1835.55	9	203.95	12.77	0.0002
	A-temperature	1142.75	1	1142.75	71.56	<0.0001
	B-pressure	102.32	1	102.32	6.41	0.0298
	C-maltodextrin	5.17	1	5.17	0.32	0.5820
	AB	123.40	1	123.40	7.73	0.0195
Survival (%)	AC	7.61	1	7.61	0.48	0.5058
	BC	2.14	1	2.14	0.13	0.7218
	A^2	320.76	1	320.76	20.09	0.0012
	B^2	3.81	1	3.81	0.24	0.6359
	C^2	91.48	1	91.48	5.73	0.0377
	Residual	159.69	10	15.97		
	Model	20.16	9	2.24	11.57	0.0003
	A-temperature	16.48	1	16.48	85.06	<0.0001
	B-pressure	0.014	1	0.014	0.072	0.7933
	C-maltodextrin	0.79	1	0.79	4.08	0.0711
	AB	0.072	1	0.072	0.37	0.5551
Moisture (%)	AC	0.86	1	0.86	4.43	0.0616
	BC	0.26	1	0.26	1.34	0.2742
	A^2	0.37	1	0.37	1.89	0.1996
	B^2	0.37	1	0.37	1.89	0.1996
	C^2	0.076	1	0.076	2.12	0.1765
	Residual	1.94	10	0.19		

more effective. Analysis of these models (Eq. 3) also showed that low moisture content is due to high maltodextrin conc. or application of high temperature or pressure, although the effect of temperature is significantly higher than other factors. To achieve a proper comprehension of the results, the predicted models are presented in Figure 2. The use of two-dimensional contour plots and three-dimensional surface plots of the regression model was highly recommended to obtain a graphical interpretation of the interactions [22,29].

Figure 2 depicts a three dimensional surface plot of the empirical model for moisture (%) as a function of

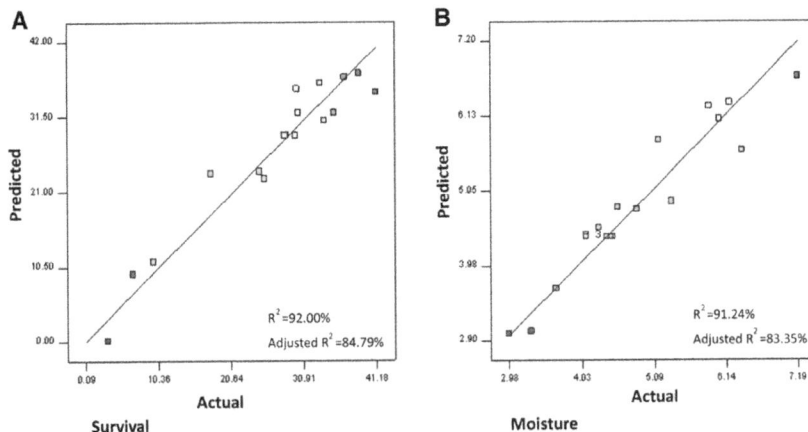

Figure 1 Predicted vs. actual plot of: (A) survival rate and (B) moisture content of *B. bifidum* powder.

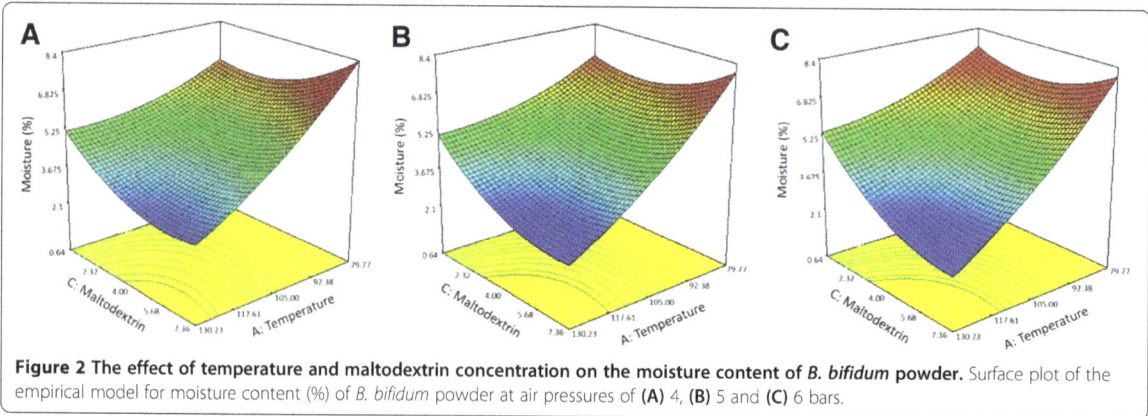

Figure 2 The effect of temperature and maltodextrin concentration on the moisture content of *B. bifidum* powder. Surface plot of the empirical model for moisture content (%) of *B. bifidum* powder at air pressures of **(A)** 4, **(B)** 5 and **(C)** 6 bars.

three factors. Maltodextrin conc. and temperature were used for the RSM plots of moisture (%), while air pressure was increased from 4 bar to 5 bar and then 6 bar from left to right. As shown in Figure 2, at all air pressures, the lowest moisture was achieved at the highest concentrations of maltodextrin (7.36) and temperature (130.23). The results imply the need for application of more maltodextrin for having minimum moisture at the highest temperature. According to the surface plots, at the lowest maltodextrin conc. (0.64) and temperature (79.77) the moisture (%) increased by decreasing the air pressure from left to right. The moisture decreased when at the highest temperature (130.23), maltodextrin conc. increased, and vice versa. It was also true while at the highest conc. of maltodextrin (7.36), the temperature increased to its highest level.

However, at the lowest temperature (79.77), specifically at air pressure ≥5, decreasing the maltodextrin to 4%, resulted in lower moisture content, which may have been due to the more inhibitory effect of the maltodextrin concentration at air pressure ≥5. These results indicate that the measure of maltodextrin was critical for moisture of powder, which depends on inlet air temperature and air pressure.

The dependence of the survival of *B. bifidum* on temperature and air pressure at 4% maltodextrin is depicted in Figure 3. The survival rate of *B. bifidum* increased linearly as pressure was increased from 4 to 6 at temperature ≤105°C. At temperature >105°C, survival of *B. bifidum* increased linearly as pressure decreased from 6 to 4 bar. Therefore the effect of pressure on survival of *B. bifidum* depends on the operational temperature. A curvature type relationship existed between the survival of *B. bifidum* and the temperature at the lowest pressure (4 bar), survival of *B. bifidum* increased by increasing the temperature toward 105°C. Furthermore increasing the temperature resulted in lower bacterial survival rate. As shown in Figure 3, the highest survival rate of *B. bifidum* was achieved at high pressure (6 bar) and low temperature (79.77).

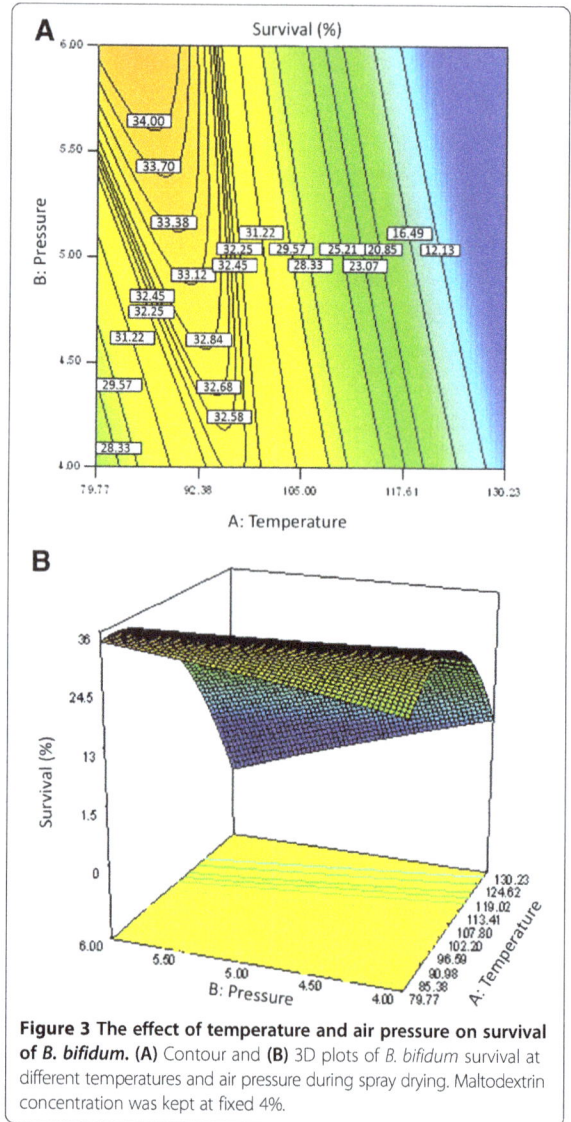

Figure 3 The effect of temperature and air pressure on survival of *B. bifidum*. (A) Contour and **(B)** 3D plots of *B. bifidum* survival at different temperatures and air pressure during spray drying. Maltodextrin concentration was kept at fixed 4%.

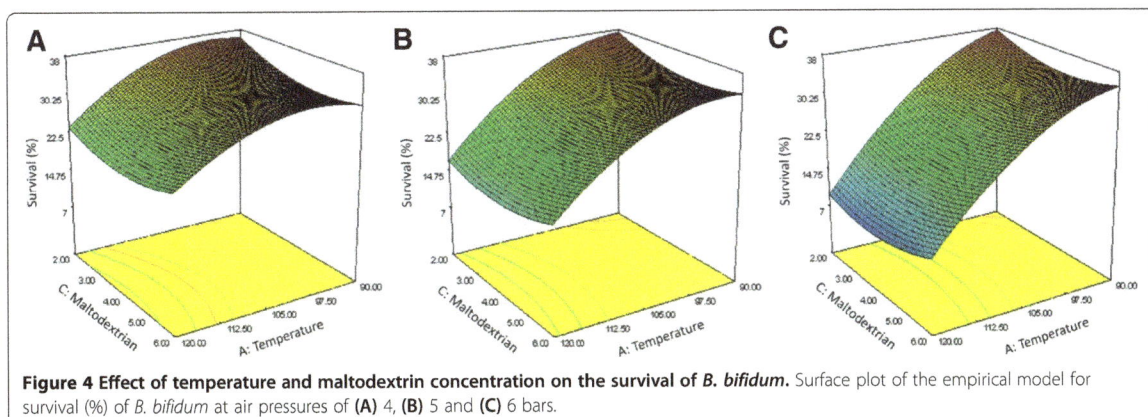

Figure 4 Effect of temperature and maltodextrin concentration on the survival of *B. bifidum*. Surface plot of the empirical model for survival (%) of *B. bifidum* at air pressures of **(A)** 4, **(B)** 5 and **(C)** 6 bars.

Figure 4 shows the effect of temperature and maltodextrin concentration on the survival of *B. bifidum*. The air pressure ranged from 4 bar to 6 bar from left to right. At the lowest temperature, particularly at air pressure ≥5, the survival rate was decreased by increasing the maltodextrin concentration to 5%. These results suggests maltodextrin content could highly affect survival of *B. bifidum* and low maltodextrin content could result to higher humidity of probiotic powder. Hence, maltodextrin concentration higher than 5% is highly recommended.

Optimization
A simultaneous optimization technique was used for optimization of multiple responses by RSM. The objective of response surface optimization is to find a desirable location in the design space. Various optimum conditions can be considered, but the main goal of current experiment was to achieve maximal bacterial survival rate and keeping the moisture at as low as possible. According to numerical optimization by Design-Expert 7.0.0, the optimum was obtained by using the following spray drying conditions: inlet air temperature of 111.15°C, air pressure of 4.5 bar and maltodextrin conc. of 6.0%. Under these conditions, the survival of *B. bifidum* was 28.38% while the moisture content of the powder remained at 4.05%. These values are all in agreement with the results obtained from the three-dimensional surface plots.

Table 4 presents the results confirmation test and shows that verification experiments and predicted values from fitted correlations were in close agreement at a 95% confidence interval. These results confirmed the validity of the models.

The role of other culture media substances during spray draying
The main goal of current study was to achieve a high bacterial survival rate using cost effective media suitable for industrial scale production of probiotic powder. Both sucrose and glucose showed similar effect on bacterial growth but glucose did not have the protective effect of sucrose during spray drying. Previous studies used RSM as the carbon source for bacterial growth and also key protective substance in spray drying of bacteria. In current study RSM was replaced by inexpensive permeate. It owns all beneficial features of RSM and also contains vitamins like thiamine, riboflavin and niacin which are required for the growth of *B. bifidum*. Permeate was found to be the ideal medium for spray drying due to its protective proteins which prevent bacterial damage by stabilizing cell membrane components [30]. In addition, its calcium may form a protective layer. The solid ratio index was 20% for permeate, maltodextrin, sucrose and yeast extract had the best effect in bacterial count which is consistent with those reported by previous studies [31].

Different types of probiotic adherent fibers such as fructo-oligosaccharide (FOS) and galacto-oligosaccharide (GOS) are usually used as a carrier in the culture medium of bifidobacteria and lactobacilli during spray and freeze drying. Maltodextrin was used in the culture medium as the adhesion agent. Despite the structural

Table 4 Optimum process and validation experiment results at 95% confidence interval

Responses	Target	Predicted results	Confirmation test results	95% CI low	95% CI high
Survival (%)	Maximize	28.38	29.78	23.95	32.83
Moisture (%)	Minimize	4.05	4.26	3.56	4.54

and functional similarities of maltodextrinwith dextrose, maltodextrin protects bacteria much better than Polydextrose at the high temperature and pressure and has the advantage of cost-effectiveness compared to inulin [32]. It has also been considered as prebiotic which stimulates probiotic growth.

Role of spray dryer factors
The results showed that air temperature had the main effect on residual moisture of bacterial products, as well as bacterial survival rate. Since bacteria are exposed to outlet temperature in different parts of spray dryer, it should not be above 75°C which causes serious damage to susceptible bacteria during spray drying process. Also it should not be too low (below 60°C) which could end up with high moisture content (up 7%). Protective effects of polysaccharides are due to the ability of the sugars to form a high viscous glassy matrix during dehydration. Moisture uptake would decrease the glass transition temperatures of the system, and consequently a transition of the glass state of sugar towards the rubbery state (denitrification) could occur which might decrease the stability of spray dried powder. Therefore, the best moisture content of 4-7%, was achieved in the outlet temperature of 60-80°C.

Conclusions
Statistical modeling and optimization of spray drying of *Bifidobacterium bifidum* PTCC 1644 was investigated. The thermal compliances of an acid-bile-adopted probiotic strain was increased to 75°C using induced environmental stress condition. Permeate and maltodextrin were used as the protecting agents instead of reconstituted skim milk reported by other researchers. The RSM-CCD was used for statistical analysis and optimization of the process. The effect of inlet air temperature, air pressure and maltodextrin concentrations on survival and moisture of spray dried *B. bifidum* were assessed. Two quadratic models for the responses were developed. Temperature had the most significant effect on spray drying of *B.bifidum*. Maximum survival rate of 28.38% and minimum moisture content of 4.05% was achieved at $T = 111.15°C$, $P = 4.5$ bar and maltodextrin content of 6%.

Powders of live beneficial probiotic bacterial cultures could be achieved by preadaptation of the individual strains to gastrointestinal as well as other environmental factors and further addition of selected protective polysaccharides into the culture media before spray drying.

Competing interests
The authors declare that they have no competing interests.

Authors' contributions
ZS carried most of the experimentals as her MSc thesis. MRF was the supervisor of the thesis and proposed the research subject and contributed in writing the manuscript. MA was the consultant of the thesis and has

contributed in writing. SMM has done the statistics. KG has supervised the spray drying work. All authors read and approved the final manuscript.

Acknowledgment
The authors wish to thank the Pharmaceutical Sciences Research Center of the Tehran University of Medical Sciences for partially financing this project The authors are grateful to Stat-Ease, Minneapolis, MN, USA, for the provision of the Design-Expert 7.1.4 package.

Author details
[1]Department of Chemical Engineering, Islamic Azad University-Tehran South Branch, Tehran, Iran. [2]Probiotic Research Laboratory, Department of Drug and Food Control, Pharmaceutical Sciences Research Center, Faculty of Pharmacy, Tehran University of Medical Sciences, Tehran, Iran. [3]Biotechnology Group, Chemical Engineering Department, Tarbiat Modares University, Tehran, Iran. [4]Aerosol Research Laboratory, Department of Pharmaceutics, Faculty of Pharmacy, Tehran University of Medical Sciences, Tehran, Iran.

References
1. Anal AK, Singh H. Recent advances in microencapsulation of probiotics for industrial applications and targeted delivery. Trends Food Sci Tech. 2007;18:240–51.
2. Agrawal R. Probiotics: an emerging food supplement with health benefits. Food Biotechnol. 2005;19:227–46.
3. Dave RI, Shah NP. Evaluation of media for selective enumeration of S. thermophilus, L. delbrueckii ssp. bulgaricus, L. acidophilus, and bifidobacteria. J Dairy Sci. 1996;79:1529–36.
4. Fazeli MR, Hajimohammadali M, Moshkani A, Samadi N, Jamalifar H, Khoshayand MR Vaghari E, et al. Aflatoxin B1 binding capacity of autochthonous strains of lactic acid bacteria. J Food Protect. 2009;72:189–92.
5. Fazeli MR, Toliyat T, Samadi N, Hajjaran S, Jamalifar H. Viability of Lactobacillus acidophilus in various tablet formulations. DARU. 2006;14:172–8.
6. To BCS, Etzel MR. Spray drying, freeze drying, or freezing of three different lactic acid bacteria species. J Food Sci. 1997;62:576–8.
7. Menshutina N, Gordienko M, Voinovskiy A. Spray drying of probiotics: process development and scale-up. Drying Tech. 2010;28:1170–7.
8. Gardiner GE, O'Sullivan E, Kelly J, Auty MAE, Fitzgerald GF, Collins JK, et al. Comparative survival rates of human-derived probiotic Lactobacillus paracasei and L. salivarius strains during heat treatment and spray drying. Appl Environ Microbiol. 2000;66:2605–12.
9. Ananta E, Volkert M, Knorr D. Cellular injuries and storage stability of spray dried Lactobacillus rhamnosus GG. Int Dairy J. 2005;15:399–409.
10. Brodhead J, Rhodes CT. The drying of pharmaceuticals. Drug Dev Ind Pharm. 1992;12:1169–206.
11. Silva J, Carvalho AS, Teixera P, Gibbs P. Effect of stress on cells of Lactobacillus delbrueckii spp. bulgaricus. J Food Tech. 2005;3:479–90.
12. Roos YH. Importance of glass transition and water activity to spray drying and stability of dairy powders. Lait. 2002;82:475–84.
13. Jouppila K, Roos YH. Glass transitions and crystallization in milk powders. J Dairy Sci. 1994;77:2907–15.
14. Heidebach T, Först P, Kulozik U. Influence of casein-based microencapsulation on freeze-drying and storage of probiotic cells. J Food Eng. 2010;98:309–16.
15. Jamalifar H, Bigdeli B, Nowroozi J, Zolfaghari HS, Fazeli MR. Selection for autochthonous bifidobacterial isolates adopted to simulated gastrointestinal fluid. DARU. 2010;18:57–63.
16. Jewell JB, Kashket ER. Osmotically regulated transport of prolin by Lactobacillus acidophilus IFO3532. Appl Environ Microbiol. 1991;57:2829–33.
17. Johnson JAC, Etzel MR. Properties of Lactobacillus helveticus CNRZ-32 attenuated by spray-drying, freeze-drying, or freezing. J Dairy Sci. 1995;78:761–8.
18. Santhiya D, Ting YP. Bioleaching of spent refinery processing catalyst using Aspergillus niger with high yield oxalic acid. J Biotechnol. 2005;116:171–84.
19. Chauhan K, Trivedi U, Patel KC. Statistical screening of medium components by lackett–Burman design for lactic acid production by Lactobacillus sp. KCP01 using date juice. Bioresour Technol. 2007;98:98–103.
20. Mehrabani JV, Noaparast M, Mousavi SM, Dehghan R, Ghorbani A. Process optimization and modelling of sphalerite flotation from a low-grade

Zn–Pboreusing response surface methodology. Sep Purif Technol. 2010;72:242–9.

21. Liu RS, Tang YJ. Melanosporum fermentation medium optimization by Plackett–Burman design coupled with Draper–Lin small composite design and desirability function. Bioresour Technol. 2010;101:3139–46.

22. Majumder A, Goyal A. Enhanced production of exocellular glucansucrose from *Leuconostoc dextranicum* NRRL B-1146 using response surface method. Bioresour Technol. 2008;99:3685–91.

23. Montgomery DC. Design and Analysis of Experiments. 4th ed. New York: John Wiley & Sons; 1991.

24. Myers RH, Montgomery DC. Response surface methodology. 3rd ed. New York: John Wiley & Sons; 2002.

25. Bas D, Boyaci IH. Modeling and optimization I: Usability of response surface methodology. J Food Eng. 2007;78:836–45.

26. Bezera MA, Santelli RE, Oliveira EP, Villar LS, Escaleira LA. Review response surface methodology (RSM) as a tool for optimization in analytical chemistry. Talanta. 2008;76:965–77.

27. RehCh N, Bhat SH, Berrut S. Determination of water content in powdered milk. Food Chem. 2004;86:457–64.

28. Tanyildizi MS, Ozer D, Elibol M. Optimization of a-amylase production by *Bacillus sp.* using response surface methodology. Process Biochem. 2005;40:2291–6.

29. Sharma S, Malik A, Satya S. Application of response surface methodology (RSM) for optimization of nutrient supplementation for Cr (VI) removal by *Aspergillus lentulus AML05*. J Hazard Mater. 2009;164:1198–204.

30. Teixeira PC, Castro MH, Malcata FX, Kirby RM. Survival of *Lactobacillus-Delbrueckii ssp. bulgaricus* following spray-drying. J Dairy Sci. 1995;78:1025–31.

31. Corcoran BM, Ross RP, Fitzgerald G, Stanton C, Corcoran BM, Ross RP, et al. Comparative survival of probiotic lactobacilli spray dried in the presence of prebiotic substances. J Appl Microbiol. 2004;96:1024–39.

32. Bielecka M, Majkowska A. Effect of spray drying temperature of yoghurt on the survival of starter cultures, moisture content and sensoric properties of yoghurt powder. Nahrung. 2000;44:257–60.

Cardanol isolated from Thai Apis mellifera propolis induces cell cycle arrest and apoptosis of BT-474 breast cancer cells via p21 upregulation

Sureerat Buahorm[1], Songchan Puthong[2], Tanapat Palaga[3], Kriengsak Lirdprapamongkol[4], Preecha Phuwapraisirisan[5], Jisnuson Svasti[4] and Chanpen Chanchao[6*]

Abstract

Background: Cardanol was previously reported to be an antiproliferative compound purified from Thai *Apis mellifera* propolis. By morphology, it could induce the cell death to many cancer cell lines but not the control (non-transformed human foreskin fibroblast cell line, Hs27). Here, it was aimed to evaluate the molecular effects of cardanol on breast cancer derived cell line (BT-474).

Methods: Morphological changes in BT-474 cells induced by cardanol compared to doxorubicin were evaluated by light microscopy, cytotoxicity by using the 3- (4, 5-dimethyl-thiazol-2-yl) 2, 5-diphenyl-tetrazolium bromide (MTT) assay, induction of cell cycle arrest and cell death by flow cytometric analysis of propidium iodide and annexin-V stained cells, and changes in the expression level of genes involved in the control of apoptosis and the cell cycle by quantitative reverse transcriptase-PCR (qRT-PCR) and western blot analyses.

Results: It revealed that cardanol induced a time- and dose-dependent cytotoxicity along with cell shrinkage and detachment from substratum. Cardanol caused cell cycle arrest at the G_1 subphase (as opposed to at the G_2/M subphase seen with doxorubicin) and cell death by late apoptosis, with both late apoptosis (27.2 ± 1.1 %) and necrosis (25.4 ± 1.4 %) being found in cardanol treated cells after 72 h, compared to a lower proportion of apoptosis (4.3 ± 0.4 %) and higher proportion of necrosis (35.8 ± 13.0 %) induced by doxorubicin. Moreover, cardanol changed the transcript expression levels of genes involved in the control of apoptosis (increased *DR5* and *Bcl-2* expression and decreased *Mcl-1*, *MADD* and *c-FLIPP*) and cell division (increased p21 and E2FI and decreased cyclin D1, cyclin E, CDK4 and CDK2 expression), as well as increasing the level of p21 p-ERK, p-JNK and p-p38 and decreasing cyclin D. This accounts for the failure to progress from the G_1 to the S subphase.

Conclusion: Cardanol is a potential chemotherapeutic agent for breast cancer.

Keywords: *Apis mellifera*, Cardanol, Cell arrest, Cell death, p21, Propolis

* Correspondence: chanpen@sc.chula.ac.th
[6]Department of Biology, Faculty of Science, Chulalongkorn University, 254 Phayathai Road, Bangkok 10330, Thailand
Full list of author information is available at the end of the article

Background

Propolis, one of honeybee products, has mostly been used in traditional medicine. As known, the components and properties of propolis mainly depend on the geographic location and bee species. For example, the propolis derived from bees foraging on poplar (*Populus nigra* L.) was found to consist of plant resin (50 %), wax (30 %), oil (10 %), pollen (5 %) and other components (5 %) [1].

Propolis has been reported to show many bioactivities, including antibacterial, antiviral, anti-inflammatory and antioxidant activities [2–5]. These reports have typically presented the potential of propolis in the form of either crude or purified extracts/compounds and assayed in either an in vitro or an in vivo model. Also, it was linked to the regulation of gene expression in many types of cells like macrophages, spleenocyte cells and human monocytes [6, 7].

Interestingly, propoelix™, a water-soluble extract of propolis, has been used successfully in the treatment of patients with dengue hemorrhagic fever [8]. In addition, propolis has been reported to be a very rich source of polyphenolic compounds, flavonoids and fatty acids [9]. For example, baccharin isolated from Brazillian propolis and its analogs were able to inhibit aldo-keto reductase 1C3 (AKR1C3), which is involved in castration resistant prostate cancer [10]. The administration of caffeic acid phenethyl ester (CAPE) at 5 μM/kg in mice by intraperitoneal injection showed anti-depressant activity in mice receiving chronic unpredictable stress for 21 consecutive days. Downregulation of p38MAPK phosphorylation by CAPE, which contributed to enhance glucocorticoid receptor function, has also been reported [11].

The molecular mechanism of those active compounds has been revealed, or at least in part. For example, CAPE (25 μM) induces apoptosis in the HeLa cervical cancer cell line (ME 180) and induces cell cycle arrest at the S and G_2/M subphases. The expression level of the E2F-1 target gene, cyclin A, cyclin E, apoptosis protease activating of factor-1 (Apaf-1) and myeloid leukemia cell differentiation protein (Mcl-1) were upregulated but cyclin B was down-regulated [12].

In addition, chrysin significantly reduced the serum levels of the pro-inflammatory cytokines IL-1β and IL-6 in high fat diet/streptozotocin -induced type 2 diabetic rats. Since these pro-inflammatory cytokines, along with especially TNF-α, have an important function in insulin resistance and inflammatory responses, chrysin could be a new target for the treatment of type 2 diabetes [13].

Cardanol, a phenolic compound found in members of the cashew tree (Anacardiaceae) family, has been associated with diverse biological effects, such as antiproliferative, antimicrobial and antioxidant activities [14–17].

However, the molecular mode of action of cardanol is unknown. In this research, the BT-474 cell line, as an in vitro breast cancer model, was focused because it is the leading cause of death in Thai women [18]. Here, the induction of cell cycle arrest as well as program cell death was reported. The change in the expression level of genes that control these functions was also investigated. Finally, a molecular mechanism of cardanol action on the BT-474 cell line is proposed.

Methods

Preparation of propolis

Propolis from *Apis mellifera* was collected from the hives at a bee farm in Pua district, Nan province, Thailand in January, 2012. It was wrapped in aluminum foil and kept in the dark at −20 °C until used. The extraction and enrichment to apparent homogeneity of cardanol from the propolis, along with the one-dimensional thin layer chromatography (1D-TLC), was performed as previously reported [14].

Cell culture

The BT-474 cells (ATCC no. HTB 20) was cultured in complete medium (CM) comprised of Roswell Park Memorial Institute (RPMI) 1640 medium containing 5 % (v/v) fetal calf serum. Cells were seeded at 1×10^5 cells/5 ml CM/ 25-cm^2 flask and incubated at 37 °C with 5 % (v/v) CO_2. Cells were re-passaged when they reached 70–80 % confluency.

Cytotoxicity

Cytotoxicity was evaluated indirectly from MTT assay. Thus, the results are influenced by changes in the average cell proliferation rate and/or cell viability, and the reduction in the total number of viable cells is herein referred to as the cytotoxicity without delineation of these two components. BT-474 cells (5 10^3 cells in 198 μl) were seeded in each well of a 96 well plate, and incubated at 37 °C with 5 % (v/v) CO_2 for 24 h. Then 2 μl of cardanol or doxorubicin, dissolved in dimethylsulfoxide (DMSO) to a concentration of 10000, 1000, 100, 10, 1 and 0.1 μg/ml for cardanol and 50 μg/ml for doxorubicin, was added to the wells in triplicate, along with DMSO only (2 μl/well) as the solvent (no treatment) control. The cells were then incubated for 72 h before 10 μl of 5 mg/ml of MTT solution was added to each well and incubated for another 4 h. After that, the media was removed and replaced with 150 μl of DMSO and 25 μl of 0.1 M glycine and gently aspirated to lyse the cells and dissolve the formazan crystals. The absorbance was then measured at 540 nm (A_{540}) by a microplate reader. Setting the total number of viable cells in the control culture to be 100 %, the relative percentage of viable cells was calculated from Eq. (1):

$$\text{Relative number of viable cells} = (A_{540} \text{of sample} / A_{540} \text{of control}) \times 100 \quad (1)$$

The concentration of the test compound that caused a 50 % maximal inhibition of the viable cell number (IC_{50}) was derived from the graphical plot of the relative number of viable cells *vs.* test compound concentration.

Growth curve of BT-474 cells

BT-474 cells treated with solvent only (control) or with cardanol at the IC_{50} value (15.6 ± 1.76 µg/ml) were assayed for the relative number of viable cells using the MTT assay after 1, 2, 3, 5 and 7 d of culture. The graph of relative number of viable cells *vs.* time was drawn, where the trend line was compared to the control cell line.

Cell morphology

BT-474 cells (2×10^5 cells/ml) were cultured in CM with the addition of (i) the DMSO solvent only (Control), (ii) 30 µg/ml of cardanol and (iii) 0.5 µg/ml of doxorubicin (positive control). The morphology of the cells was observed after 0, 24, 48, 72 and 96 h incubation using inverted light microscope (Ziess, Jena) connected to a digital camera (Canon EOS 7D, Tokyo).

Detection of apoptosis and necrosis

BT-474 cells ($3–5 \times 10^6$ cells/ml) were cultured in CM with the addition of (i) the DMSO solvent only (Control), (ii) 30 µg/ml of cardanol and (iii) 0.5 µg/ml of doxorubicin (positive control). After the indicated time in culture (24–72 h) the cells were harvested by centrifugation ($3000 \times g$, 4 °C for 10 min), washed in 1 ml of cold 1 x phosphate buffer saline (PBS) and harvested as before. The pellet was resuspended in 50 µl of $1 \times$ binding buffer pH 7.4 (10 mM Hepes, 140 mM NaCl and 2.5 mM $CaCl_2$) and stained with the addition 1 µl of annexin V (Alexa Fluor 488 conjugate, Life Technologies, Carlsbad, CA) and 5 µl of 1 mg/ml propidium iodide (PI) solution (Sigma Aldrich, St. Louis, MO) in the dark at room temperature (RT) for 30 min. Cells were then analyzed by flow cytometry on a FC 500 MPL cytometer (Beckman Coulter, Brea, CA) recording 2 events (cells).

Detection of cell cycle arrest

BT-474 cells ($1–100 \times 10^6$ cells/ml) were cultured in CM with the addition of (i) the DMSO solvent only (Control), (ii) 30 µg/ml of cardanol and (iii) 0.5 µg/ml of doxorubicin (positive control) for 24, 48 and 72 h and then harvested and washed as above. The cell pellet was resuspended and fixed in 500 µl of cold PBS and 200 µl of 70 % (v/v) ethanol at −20 °C overnight or on ice for

4 h. Cells were then harvested and washed as above and the pellet resuspended in 250 µl of PBS with 0.1 mg/ml RNAse and incubated at 37 °C for 30 min. After harvesting, the cells were resuspended in 12.5 µl of 1 mg/ml PI and incubated at RT in the dark for 30 min before being analyzed by flow cytometry on a FC 500 MPL cytometer (Beckman Coulter) recording 2 events per sample. The obtained linear fluorescence profile was interpreted in terms of the (1) sub G_1 phase (apoptotic cells), (ii) G_1 phase (diploid chromosome content), (iii) S phase (DNA synthesis) and (iv) G_2/M subphase (double diploid).

Change in gene expression levels
Transcript expression levels

BT474 cells were cultured in CM with the addition of (i) the DMSO solvent only (Control), (ii) 30 µg/ml of cardanol and (iii) 0.5 µg/ml of doxorubicin (positive control) for 72 h, and then harvested. Total RNA was then extracted from them using the RNeasy Plus Mini Kit (Qiagen, Hilden) as per the suppliers protocol. The extracted RNA was eluted in 20 µl of RNase-free H_2O and the absorbance at 260 and 280 nm (A_{260} and A_{280}, respectively) was measured. The concentration of RNA was calculated from Eq. (2),

$$\text{Concentration of RNA (µg/ml)} = (A_{260}) \times \text{dilution factor} \times (40). \quad (2)$$

The purity of the extracted RNA was estimated from the A_{260}/A_{280} ratio. The RNA samples were stored at −20 °C until use.

The transcript expression levels of the selected genes were then assayed by single-stage qRT-PCR. Two groups of genes were selected for screening. The first group were the death receptor group of the apoptosis regulated genes *b-cell lymphoma-2* (*Bcl-2*), *Mcl-1*, *mitogen activating protein-kinase activating death domain* (*MADD*), *cellular FLICE-like inhibitory protein* (*c-FLIP*) and *human death receptor 5* (*DR5*). The second group were the cell cycle regulating genes of *p21*, *cyclin D1*, *cyclin E*, *cyclin A*, *cyclin-dependent kinase 4* (*CDK4*), *CDK6* and *CDK2*.

The reaction mixture was prepared using the One Step SYBR PrimeScript RT-PCR Kit II (Takara, Tokyo) as per the manufacturer's protocol. Each qRT-PCR reaction mixture (20 µl final volume) contained total RNA (10 ng), 10 µl of 2x one step SYBR RT-PCR buffer, 1 µl of Prime Script 1 step enzyme mix, 0.5 µl of each gene fragment specific forward and reverse PCR primer (20 µM stock) and RNase-free d-H_2O. The respective forward and reverse primers are listed in Table 1. The PCR thermocycling was performed at 95 °C for 15 min, followed by 40 cycles of 94 °C for 15 s, x °C for 30 s and 72 °C for 30 s, where x is gene specific and is given in Table 1. The relative expression level of each gene was

Table 1 Forward and reverse primers (5' → 3') used in the qRT-PCR

Gene	Nucleotide sequence of F primer	Nucleotide sequence of R primer	Annealing temp. (°C)	Reference
ß-actin	GACCTGACTGACTACCTCATGA	AGCATTTGCGGTGGACGATGGAG	55	Lirdprapamongkol et al. [20]
MADD	TCAACCCACTCATCTATGGCAATG	GCGGAATTGAAGAACCGTACCA	60	Li et al. [36]
c-FLIP	CCAGAGTGTGTATGGTGTGGAT	TCTCCCATGAACATCCTCCTGAT	60	Li et al. [36]
Bcl-2	TGGGATGCGGGAGATGTG	CGGGATGCGGCTGGAT	60	Li et al. [36]
Mcl-1	AGCAGAGGAGGAGGAGGAC	GCCTGCTCCCGAAGGTA	55	Lirdprapamongkol et al. [20]
DR5	TGCTGCTCAAGTGGCGC	GGCATCCAGCAGATGGTTG	60	Pillai et al. [37]
P21	CACTCCAAACGCCGGCTGATCTTC	TGTAGAGCGGGCCTTTGAGGCCCTC	55	Weglarz et al. [38]
E2F1	GCCACTGACTCTGCCACCA	GGACAACAGCGGTTCTTGCT	60	Galanti et al. [39]
Cyclin A	GAAGACGAGACGGGTTGCA	AGGAGGAACGGTGACATGCT	60	Galanti et al. [39]
Cyclin D1	AATGACCCCGCACGATTTC	TCAGGTTCAGGCCTTGCAC	60	Ullmannova et al. [40]
Cyclin E	TTCTTGAGCAACACCCTCTTCTGCAGCC	TCGCCATATACCGGTCAAAGAAATCTTGTGCC	58	Potemski et al. [41]
CDK2	TTTGGAGTCCCTGTTCGTAC	TGCGATAACAAGCTCCGTCC	58	Chiang et al. [42]
CDK4	CTTTGACCTGATTGGGCTGC	GGAGAGGTGGGAGGGGAATG	58	Chiang et al. [42]
CDK6	TCTTGCTCCAGTCCAGCTAC	AGCAATCCTCCACAGCTCTG	60	Ullmannova et al. [40]

normalized to the expression level of the ß-actin gene as an internal control. The crossing point (Cp) was used to calculated the relative gene expression level as per Eq. (3),

$$\text{Relative expression level} = 2^{(\text{Cp actin}-\text{Cp target})}. \quad (3)$$

The Cp value is correlated to the amount of the initial template and so indicates the expression of the target mRNA [19].

Protein expression levels

Changes in the expression level of selected proteins were evaluated by western blot analysis following the protocol of Lirdprapamongkol et al. [20] with slight modification. BT-474 cancer cells (2×10^5 cells/ml) were cultured in CM with the addition of (i) the DMSO solvent only (Control), (ii) cardanol at the 2x IC_{50} concentration (30 µg/ml) and (iii) 0.5 µg/ml of doxorubicin (positive control) for 24 h. Cells were then harvested and lysed in 150 µl of radioimmunoprecipitation assay buffer, which contained 1x halt protease phosphatase and phosphatase inhibitor cocktail with EDTA (Thermo Scientific, Waltham, MA), on ice. The concentration of protein in the lysate was measured by the Bradford assay.

Twenty µg of protein was loaded per well of a sodium dodecyl sulfate polyacrylamide gel (SDS-PAGE) with a 7 and 4 % (w/v) acrylamide separating and stacking gel, respectively. After electrophoresis at 15 mA for 105 min, the protein was transferred to immobilon-P nylon membrane (Millipore, Billerica, MA) by electroblotting at 100 V for 90 min. The membrane was later blocked with 3 % (w/v) bovine serum albumin (BSA) for 1 h with gentle shaking at RT. After that, the membrane was cut and probed with the primary antibodies (Cell Signaling Technology, Danvers, MA) diluted in 3 % (w/v) BSA to 1: 1000 (all except for anti-pERK that was 1: 5000) overnight at 4 °C in the dark. The membrane was washed in 1x TBS/T pH 7.6 (20 mM Tris and 137 mM NaCl) and incubated with the diluted horseradish peroxidase-conjugated secondary antibody (Promega, Fitchburg, WI) in TBS/T containing 5 % (w/v) skim milk (1: 10000 mouse, 1: 5000 rabbit) with gentle shaking at RT for 1 h. The bound secondary antibodies were then visualized using western bright ECL reagents (Advansta, Menlo Park, CA) as per the supplier's protocol and the image was captured using an Image Quant LAS 4000 mini instrument (GE Healthcare Life Sciences, Little Chalfont).

Statistical analysis

Data are expressed as the mean ± one standard deviation (1 S.D.), derived from triplicate replications in each experiment. The data were analyzed by one way analysis of variance (ANOVA) followed by Tukey's test of multiple comparisons to test for the significance of differences in the means. Significance was accepted at the $p < 0.05$ level. All analyses were performed using the SPSS program version 19.0.

Results
Cardanol isolation

Starting with 90 g of *Apis mellifera* propolis, 1.54 g of crude dichloromethane extract (CDE) was obtained and then further fractionated by successive quick column and adsorption column chromatography (CC). The obtained cardanol (0.52 mg) was confirmed from its 1D-TLC derived R_f value [14] and from its mass spectrometry derived spectrum. The IC_{50} value for the cytotoxicity against

BT-474 cells was calculated to be 15.6 ± 1.76 μg/ml (Fig. 1), which was close to the 14.0 ± 1.0 μg/ml previously reported on this cell line [14].

In order to confirm that the BT-474 cells were healthy under these culture conditions and were responsive to cardanol, the growth of BT-474 cells in CM with either DMSO only (solvent control) or with various concentrations of cardanol (0.001–100 μg/ml) was evaluated, and is shown in terms of relative to the initial amount as 100 % (Fig. 1). Among the four phases of a usual growth curve, the total number of viable cells was recorded from the lag phase to the log (exponential growth) phase because treated cells at any cardanol concentration started to die at the end of the log phase. Overall, the inhibition by cardanol was time- and dose-dependent manner.

Morphological changes in BT-474 cells
The morphology of the control BT-474 cells (Fig. 2a) showed no major changes over the 96 h culture period (except for the increased cell density) with most cells being alive, attached to the substratum and flat in appearance. However, the morphology of the cardanol treated cells (IC_{50} concentration of 15.6 ± 1.76 μg/ml) was different, with unattached cells being observed after 48 h incubation, whilst the attached cells had started to shrink and large clumps of cells were observed at 72 h after treatment with markedly lower cell numbers being visible after 96 h (Fig. 2b).

Doxorubicin treatment (0.5 μg/ml) induced broadly similar changes in the BT-474 morphology as those induced by cardanol, except smaller clumps of custard apple shaped cells and a lower number of viable cells was observed (Fig. 2c).

Induction of apoptosis and necrosis
The induction of apoptosis and necrosis in BT-474 cells was determined by the distribution of annexin V and PI stained cells using flow cytometry. Representative flow cytometry dot plots are shown in Additional file 1: Figure S1 in the supplementary information (SI),

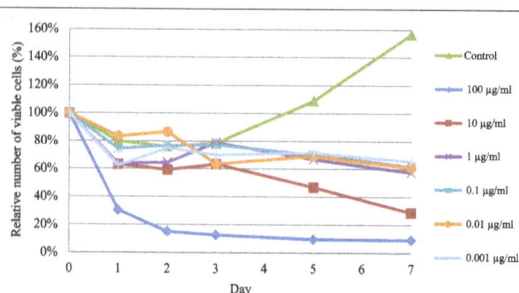

Fig. 1 Growth curve of the solvent only (Control) and cardanol treated (0.001–199 μg/ml) BT-474 cell line. Data are shown as the mean ± 1SD, derived from three independent repeats

whilst the analysis of all three replications is summarized in Fig. 3. The control cells remained largely viable (98 % at 24 h to 78 % at 72 h) with very few apoptotic cells. In contrast, the cardanol (30 μg/ml) treated cells were dead by late apoptosis at 72 h of incubation (27.2 ± 1.1 %), whereas the doxorubicin (0.5 μg/ml) treated cells had mostly died by necrosis from 48 h of incubation (29.9 ± 2.9 %) and this proportion was higher (35.8 ± 13.0 %) after 72 h of incubation. Significant difference between the control and treated cells in both groups could be noticed after 48 h of exposure.

Cell cycle arrest
The cell cycle position, in terms of the interphase subphases G_1, S and G_2/M, were identified by the DNA content as determined by flow cytometric analysis of PI stained cells. Representative histograms (PI fluorescence *vs.* number of cells) are shown in Additional file 2: Figure S2 (SI) and a summary of all the data is shown in Table 2.

For the control cells after 24–72 h culture, around 17–19.3 % of the cells were in the G_2/M phase and 66–71.5 % in the G_1 phase of the cell cycle. Cardanol (30 μg/ml) treatment increased the proportion of cells in the G_1 subphase of the cell cycle compared to the control cells at all three time points, from 66.2 to 72.9 %, 67.2 to 74.6 % and 71.5 to 80.7 % at 24, 48 and 72 h, respectively. Thus, cardanol appeared to induce the cell cycle arrest of BT-474 cells at the G_1 subphase. Furthermore, 0.5 μg/ml doxorubicin increased the proportion of cells in the G_2/M subphase of the cell cycle compared to the control at all three time points, from 19.3 to 20.6 %, 20.1 to 30.0 %, and 17.0 to 41.3 % at 24, 48 and 72 h, respectively. Thus, doxorubicin induced cell cycle arrest of BT-474 cells at the G_2/M subphase.

Changes in gene transcript expression levels
Since 30 μg/ml cardanol induced the late apoptosis of BT-474 cells after 72 h of incubation, total RNA was extracted from BT-474 cells at this period and the transcript level of genes in the apoptosis and cell cycle regulating groups were evaluated by single stage qRT-PCR.

Within the apoptosis regulating genes evaluated, cardanol (30 μg/ml) treatment increased the transcript expression level of *DR5* and *Bcl-2* significantly at $p < 0.01$ but decreased significantly that of *Mcl-1* ($p < 0.01$), *MADD* ($p < 0.01$) and *c-FLIP* ($p < 0.05$). Doxorubicin (0.5 μg/ml) up-regulated the transcript expression level of *Bcl-2* significantly at $p < 0.01$ but down-regulated significantly that of *Mcl-1* ($p < 0.01$), *MADD* ($p < 0.01$), *c-FLIP* ($p < 0.05$) and *DR5* ($p < 0.05$) (Fig. 4a). A significant difference at either $p < 0.01$ or $p < 0.05$ levels was compared between the control and treated cells.

For the cell cycle regulation group of genes evaluated, 30 μg/ml cardanol increased the transcript expression

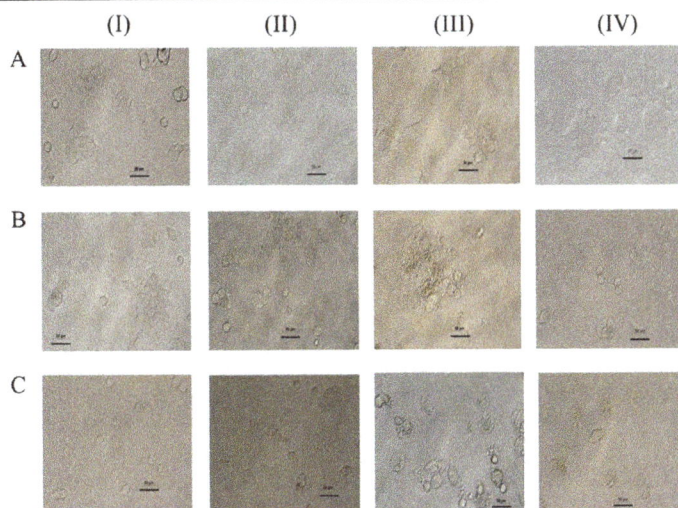

Fig. 2 Morphology of the **a** control BT-474 cells and those treated with **b** cardanol at the IC$_{50}$ concentration (15.6 ± 1.76 µg/ml) and **c** doxorubicin (0.5 µg/ml) for (I) 24 h, (II) 48 h, (III) 72 h and (IV) 96 h of incubation. The scale bar represents 50 µM. The arrow indicates custard apple shaped cells. All images were magnified at 200 x and are representative of at least 3 such fields of view per sample and three independent repeats

level of *p21* and *E2F1* but decreased that of *cyclin D1*, *cyclin E*, *CDK4* and *CDK2* significantly at $p < 0.01$, whilst 0.5 µg/ml doxorubicin up-regulated significantly *E2F1*, *p21*, *cyclin A*, *CDK6* and *CDK2* transcript expression levels (Fig. 4b). A significant difference at $p < 0.01$ level was compared between the control and treated cells.

Changes in protein expression levels by western blot analysis

The protein expression levels of ERK, JNK and p38 MAPK plus their phosphorylated (active) forms (p-ERK, p-JNK and p-P38), as well as p21 and cyclin D1 in BT-474 cells was evaluated after a 24 h incubation with or without 30 µg/ml cardanol or 0.5 µg/ml doxorubicin (Fig. 5). Cardanol activated ERK, JNK and p38 MAPK, as seen by the increased expression levels of the phosphorylated forms of these three proteins. The increased phosphorylation of ERK, JNK and p38 MAPK, and so their active enzyme levels, is likely to have caused the increased the p21 and cyclin D1 expression levels. Overall, the results strongly suggested that the G$_1$ subphase arrest induced by cardanol was mediated by activation of the MAPK-p21 pathway.

Discussion

Bees collect nectar, bee pollen and resin from different plants and so many compounds can found in bee products. For example, α-pinene was reported to be the major compound in European propolis, and it originated from many plant species, including coniferous species like *Cupressus sempervirens* [21]. Moreover, galangin, chrysin and pinocembrin were found to be the main

compounds in Serbian propolis, and were similar to the composition of the resin in poplar trees that are widely distributed in Europe [22]. The propolis from Hungary, Bulgaria, France and Northern Italy were all found to contain resin from poplar trees as well, although the major compounds found in those propolis types were the non-terpenic compounds of benzyl alcohol and benzyl benzoate [23]. Benzyl benzoate was not detected in the volatile oils of poplar buds, although this might reflect differences in the volatiles of different poplar subspecies. Thus, the bud exudates of even of the same species can demonstrate quantitative variability.

Cardanol inhibited the growth of BT-474 cells in a time- and dose-dependent manner (Fig. 1), which is broadly consistent with other reports. For example, the CEE of propolis harvested from many regions in Korea inhibited the angiogenesis, as in tube formation of human umbilical vein endothelial cells (HUVECs), in a dose-dependent manner (6.25–25 µg/ml) [24]. In addition, the CEE of propolis from the Uijeongbu and Pyoseon regions significantly suppressed the proliferation of HUVECs in a dose dependent manner (3.13–25 µg/ml) [24].

Considering the induction of apoptosis by cardanol (Fig. 3 and Additional file 1: Figure S1), cardanol killed BT-474 cells at the late apoptosis (apoptosis and necrosis) stage, which was somewhat similar to doxorubicin, a currently used chemotherapeutic drug, although the later had a higher proportion of necrotic cells. The induction of apoptosis like this is commonly found in compounds purified from natural products, including chemotherapeutic drugs. In addition to propolis, Tualang honey induced late apoptosis in human breast adenocarcinoma (MCF-7 and

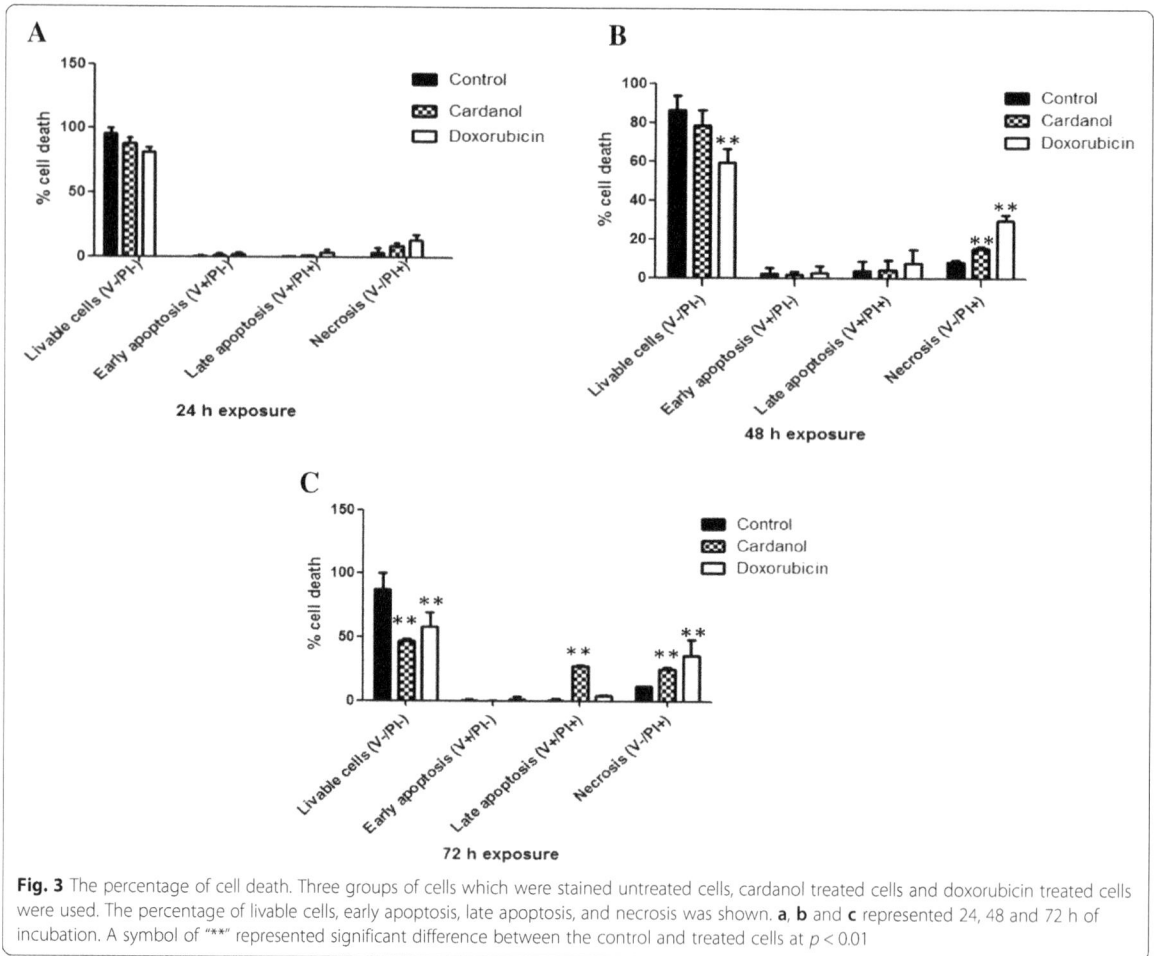

Fig. 3 The percentage of cell death. Three groups of cells which were stained untreated cells, cardanol treated cells and doxorubicin treated cells were used. The percentage of livable cells, early apoptosis, late apoptosis, and necrosis was shown. **a**, **b** and **c** represented 24, 48 and 72 h of incubation. A symbol of "**" represented significant difference between the control and treated cells at $p < 0.01$

MDA-MB-231) and cervical (HeLa) cancer cell lines with an EC_{50} value of 2.4–2.8 % (v/v) [25]. MDA-MB-231 cells treated with Tualang honey at 24 h showed the highest percentage of late apoptosis at 37.8 %, while for MCF-7 and Hela cells it was 55.6 and 56.2 %, respectively [25].

The mechanism of induction of apoptotic cells has many pathways. In this study, cardanol increased the transcript expression level of the *Bcl-2* and *DR5* apoptosis-related genes but decreased that of *Mcl-1*, *c-FLIP* and

MADD (Figs. 4 and 5), somewhat similar to doxorubicin (positive control). The DR5 protein is an apoptosis inducing membrane receptor for TNF-related apoptosis-inducing ligand, where apoptosis in human renal cancer cells is induced by up-regulation of *DR5* and down-regulation of *c-FLIP* [26]. In addition, the combined treatment with rosiglitazone and TNF-α-related apoptosis inducing ligand (TRAIL) could induce apoptosis in renal cancer cells via induction of *Bcl-2* overexpression [26]. Similarly acrolein can effectively sensitize human renal

Table 2 Summary of the percentage of cells in each interphase subphase of the cell cycle

Subphase	Control			Cardanol treated cells			Doxorubicin treated cells		
	24 h	48 h	72 h	24 h	48 h	72 h	24 h	48 h	72 h
Early G$_1$	1.1 ± 0.7	1.3 ± 0.9	1.1 ± 1.0	1.7 ± 1.2	2.5 ± 0.6	2.0 ± 1.3	2.0 ± 0.9	3.5 ± 1.1	5.3 ± 3.9
G$_1$	66.2 ± 11.4	67.2 ± 6.3	71.5 ± 8.7	72.9 ± 10.2	74.6 ± 3.4	80.7 ± 4.1	59.5 ± 11.5	46.9 ± 3.4	31.8 ± 7.9
S	10.2 ± 1.1	7.7 ± 0.5	7.3 ± 1.7	8.5 ± 4.5	6.5 ± 7.2	5.8 ± 2.2	13.9 ± 1.8	14.4 ± 7.2	14.0 ± 2.2
G$_2$/M	19.3 ± 10.2	20.1 ± 6.5	17.0 ± 8.2	14.3 ± 6.7	13.2 ± 8.2	9.2 ± 5.8	20.6 ± 10.4	30.0 ± 8.2	41.3 ± 1.4

Data are shown as the mean ± 1 SD, derived from three independent repeats

A

B

Fig. 4 The change in transcript expression levels of genes in the **a** death receptor group (apoptosis regulating) and **b** cell cycle regulating genes (transcription factors important for the cell cycle). BT-474 cells were cultured for 72 h in CM with the addition of DMSO only (Control) or 30 µg/ml cardanol or 0.5 µg/ml doxorubicin. Data are shown as the mean ± 1 SD, derived from three independent repeats. Significant difference between the control and treated cells are shown at the (**) $p < 0.01$ and (*) $p < 0.05$ levels

Fig. 5 Western blot analysis of protein expression levels in BT-474 cells after incubation in CM with the addition of DMSO only (Control) or with 30 µg/ml cardanol or 0.5 µg/ml doxorubicin for 24 h. Unphosphorylated and phosphorylated forms (p-) of the ERK, p38 and JNK proteins are shown. The blot shown is representative of those seen from 3 independent repeats

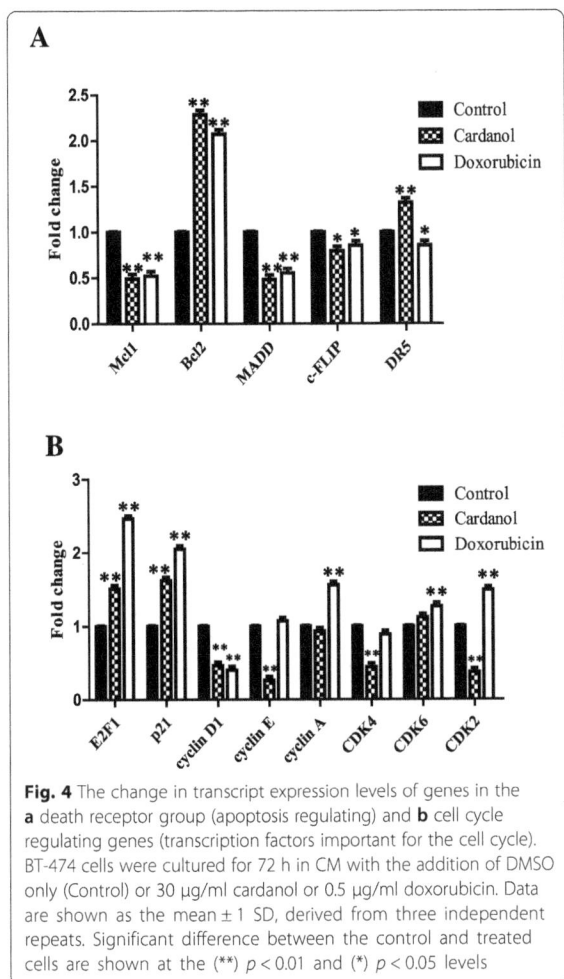

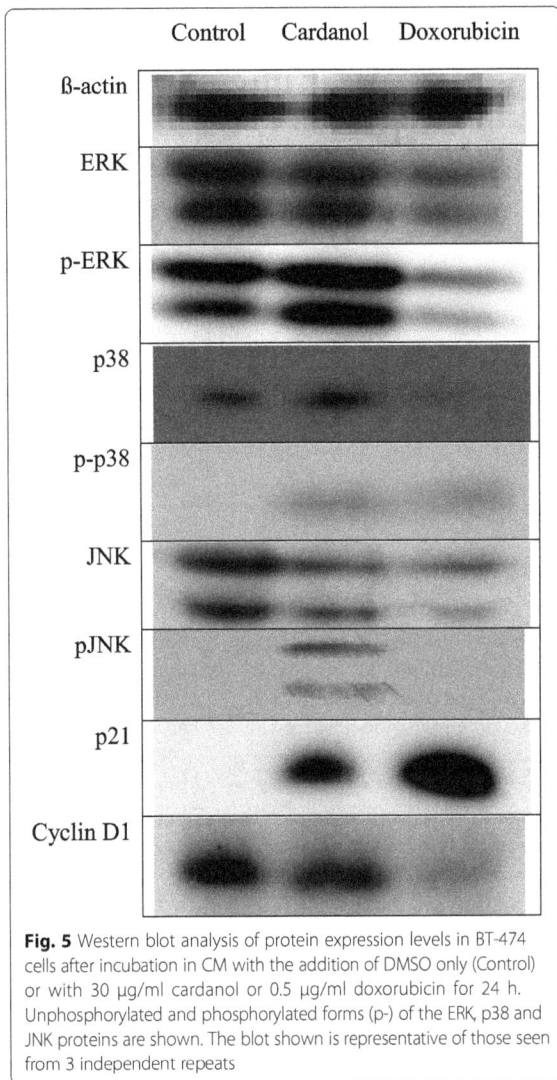

Caki cells to TRAIL-induced apoptosis through down-regulating *Bcl-2* and up-regulating *DR5*, mediated via generation of reactive oxygen species and induction of the C/EBP homologous protein [27]. Thus, lowering the TRAIL resistance or increasing the damage of tumor cells could help in cancer therapy. Moreover, the knockdown of *MADD* and *c-FLIP* reduced the resistance to TRAIL-induced apoptosis in SKOV-3 ovarian cancer cells to 64.2 ± 3.0 % [27].

The Mcl-1 protein is an anti-apoptotic member in the *Bcl-2* family of apoptosis regulating proteins. Benzyl isothiocyanate, an anti-cancer agent, causes G_2/M cell cycle arrest and apoptosis in human leukemia cell lines via the down-regulation of *Mcl-1* [28].

Cardanol appears to arrest BT-474 cells at the G_1 subphase of the cell cycle, somewhat similar to the effect of propolin H from Taiwanese propolis that arrested the human lung carcinoma H460 cell line in the G_1 subphase. Treatment of H460 cells with 40 µM of propolin

H increased the proportion of cells in the G_1 subphase from 57.8 to 75.1 % [29].

Cancer cells display an uncontrolled growth and present abnormal gene expression profiles. The expression level of regulating genes, such as cyclin and CDKs, are typically higher and so induce the cell cycle to move to the next phase. With respect to the effect of cardanol on BT-474 cells, it affected the expression of many genes important for the cell cycle, such as decreasing p21, cyclin D1, cyclin E, CDK2 and CDK4 expression levels and increasing that for p21 and E2F1. These results are in accord with those for CAPE at a concentration of 2.5–80 mg/l that increased the proportion of cells in the G_1 subphase in a dose-dependent manner, and also increased the expression of beta-catenin and decreased the expression of cyclin D1 and c-myc [30]. In addition, a 24 h exposure to CAPE

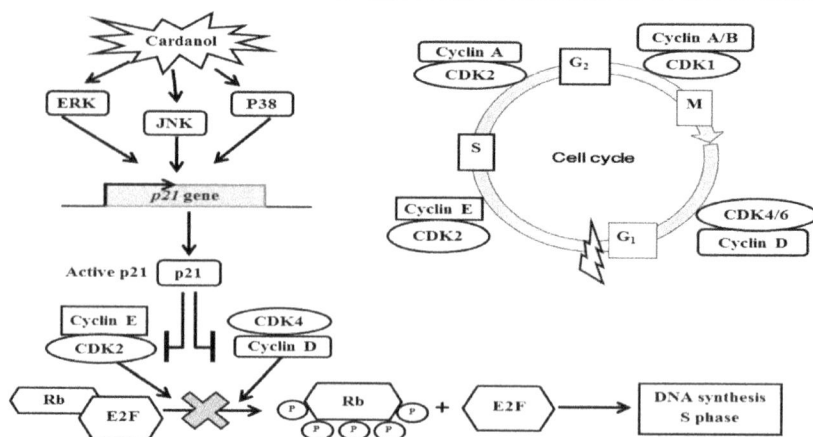

Fig. 6 A model of the mechanism of action of cardanol to induce cell cycle arrest at the G_1 subphase and cell death in BT-474 cancer cells

(50 µg/ml) inhibited the growth of C6 glioma cells, inducing cell cycle arrest at the G_1 subphase after a 24 h incubation, decreasing the CDK2/cyclin E and CDK4/cyclin D activity and inhibiting Rb phosphorylation by increasing p21, p27 and p16 expression [31].

The potential induction of the G_1 cell cycle arrest by cardanol via increasing p21, p-p38 MAPK, p-JNK and p-ERK protein levels was similar to isothiocyanate sulforaphane, a chemotherapeutic drug. The mechanism of SFN on human colon carcinoma HT-29 cells was reported to be mediated via inducing expression of $p21^{CIP1}$ and cyclin D1 through activating the MAPK pathways, including ERK, JNK and p38 [32].

In this report, doxorubicin was used as positive control since its action is already well reported [33]. It is an anthracyline drug extracted from *Streptomyces peucetius var caesivs* and has been used for treatment of diverse cancers, including breast, lung, gastric, ovarian, thyroid, non-Hodgkin's and Hodgkin's lymphoma. The mechanism of action of this drug on cancer inhibition has been described in two pathways. First, it binds to DNA and disrupts topoisomerase II-mediated DNA repair. Second, it produces free radicals and damages the cell membrane, DNA and protein leading to cell death. The data of this research supported the effect of doxorubicin on the BT-474 cell line with a cell cycle arrest at the G_2/M subphase, up-regulated transcript expression levels of *Bcl-2, E2F1, p21, cyclin A, CDK6* and *CDK2* and downregulated expression of *Mcl-1, MADD, c-FLIP* and *cyclin D1*. Thus, doxorubicin is likely to act via inhibiting DNA synthesis through increased p21 and cyclin D1 activities. Moreover, doxorubicin decreased the expression level of the anti-apoptotic genes *Mcl-1* and *c-FLIP*.

In summary, the proposed mechanism of how cardanol could inhibit the growth of BT-474 cells is shown in Fig. 6. In this model, cardanol increases the phosphorylation of ERK, JNK and p38 MAPK leading to p21 activation. Then, the active p21 suppressed CDK4/cyclin D and cyclin E/CDK2 and so prevented the hyperphosphorylation of the retinoblastoma protein. This led to the obstruction of DNA synthesis and prevented the movement of cells into and from the S subphase, causing the G_1 subphase arrest.

However, the data mentioned above were from in vitro only. In the future, primary normal cell culture and animal models must be performed before going forward to human testing. As known, in vitro cultured cells can not represent the whole organism due to lack of precise control of physicochemical surrounding, physiological conditions and so on [34].

In addition, it should be aware of an agent with both anticancer and antioxidant activities. Recently, it has been contradictorily reported whether such compound could be applied to the treatment of cancer [35].

Conclusion

Cardanol, purified from *Apis mellifera* propolis from Nan province, Thailand, had a cytotoxic activity (IC_{50} value of 15.6 ± 1.76 µg/ml) against the BT-474 cell line. The inhibition by cardanol was time- and dose-dependent manner. Morphologically, cardanol treated cells revealed a loss of adhesion and cell shrinking with the formation of large clumps and a reduced number of viable cells. After 72 h, significant numbers of cells were dead by late apoptosis. The change in transcript and protein expression levels of genes involved in apoptosis induction and cell proliferation strongly suggested that the MAPK regulated p21-mediated G_1 phase cell cycle arrest was a mechanism underlying the growth inhibitory effect of cardanol on BT-474 cells.

Additional files

Additional file 1: Program cell death of BT-474 cells. A, B and C represented untreated cells as control, 30 μg/ml cardanol treated cells and 0.5 μg/ml doxorubicin treated cells while I, II and III represented 24, 48 and 72 h of incubation, respectively. Duplication of experiments was done. This figure was from one replication only. (DOCX 91 kb)

Additional file 2: The cell cycle arrest of BT-474 cells. (A) Control, (B) 30 μg/ml cardanol treated and (C) 0.5 μg/ml doxorubicin treated cells after (I) 24 h, (II) 48 h and (III) 72 h of incubation. Histograms shown are derived from 2 events (cells) and are representative of three independent repeats. (DOCX 235 kb)

Competing interests
The authors declare that they have no competing interests.

Authors' contributions
SB conducted the experiments. SP helped in cell culture. TP provided the convenience in using real-time PCR machine and flow cytometry. KL provided advice in western blot analysis. PP provided overall advice in chemistry. JS gave valuable comments and suggestions on the manuscript. CC designed the experiments, provided overall advice in biology and wrote the manuscript. All authors read and approved the final manuscript.

Author details
[1]Program in Biotechnology, Faculty of Science, Chulalongkorn University, 254 Phayathai Road, Bangkok 10330, Thailand. [2]Institute of Biotechnology and Genetic Engineering, Chulalongkorn University, 254 Phayathai Road, Bangkok 10330, Thailand. [3]Department of Microbiology, Faculty of Science, Chulalongkorn University, 254 Phayathai Road, Bangkok 10330, Thailand. [4]Laboratory of Biochemistry, Chulabhorn Research Institute, Vipawadee Rangsit Highway, Bangkok 10210, Thailand. [5]Department of Chemistry, Faculty of Science, Chulalongkorn University, 254 Phayathai Road, Bangkok 10330, Thailand. [6]Department of Biology, Faculty of Science, Chulalongkorn University, 254 Phayathai Road, Bangkok 10330, Thailand.

References
1. Burdock GA. Review of the biological properties and toxicity of bee propolis (propolis). Food Chem Toxicol. 1998;36:347–63.
2. Popova M, Dimitrova R, Al-Lawati HT, Tsvetkova I, Najdenski H, Bankova V. Omani propolis: chemical profiling, antibacterial activity and new propolis plant sources. Chem Cent J. 2013;7:158.
3. Diaz-Carballo D, Ueberl K, Kleff V, Ergun S, Malak S, Freistuehler M, et al. Antiretroviral activity of two polyisoprenylated acylphloroglucinols, 7-epi-nemorosone and plukenetione A, isolated from Caribbean propolis. Int J Clin Pharm Th. 2010;48:670–7.
4. Hu F, Hepburn HR, Li Y, Chen M, Radloff SE, Daya S. Effects of ethanol and water extracts of propolis (bee glue) on acute inflammatory animal models. J Ethnopharmacol. 2005;100:276–83.
5. Sulaiman GM, Al Sammarrae KW, Ad'hiah AH, Zucchetti M, Frapolli R, Bello E, et al. Chemical characterization of Iraqi propolis samples and assessing their antioxidant potentials. Food Chem Toxicol. 2011;49:2415–21.
6. Orsatti CL, Missima F, Pagliarone AC, Sforcin JM. Th1/Th2 cytokines' expression and production by propolis-treated mice. J Ethnopharmacol. 2010;129:314–8.
7. Bufalo MC, Bordon-Graciani AP, Conti BJ, De Assis GM, Sforcin JM. The immunomodulatory effect of propolis on receptors expression, cytokine production and fungicidal activity of human monocytes. J Pharm Pharmacol. 2014;66:1497–504.
8. Soroy L, Bagus S, Yongkie IP, Djoko W. The effect of a unique propolis compound (Propoelix™) on clinical outcomes inpatients with dengue hemorrhagic fever. Infect Drug Resist. 2014;7:323–9.
9. Lotfy M. Biological activity of bee propolis in health and disease. Asian Pac J Cancer Prev. 2006;7:22–31.
10. Zang T, Verma K, Chen M, Jin Y, Trippier PC, Penning TM. Screening baccharin analogs as selective inhibitors against type 5 17β-hydroxysteroid dehydrogenase (AKR1C3). Chem Biol Interact. 2014; doi:10.1016/j.cbi.2014.12.015.
11. Lee MS, Kim YH, Lee BR, Kwon SH, Moon WJ, Hong KS, et al. Novel antidepressant-like activity of caffeic acid phenethyl ester is mediated by enhanced glucocorticoid receptor function in the hippocampus. Evid-Based Compl Alt Med. 2014; doi:10.1155/2014/646039.
12. Hsu TH, Chu CC, Hung MW, Lee HJ, Hsu HJ, Chang TC. Caffeic acid phenethyl ester induces E2F-1-mediated growth inhibition and cell-cycle arrest in human cervical cancer cells. FEBS J. 2013;280:2581–93.
13. Ahad A, Ganai AA, Mujeeb M, Siddiqui WA. Chrysin, an anti-inflammatory molecule, abrogates renal dysfunction in type 2 diabetic rats. Toxicol Appl Pharm. 2014; doi:10.1016/j.taap.2014.05.007.
14. Teerasripreecha D, Puthong S, Kimura K, Okuyama M, Mori H, Kimura A, et al. In vitro antiproliferative/cytotoxic activity on cancer cell lines of a cardanol and a cardol enriched from Thai Apis mellifera propolis. BMC Complement Altern Med. 2012;12:27.
15. Ola A. Molecular identification and anticancer activity of alkylphenol from cashew nut shell oil (Anacardium occidantale) grown in Timor Island. Indonesian J Pharm. 2008;19:137–44.
16. Gopalakrishnan S, Nevaditha NT, Mythili CV. Antibacterial activity of azo compounds synthesized from the natural renewable source, cardanol. J Chem Pharm Res. 2011;3:490–7.
17. Trevisan MT, Pfundstein B, Haubner R, Wurtele G, Spiegelhalder B, Bartsch H, et al. Characterization of alkyl phenols in cashew (Anacardium occidentale) products and assay of their antioxidant capacity. Food Chem Toxicol. 2006;44:188–97.
18. Suwisith N, Hanucharurnkul S, Dodd M, Vorapongsathorn T, Pongthavorakamol K, Asavametha N. Symptom clusters and functional status of women with breast cancer. Thai J Nurs Res. 2008;12:153–65.
19. Livak KJ, Schmittgen TD. Analysis of relative gene expression data using real-time quantitative PCR and the $2^{-\Delta\Delta CT}$ method. Methods. 2001;25:402–8.
20. Lirdprapamongkol K, Sakurai H, Abdelhamed S, Yokoyama S, Athikomkulchai S, Viriyaroj A, et al. Chrysin overcomes TRAIL resistance of cancer cells through Mcl-1 downregulation by inhibiting STAT3 phosphorylation. Int J Oncol. 2013;43:329–37.
21. Milos M, Radonic A, Mastelic J. Seasonal variation in essential oil compositions of Cupressus sempervirens L. J Essent Oil Res. 2002;14:222–3.
22. Ristivojevic P, Trifkovic J, Gasic U, Andric F, Nedic N, Tesic Z, et al. Ultra high-performance liquid chromatography and mass spectrometry (UHPLC–LTQ/Orbitrap/MS/MS) study of phenolic profile of Serbian poplar type propolis. Phytochem Anal. 2015;26:127–36.
23. Bankova V, Popova M, Trusheva B. Propolis volatile compounds: chemical diversity and biological activity: a review. Chem Cent J. 2014;8:28.
24. Park SI, Ohta T, Kumazawa S, Jun M, Ahn MR. Korean propolis suppresses angiogenesis through inhibition of tube formation and endothelial cell proliferation. Nat Prod Commun. 2014;9:555–60.
25. Fauzi AN, Norazmi MN, Yaacob NS. Tualang honey induces apoptosis and disrupts the mitochondrial membrane potential of human breast and cervical cancer cell lines. Food Chem Toxicol. 2011;49:871–8.
26. Kim YH, Jung EM, Lee TJ, Kim SH, Choi YH, Park JW, et al. Rosiglitazone promotes tumor necrosis factor-related apoptosis-Inducing ligand-induced apoptosis by reactive oxygen species-mediated up- regulation of death receptor 5 and down-regulation of c-FLIP. Free Radical Biol Med. 2008;44:1055–68.
27. Yang ES, Woo SM, Choi KS, Kwon TK. Acrolein sensitizes human renal cancer Caki cells to TRAIL-induced apoptosis via ROS-mediated up-regulation of death receptor-5 (DR5) and down-regulation of Bcl-2. Exp Cell Res. 2011;317:2592–601.
28. Zhou T, Li G, Cao B, Liu L, Cheng Q, Kong H, et al. Downregulation of Mcl-1 through inhibition of translation contributes to benzyl isothiocyanate induced cell cycle arrest and apoptosis in human leukemia cells. Cell Death Dis. 2013;4:1–11.
29. Weng MS, Liao CH, Chen CN, Wu CL, Lin JK. Propolin H from Taiwanese propolis induces G_1 arrest in human lung carcinoma cells. J Agric Food Chem. 2007;55:5289–98.
30. He YJ, Liu BH, Xiang DB, Qiao ZY, Fu T, He YH. Inhibitory effect of caffeic acid phenethyl ester on the growth of SW480 colorectal tumor cells involves beta-catenin associated signaling pathway down-regulation. World J Gastroentero. 2006;12:4981–5.
31. Kuo HC, Kuo WH, Lee YJ, Lin WL, Chou FP, Tseng TH. Inhibitory effect of caffeic acid phenethyl ester on the growth of C6 glioma cells in vitro and in vivo. Cancer Lett. 2006;234:199–208.

32. Shen G, Xu C, Chen C, Hebbar V, Kong AN. p53-independent G_1 cell cycle arrest of human colon carcinoma cells HT-29 by sulforaphane is associated with induction of p21CIP1 and inhibition of expression of cyclin D1. Cancer Chemother Pharmacol. 2006;57:317–27.

33. Thorn CF, Oshiro C, Marsh S, Hernandez-Boussard T, McLeod H, Klein TE, et al. Doxorubicin pathways: pharmacodynamics and adverse effects. Pharmacogenet Genomics. 2011;21:440–6.

34. Shetab-Boushehri SV, Abdollahi M. Current concerns on the validity of in vitro models that use transformed neoplastic cells in pharmacology and toxicology. Int J Pharmacol. 2012;8:594–5.

35. Abdollahi M, Shetab-Boushehri SV. Is it right to look for anti-cancer drugs amongst compounds having antioxidant effect? DARU. 2012;20:61.

36. Li LC, Jayaram S, Ganesh L, Qian L, Rotmensch J, Maker AV, et al. Knockdown of MADD and c-FLIP overcomes resistance to TRAIL-induced apoptosis in ovarian cancer cells. Am J Obstet Gynecol. 2011; doi:10.1016/j.ajog.2011.05.035.

37. Pillai MR, Collison LW, Wang X, Finkelstein D, Rehg JE, Boyd K, et al. On the plasticity of regulatory T cell function. J Immunol. 2011;187:4987–97.

38. Weglarz L, Molin I, Orchel A, Parfiniewicz B, Dzierzewicz Z. Quantitative analysis of the level of p53 and p21(WAF1) mRNA in human colon cancer HT-29 cells treated with inositol hexaphosphate. Acta Biochim Pol. 2006;53:349–56.

39. Galanti G, Fisher T, Kventsel I, Shoham J, Gallily R, Mechoulam R, et al. Delta 9-tetrahydrocannabinol inhibits cell cycle progression by downregulation of E2F1 in human glioblastoma multiforme cells. Acta Oncol. 2008;47:1062–70.

40. Ullmannova V, Stockbauer P, Hradcova M, Soucek J, Haskovec C. Relationship between cyclin D1 and p21Waf1/Cip1 during differentiation of human myeloid leukemia cell lines. Leuk Res. 2003;27:1115–23.

41. Potemski P, Pluciennik E, Bednarek AK, Kusinska R, Dorota JK, Grazyna PW, et al. Cyclin E expression in operable breast cancer quantified using real-time RT–PCR: a comparative study with immunostaining. Jpn J Clin Oncol. 2006;33:142–9.

42. Chiang PCL, Su CP, Shiow LK, Ching HT, Lin K, Mao TW, et al. Antroquinonol displays anticancer potential against human hepatocellular carcinoma cells: a crucial role of AMPK and mTOR pathways. Biochem Pharmacol. 2010;79:162–71.

Clinical results with two different pharmaceutical preparations of riboflavin in corneal cross-linking: an 18-month follow up

Hassan Hashemi[1*], Mohammad Amin Seyedian[1], Mohammad Miraftab[1], Hooman Bahrmandy[1], Araz Sabzevari[1] and Soheila Asgari[2]

Abstract

Background: Comparison of long-term clinical results of two different pharmaceutical formulations used in corneal cross-linking (CXL) in keratoconus patients.

Methods: Sixty eyes of 60 keratoconus patients underwent CXL in two groups. We used riboflavin preparations from Sina Darou, Iran in group A, and Streuli Pharma, Switzerland in group B. Here we made inter-group comparison of changes in vision, refraction, Pentacam indices, corneal biomechanical indices, and endothelial cell count (ECC) 18 months after CXL.

Results: Since four patients were lost to follow-up, 56 eyes (28 eyes in each group) were compared. Mean improvement in uncorrected visual acuity (UCVA) was 0.31 ± 0.65 LogMAR (P = 0.014) in group A and 0.24 ± 0.62 LogMAR (P = 0.082) in group B. Best corrected visual acuity (BCVA) remained quite unchanged in both groups (P = 0.774). Mean spherical refractive error reduced by 0.45 ± 1.15 diopter (D) (P = 0.041) in group A and 0.27 ± 1.73 D (P = 0.458) in group B (P = 0.655). Cylinder error and spherical equivalent had a similar trend without any change. Max-K (P = 0.006) and mean-K (P = 0.044) decreased significantly more in group A compared to group B. The reduction in CCT was significantly more in group A than group B (P = 0.004). Q-value was quite unchanged in both groups (P = 0.704). The inter-group difference in CH reduction was borderline significant statistically (P = 0.057). Changes in corneal resistance factor and endothelial cell count were not significantly different between two groups (P = 0.117 and P = 0.229).

Conclusion: Clinical results of CXL with the domestic preparation of riboflavin are similar to that achieved with the Swiss made product in some aspects, and it is the preferred brand in some other aspects. This study will continue to report longer follow-up results.

Trial registration: IRCT201212034333N2

Keywords: Keratoconus, Cross linking, Riboflavin, Sina Darou, Streuli Pharma, Clinical trial

Background

Collagen cross linking with riboflavin (CXL) was first developed by Wollensak et al. [1] to stop the progression of keratoconus. In this procedure, riboflavin plays an important role because it absorbs UVA and it reduces cell damage [1]. The riboflavin preparation used in Iran is a product of Streuli Pharma, a Swiss company. Export company of Sina Darou has manufactured this product in Iran with the same formulation and amount of active substance as the Swiss equivalent, and we have studied its clinical results in patients treated with CXL. In the preliminary report [2], we demonstrated that 6-month changes in vision, refraction, K-reading, corneal biomechanics, and endothelial cell count parameters were not significantly different between the two groups, and clinical results achieved with these formulations are similar. Here we compare 18-month results between these two

* Correspondence: hhashemi@norc.ac.ir
[1]Noor Ophthalmology Research Center, Noor Eye Hospital, No. 96 Esfandiar Blvd., Vali'asr Ave, Tehran, Iran
Full list of author information is available at the end of the article

preparations, so that we can comment on their clinical use with better certainty.

Methods

The complete study methodology has previously been described [2]. In brief, we enrolled 60 eyes of 60 keratoconus patients (30 eyes in each group) in this parallel non-randomized clinical trial. The Iranian preparation of riboflavin 0.1% (Sina Darou, Iran) was used in the first group (group A), and the Swiss preparation of riboflavin 0.1% (Streuli Pharma, Uznach, Switzerland) was used in the second group (group B) during the procedure. Inclusion criteria were the diagnosis of progressive keratoconus on clinical exam which is confirmed paraclinically, age between 15 and 35 years, keratometry less than 55.0 diopter (D), and a minimum central corneal thickness (CCT) of 400 microns (μm).

First the study methods and objectives were explained to the subjects, and they were enrolled in the study after obtaining written informed consents. The study was approved by Noor Review Board. Iranian Registry of Clinical Trials also approved the study (registration number: IRCT201212034333N2).

The surgical procedure has already been described [3]. After local anesthesia, 3 or 4 strips 2 millimeter wide, and about 1 millimeter apart were removed from the central 7 millimeter of the cornea, leaving the corneal epithelial intact in-between. Another epithelium strip was removed horizontally from the inferior third of the cornea. Then, riboflavin 0.1% drops in 20% dextran were instilled onto the corneal surface for half an hour at 3 minute intervals. After ensuring of the presence of riboflavin and observing a yellow Tyndall effect in the anterior chamber, irradiation at a wavelength of 370 nanometer and power of 3 mW/cm^2 was commenced from a distance of 5 cm. Irradiation was done using the UVX system (IROC, Zürich, Switzerland). Riboflavin instillation continued every three minutes during the 30 minutes of irradiation. At the end of this stage, the corneal surface was rinsed with sterile balanced saline solution, a soft bandage contact lens (Night & Day, Ciba Vision, Duluth, GA) was applied, and chloramphenicol 0.5% eye drop was instilled. Postoperative medication included chloramphenicol 0.5% eye drops four times daily, betamethasone 0.1%, and preservative free artificial tears (Hypromelose) as required. Patients were examined on day 1 and 3 after the procedure, and the lens was removed the epithelium had healed. After removing the lens, chloramphenicol was discontinued, and betamethasone was continued twice daily for another week. When the epithelium was not healed, daily visits were continued until complete healing. No case of intraoperative or postoperative complication was observed.

Paraclinical tests included the assessment of uncorrected and best spectacle corrected visual acuity (UCVA and BCVA) using the Snellen chart, and determining the spherical equivalent (SE) using a Retinoscope (HEINE BETA 200, Germany). We also checked corneal topographic indices using Pentacam (Oculus Optikgerate GmbH, Germany), corneal biomechanical parameters using the Ocular Response Analyzer (ORA; Reichert Ophthalmic Instruments, Buffalo, USA), and the endothelial cell count (ECC) with a non-contact specular microscope (Konan Medical, Hyogo, Japan).

The trend of changes was compared between the two groups using repeated measures analysis of variance, and intra-group differences between before and 18 months after the procedure was assessed using the paired t test. We chose a significance level of 0.05.

Results

Since 2 patients from each group did not show up on the 18 month follow-up exam, 56 eyes of 56 keratoconus patients treated with CXL (28 eyes in each group) were compared. Their mean age was 24.32 ± 4.59 years, and 65% were male. Patients were treated with Iranian riboflavin (group A) and Swiss riboflavin (group B) in two groups of 28 people. Since the study had a non-randomized approach, preoperative values of all parameters were compared between the two groups, and there was no significant difference in any case.

At 18 months, mean UCVA improved similarly (P = 0.684) by 0.31 ± 0.65 LogMAR (P = 0.014) in group A and 0.24 ± 0.62 LogMAR (P = 0.082) in group B. BCVA remained unchanged in both groups (P = 0.774). Mean spherical refractive error reduced by 0.45 ± 1.15 D (P = 0.041) in group A and 0.27 ± 1.73 D (P = 0.458) in group B (P = 0.655). Cylinder error and spherical equivalent had a similar trend without any change (Table 1).

Despite similar 6 month trends between the two groups, the 18-month decrease in max-K was 1.44 ± 1.31 D (P < 0.001) in group A and 0.52 ± 0.82 D (P = 0.007) in group B, and the inter-group difference in was statistically significant in this regard (P = 0.006). Mean-K decrease was 1.33 ± 1.19 (P < 0.001) and 0.69 ± 1.00 (P = 0.004) in groups A and B, respectively; the difference was statistically significant (P = 0.044). CCT decreased significantly more (P = 0.004) in group A (47.00 ± 33.10 μm, P < 0.001) than group B (22.32 ± 20.87 μm, P < 0.001). Q-value remained quite unchanged in group A and became slightly prolate in group B; the inter-group difference was not statistically significant (P = 0.704) (Table 2).

The inter-group difference in corneal hysteresis (CH) decrease was borderline significant (P = 0.062). Corneal resistance factor (CRF) decrease was not significantly different between the two groups (P = 0.242). Mean ECC decreased similarly in both groups (P = 0.598) (Table 3).

Table 1 Trend of changes in vision and refraction parameters in the two groups of keratoconus patients treated with Iranian and Swiss preparations of riboflavin

	Riboflavin	No of eyes	Pre operation	6 months after surgery	18 months after surgery	P-value[*]	P-value[**]
UCVA (logMAR)	Sina Darou, Iran	28	0.77 ± 0.66	0.45 ± 0.36	0.44 ± 0.41	0.014	0.684
	Streuli Pharma, Switzerland	28	0.89 ± 0.56	0.79 ± 0.53	0.66 ± .47	0.082	
BCVA (logMAR)	Sina Darou, Iran	28	0.20 ± 0.19	0.19 ± 0.13	0.17 ± 0.13	0.710	0.774
	Streuli Pharma, Switzerland	28	0.22 ± 0.20	0.20 ± 0.23	0.22 ± 0.22	0.880	
Sphere (diopter)	Sina Darou, Iran	28	−1.36 ± 2.18	−1.42 ± 2.36	−1.15 ± 2.25	0.041	0.655
	Streuli Pharma, Switzerland	28	−1.69 ± 1.92	−1.73 ± 2.48	−1.59 ± 2.69	0.458	
Cylinder (diopter)	Sina Darou, Iran	28	−2.67 ± 1.83	−2.36 ± 1.79	−2.40 ± 1.77	0.827	0.642
	Streuli Pharma, Switzerland	28	−2.64 ± 1.91	−2.95 ± 1.97	−2.33 ± 2.16	0.332	
Spherical equivalent (diopter)	Sina Darou, Iran	28	−2.69 ± 2.44	−2.60 ± 2.85	−2.35 ± 2.52	0.093	0.875
	Streuli Pharma, Switzerland	28	−3.01 ± 2.29	−3.20 ± 2.80	−2.76 ± 3.12	0.230	

*Intra-group comparison of parameters before and 18 months after the procedure using paired t test.
**Inter-group comparison of parameters' trend of changes using repeated measures ANOVA.

Discussion

CXL slows down or halts the progression of keratoconus by forming covalent bonds in the corneal stroma that are created as an effect of free radicals. In this process, UV-irradiated riboflavin produces free radicals, and riboflavin concentration influences the level of UV absorption and strengthening reactions in the cornea. In-vivo, riboflavin can increase UV absorption up to 95% [4]. This is while UV absorption in the cornea is only 25-35% without riboflavin [5]. With riboflavin concentrations between 0 to 0.04%, UV absorption increases linearly, but has no further effect [6]. Thus, using riboflavin is one of the main pillars of the treatment.

In the 6-month report [2], we compared preliminary clinical results of treatment with Iranian and Swiss preparations of riboflavin which demonstrated the effectiveness of the Iranian preparation. Six-month changes in vision, refraction, corneal topographic and biomechanical parameters, and ECC were similar in the two groups, and no inter-group difference was found. Clinical parameters were not significantly different at 18 months either, and both preparations were similar in terms of stopping the progression of keratoconus. The two preparations were only different in terms of corneal topographic indices; better flattening was achieved with the Iranian preparation while CCT decrease was less with the Swiss product. It must be noted, however, that this study was nonrandomized, and to lessen the effect of this limitation, we performed matching using base indices.

Stability of vision and refraction parameters in the group treated with Sina Darou riboflavin indicated that disease progression had stopped. Various results have been reported after treatment with CXL. Some studies demonstrated no change [2,7,8], some observed improvement [8-10], and some showed reduced vision and increased refraction [7]. This can be due to inter-study differences in preoperative values or disease severity in the study samples. Different corneal structures in different populations can be another reason that causes such differences. Another point is that vision assessment is a

Table 2 Trend of changes in parameters measured with Pentacam compared between two groups of keratoconic patients treated with Iranian vs. Swiss preparations of riboflavin

	Riboflavin	No of eyes	Pre operation	6 months after surgery	18 months after surgery	P-value[*]	P-value[**]
Maximum keratometry (Diopter)	Sina Darou, Iran	28	49.05 ± 3.57	48.45 ± 2.79	47.74 ± 3.76	<0.001	0.006
	Streuli Pharma, Switzerland	28	48.60 ± 3.33	48.74 ± 3.56	48.06 ± 3.16	0.007	
Mean keratometry (Dipoter)	Sina Darou, Iran	28	47.14 ± 3.37	46.37 ± 2.30	45.98 ± 3.78	<0.001	0.044
	Streuli Pharma, Switzerland	28	47.07 ± 2.91	47.00 ± 3.21	46.37 ± 3.00	0.004	
Q-value	Sina Darou, Iran	28	−0.69 ± 0.38	−0.68 ± 0.39	−0.68 ± 0.57	0.651	0.704
	Streuli Pharma, Switzerland	28	−0.72 ± 0.33	−0.75 ± 0.45	−0.63 ± 0.38	0.064	
Central corneal thickness (μm)	Sina Darou, Iran	28	482.1 ± 29.7	467.5 ± 29.8	441.5 ± 45.0	<0.001	0.004
	Streuli Pharma, Switzerland	28	496.9 ± 35.6	481.5 ± 37.3	474.7 ± 41.2	<0.001	

*Intra-group comparison of parameters before and 18 months after the procedure using paired t test.
**Inter-group comparison of parameters' trend of changes using repeated measures ANOVA.

Table 3 Trend of changes in corneal biomechanical parameters and endothelial cell count compared between two groups of keratoconic patients treated with Iranian vs. Swiss preparations of riboflavin

	Riboflavin	No of eyes	Pre operation	6 months after surgery	18 months after surgery	P-value*	P-value**
Corneal hysteresis (mmHg)	Sina Darou, Iran	28	7.67 ± 1.44	6.69 ± 1.52	6.44 ± 1.37	<0.001	0.062
	Streuli Pharma, Switzerland	28	7.63 ± 2.12	7.36 ± 1.50	7.53 ± 1.66	0.701	
Corneal resistance factor (mmHg)	Sina Darou, Iran	28	6.74 ± 1.66	6.20 ± 1.24	5.88 ± 1.93	0.023	0.242
	Streuli Pharma, Switzerland	28	6.94 ± 1.97	6.94 ± 1.74	6.79 ± 1.90	0.716	
Endothelial cell count (cell/mm^2)	Sina Darou, Iran	28	2789.3 ± 160.8	2455.4 ± 312.9	2511.7 ± 271.8	<0.001	0.176
	Streuli Pharma, Switzerland	28	2731.6 ± 262.9	2470.7 ± 274.1	2574.9 ± 305.5	<0.001	

*Intra-group comparison of parameters before and 18 months after the procedure using paired t test.
**Inter-group comparison of parameters' trend of changes using repeated measures ANOVA.

subjective test which can be influenced by environmental conditions, optometrists' accuracy, and patients' condition. Thus, diverse results can be expected.

Corneal topographic changes were significantly different between the two groups. Although both groups demonstrated a significantly reduced protrusion and decreased CCT, patients achieved better corneal flattening when treated with Iranian riboflavin. The reduction in corneal thickness, however, was less in the group of patients treated with Swiss riboflavin. This could imply better intra-fibril bond formation is supported by the Iranian preparation due to better UVA absorption, and thus, keratometry is decreased. The lack of significant inter-group difference in ECC showed that despite better UV absorption, cytotoxic effects were not intensified, and there was no keratocyte loss [11,12]. Some studied have demonstrated reduced corneal thickness despite reduced keratometry and halted disease progression [13-15], and this has mostly been attributed to stages of epithelium removal and riboflavin instillation [16].

CRF reduction was similar in the two groups. The inter-group difference in CH reduction was borderline significant (P = 0.062). However, CH and CRF are not enough to show changes in corneal biomechanical properties [17], we would need to examine other indices measured with ORA to have a more accurate assessment of the effects of these two preparations.

Conclusion

Finally, based on 18-month results, apart from better flattening with the Iranian preparation and better maintenance of corneal thickness with the Swiss product, cresults in terms of clinical vision, refraction, biomechanical properties, and the endothelial cell count were comparable with these two types preparations of riboflavin. We can thus conclude that the Iranian riboflavin (Sina Darou) can be an alternative for its Swiss counterpart in CXL. This study will continue to assess the stability of results at later follow-ups.

Abbreviations
CXL: Corneal cross linking; SE: Spherical equivalent; BCVA: Best corrected visual acuity; UCVA: Uncorrected visual acuity; max K: Maximum keratometry; CCT: Central corneal thickness; ECC: Endothelial cell count; CH: Corneal hysteresis; CRF: Corneal resistance factor.

Competing interests
The authors declare that they have no competing interests.

Authors' contributions
HH has designed and supervised the project. MA, MM and HB performed the surgeries. AS and SA analyzed and interpreted the data and wrote the manuscript. HH, MA, MM and HB finalized the manuscript. All authors read and approved the final manuscript.

Author details
[1]Noor Ophthalmology Research Center, Noor Eye Hospital, No. 96 Esfandiar Blvd., Vali'asr Ave, Tehran, Iran. [2]Department of Epidemiology and Biostatistics, School of Public Health, Tehran University of Medical Sciences, International Campus (TUMS-IC), Tehran, Iran.

References
1. Wollensak G, Spoerl E, Seiler T. Riboflavin/ultraviolet-a-induced collagen crosslinking for the treatment of keratoconus. Am J Ophthalmol. 2003;135:620–7.
2. Hashemi H, Seyedian MA, Miraftab M, Bahrmandy H, Sabzevari A, Asgari S. Comparison of clinical results of two pharmaceutical products of riboflavin in corneal collagen cross-linking for keratoconus. Daru: J Faculty Pharm, Tehran Univ Med Sci. 2014;22:37.
3. Hashemi H, Seyedian MA, Miraftab M, Fotouhi A, Asgari S. Corneal Collagen Cross-linking with Riboflavin and Ultraviolet A Irradiation for Keratoconus: Long-term Results. Ophthalmology. 2013;120:1515–20.
4. Sporl E, Schreiber J, Hellmund K, Seiler T, Knuschke P. Studies on the stabilization of the cornea in rabbits. Ophthalmologe. 2000;97:203–6.
5. Tsubai T, Matsuo M. Ultraviolet light-induced changes in the glucose-6-phosphate dehydrogenase activity of porcine corneas. Cornea. 2002;21:495–500.
6. Spoerl E, Mrochen M, Sliney D, Trokel S, Seiler T. Safety of UVA-riboflavin cross-linking of the cornea. Cornea. 2007;26:385–9.
7. Asri D, Touboul D, Fournie P, Malet F, Garra C, Gallois A, et al. Corneal collagen crosslinking in progressive keratoconus: multicenter results from the French National Reference Center for Keratoconus. J Cataract Refract Surg. 2011;37:2137–43.
8. Goldich Y, Marcovich AL, Barkana Y, Mandel Y, Hirsh A, Morad Y, et al. Clinical and Corneal Biomechanical Changes After Collagen Cross-Linking With Riboflavin and UV Irradiation in Patients With Progressive Keratoconus: Results After 2 Years of Follow-up. Cornea. 2012;31:609–14.

Clinical results with two different pharmaceutical preparations of riboflavin in corneal...

163

9. Henriquez MA, Izquierdo Jr L, Bernilla C, Zakrzewski PA, Mannis M. Riboflavin/Ultraviolet A corneal collagen cross-linking for the treatment of keratoconus: visual outcomes and Scheimpflug analysis. Cornea. 2011;30:281–6.

10. Hersh PS, Greenstein SA, Fry KL. Corneal collagen crosslinking for keratoconus and corneal ectasia: One-year results. J Cataract Refract Surg. 2011;37:149–60.

11. Wollensak G, Spoerl E, Reber F, Seiler T. Keratocyte cytotoxicity of riboflavin/UVA-treatment in vitro. Eye (Lond). 2004;18:718–22.

12. Wollensak G, Spoerl E, Seiler T. Stress–strain measurements of human and porcine corneas after riboflavin-ultraviolet-A-induced cross-linking. J Cataract Refract Surg. 2003;29:1780–5.

13. Cinar Y, Cingu AK, Turkcu FM, Cinar T, Yuksel H, Ozkurt ZG, et al. Comparison of accelerated and conventional corneal collagen cross-linking for progressive keratoconus. Cutan Ocul Toxicol. 2014;33:218–22.

14. Saffarian L, Khakshoor H, Zarei-Ghanavati M, Esmaily H. Corneal Crosslinking for Keratoconus in Iranian Patients: Outcomes at 1 year following treatment. Middle East Afr J Ophthalmol. 2010;17:365–8.

15. Kanellopoulos AJ, Asimellis G. Keratoconus management: long-term stability of topography-guided normalization combined with high-fluence CXL stabilization (the Athens Protocol). J Refract Surg. 2014;30:88–93.

16. Kymionis GD, Kounis GA, Portaliou DM, Grentzelos MA, Karavitaki AE, Coskunseven E, et al. Intraoperative pachymetric measurements during corneal collagen cross-linking with riboflavin and ultraviolet A irradiation. Ophthalmology. 2009;116:2336–9.

17. Hallahan KM, Sinha Roy A, Ambrosio Jr R, Salomao M, Dupps Jr WJ. Discriminant value of custom ocular response analyzer waveform derivatives in keratoconus. Ophthalmology. 2014;121:459–68.

20

Carum induced hypothyroidism: an interesting observation and an experiment

Seyede Maryam Naghibi[1], Mohamad Ramezani[2], Narjess Ayati[1] and Seyed Rasoul Zakavi[1*]

Abstract

Carum carvi is a widely available herb that has been used as a food additive and as a medication in traditional medicine for many years. Its potential biological effects include analgesic, anti-inflammatory, anti-anxiety and antispasmodic activities. We report a patient with papillary thyroid carcinoma who were under treatment with levothyroxine and experienced an elevated TSH level by ingestion of *Carum carvi*. TSH level was increased to 60.3 mIU/L with no change in levothyroxine dosage and decreased to normal range after discontinuation of the *Carum carvi*. Observing this dramatic change in TSH level by carum ingestion, carum carvi capsules was produced and one of the researcher tried the medication on herself with a dose of 40 mg/kg/day. She had a history of hypothyroidism and was taking 100 ugr/day of levothyroxine. TSH was markedly increased 2 weeks after ingestion of Carum carvi and returned to normal range 5 months after discontinuation of it. This case report shows the effect of consumption of Carum carvi in increasing TSH level in hypothyroid patients treating with levothyroxine. The exact mechanism of action of carum carvi remains unknown.

Keywords: Thyroid, Carum carvi, TSH, Hypothyroidism

Background

Medicinal plants play a key role in several physiologic and pathologic processes in our body and there are many effects which are still to be discovered. *Carum carvi* (black zeera) from Apiaceae family has various biological effects including analgesic, anti-inflammatory, anti-anxiety and antispasmodic activities which provide pharmacological basis for its use in hyperactivity disorders of gut and airways, such as diarrhea, colic and asthma [1-9]. It seems to be a safe food additive commonly used in our daily life but its effect on thyroid hormones remains unknown.

In this study we are reporting two patients with hypothyroidism, under treatment with levothyroxine, who showed elevated TSH levels after ingestion of Carum carvi. This is the first report on effect of carum on thyroid hormones level in patients treating with levothyroxine.

Case presentation

The first case was a 24-years-old girl (weight: 44.2 kg) with advanced papillary thyroid cancer (T4N1bM1) who had a history of near total thyroidectomy, external radiotherapy of the neck and mediastinum and repeated radio-iodine therapy in the last 17 years. She had bilateral lung metastases and received 34.4 GBq of I-131 during her treatment. She was under suppressive therapy with 100 µg/day of levothyroxine. She was also taking calcium carbonate 1000 mg/day and calcitriol 0.25 µg/day. Her TSH level ranged from 0.07-0.3 mIU/L during follow up consistent with subclinical hyperthyroidism. During her last follow up, TSH and T3RIA level were found to be 60.3 µU/L and 135.9 ng/ml, respectively. Padyab Teb kits was used for measurement of TSH (interassay CV = 8.21%, Intra-assay CV = 5.41%, Padyab Teb, IRI) and T3RIA (interassay CV = 5.56%, intra-assay CV = 5.45%). The laboratory results were repeated and TSH and T3RIA level were 60.72 mIU/L and 150.2 ng/ml, respectively. She had no complaint except occasional cough and dyspnea which were due to bilateral lung metastasis. Biochemically, she was considered hypothyroid. Complete interview was done to find the reason behind the elevated TSH level during levothyroxine consumption.

* Correspondence: zakavir@mums.ac.ir
[1]Nuclear Medicine Research Center, Faculty of Medicine, Mashhad University of Medical Sciences, Mashhad, Iran
Full list of author information is available at the end of the article

The patient was not receiving any new medication and her drug regimen had not been changed during last 6 months. The only new food additive, she was receiving was *Carum carvi* seed and yarrow. Dose of levothyroxine was not changed and *Carum carvi* and yarrow consumption was stopped. After 2 months of discontinuation of *Carum carvi* and yarrow consumption, measurement of thyroid hormones was performed using the same kits in the same laboratory. The new TSH and T3RIA levels were 1.75 mIU/l and 166.07 ng/ml, respectively indicating euthyroid state. This observation was assessed by Naranjo causality index and found a "possible adverse drug reaction" (score 3) while using WHO-UMC causality scale it was considered a "probable" ADR. Written informed consent was obtained from the patient for publication of this Case report and any accompanying images.

Considering the dramatic change in TSH level by carum ingestion, *Carum carvi* capsules containing 200, 400 and 800 mg of powdered *Carum carvi* was produced in School of Pharmacy and one of the researchers with history of hypothyroidism tried to test it on her. She was a 24-years-old girl (weight = 45 kg) with a history of hypothyroidism for 5 years and had been treating with 100 μg/day of levothyroxine. TSH level was between 2.5-3.7 mIU/l in her medical records. In the first visit, all clinical signs and symptoms were assessed and none of hypothyroid symptoms were observed. Her pulse rate was 76/min and her blood pressure was 90/70 mmHg. In physical examination, she had a painless, small goiter with no palpable nodule or adenopathy. She was not taking any other medication and her mother had a history of hypothyroidism as well. Her initial TSH level before starting Carum carvi was 2.3 mIU/L, indicating euthyroidism. She started to take carum with dose of 1800 mg/day (40 mg/kg) divided in 3 doses. The dose of 40 mg/kg was 1% of the maximum safe dose of *Carum carvi* in rats. Levothyroxine was ingested in fasting state in early morning and carum capsules were used after each meal (breakfast, lunch and dinner). After 2 weeks, TSH level was 26 mIU/l and thyroid hormone levels were decreased indicating hypothyroid state (Table 1).

Vital signs remained in normal range (PR: 80 and BP: 90/70). In physical examination, no new change was observed but she suffered from dry and cold skin. She continued using carum capsules for 4 additional weeks when she started to complain from constipation. At the same time, TSH level increased to 110 mIU/L, and thyroid hormone level was further decreased (Table 1). Thyroid exam was unchanged while she was in hypothyroid state both biochemically and clinically. *Carum carvi* was discontinued and thyroid values was measured after 2 weeks and showed TSH level of 25 mIU/L. Dose of Levothyroxine was not changed and thyroid values were measured again 6 weeks after discontinuation of *Carum carvi*. The TSH level further decreased to 11 mIU/l and T4RIA level was increased to 9 ng/L (Table 1). Two months later, TSH was further decreased to 7 mIU/l with no intervention indicating subclinical hypothyroid state. The patient obtained 7 scores in Naranjo causality algorithm (probable ADR) and categorized as "certain ADR" in WHO-UMC score.

Discussion

In the present study, we observed dramatic effect of oral administration of *Carum carvi* seed on TSH level in patients with hypothyroidism. Although one of our patients had follicular thyroid cancer and the other had hypothyroidism due to autoimmune thyroiditis, both patients was receiving levothyroxine and showed marked elevation of TSH level after ingestion of carum seeds.

Carum carvi has been used traditionally as an acceptable food additive and its beneficial effect was reported in treating diarrhea, colic and asthma. Due to its antispasmodic activity, it was used in gastrointestinal disorders and as bronchodilator in hyperactive airways [1,6]. In addition, studies indicated that caraway oil probably has a protective antioxidant role in heart and kidney in patients with sepsis [10]. The mechanism of the effect of *Carum carvi* in our patients is unknown. Our first patient was receiving carum and yarrow while the second patient was receiving carum only. As the effect was similar in both patients, it seems that carum effect is more prominent than any possible effect of yarrow.

Some herbal products were reported to change thyroid metabolism. Soy consumption is related to thyroid disorders such as hypothyroidism, goiter, and autoimmune thyroid disease besides increased iodine metabolism in animal studies but the exact molecular mechanisms which might be responsible for hypothyroidism is unclear [11]. In our patients, hypothyroidism could not be related to iodine metabolism as both patients were taking levothyroxine. It was found that the peel extracts of *Mangifera indica*, *Citrullus vulgaris*, and *Cucumis melo*

Table 1 Hormonal levels in different time points after carum ingestion and discontinuation

Time	Carum ingestion			Carum discontinued	
	Beginning	2 weeks	6 weeks	8 weeks	12 weeks
TSH (mIU/L)	2.3	26	110	25	11
T4RIA (ng/L)	11	12	3.7	4.6	9
T3RIA (ng/L)	148	106	57	90	143
T3RU (%)	30	31	26	24	30

TSH = Thyroid stimulating hormone, T4RIA = T4 Radio-immuno-assay,
T3RIA = T3-Radio-immuno-assay, T3RU = T3 Resin uptake.

were thyro-stimulatory increasing the levels of both T3 and T4 which is indicative of the role of these peel extracts in ameliorating hypothyroidism [12,13]. The possible reasons for this beneficial role may be attributed to the presence of flavonoids, phenolic compounds, and ascorbic acid content of the peel extracts [12,14]. Full phytochemical analysis of both essential oil and seed extract showed the presence of many mono and sesqui-terpenes in essential oil and diverse flavonoids, isoflavo-noids, flavonoid glycosides, monoterpenoid glucosides, lignins and alkaloids and other phenolic compounds in seed extract [13,15-17]. However, none of these compounds has been specifically linked to a mechanism by which TSH elevation could be explained.

In our patient, the mechanism of TSH elevation may be attributed to prevention of absorption of levothyrox-ine in the bowel and/or its action in the receptor level. Since in our trial case, T4 and T3 levels decreased by consumption of *Carum carvi*, the most plausible explan-ation would be the interference with levothyroxine ab-sorption. This hypothesis is also supported by the observation that hypothyroidism was gradually becom-ing severe and symptoms of hypothyroidism were more prominent at the end of the experiment. Interestingly, symptoms and signs of hypothyroidism were not prom-inent in our patient early after experiment, suggesting that peripheral action of the hormone is well preserved. Moreover, this finding may suggest that Carum may have more prominent effects on blocking of T4 to T3 conversion at the hypophysis.

Many causality scoring systems have been used for evaluation of adverse drug reaction. We used Naranjo score and WHO-UMC in our patients and it was "prob-able" and "certain" ADR according to these categories, respectively [18].

The carum seeds consumption did not produce any observable toxicity based on evaluated signs and symp-toms at the dose of 40 mg/kg [3]. However, more exten-sive toxicity assessments are required to make sure that the seeds are safe at the dose of 40 mg/kg.

Conclusion

This case report shows that consumption of *Carum carvi* interfere with levothyroxine effect in hypothyroid patients and increase TSH prominently. The exact mechanism of action of *Carum carvi* is not known. Informing patients and physicians about the possible interaction of *Carum carvi* on TSH elevation would be helpful.

Abbreviations

TSH: Thyroid stimulating hormone; T3RIA: T3 radioimmunoassay; IRMA: Immuno-radio-metric-assay; GBq: Giga becquerel; CV: Coefficient of variation; ADR: Adverse drug reaction; WHO-UMC: World Health Organization- Uppsala Monitoring Center.

Competing interest

The authors declare that they have no competing interest.

Author's contributions

SMN: Study design, acquisition of the data and drafting article. MR: Study design, preparing drugs and critical revision of the article. NA: Study design, follow up and helping in drafting the article. SRZ: Initial idea, study design, acquisition of the data, analysis and critical revision of the article. All authors read and approved the manuscript.

Acknowledgement

The authors wish to thanks Mrs. Fateme Khani for her assistance in performing the study. The authors received no grant or financial support for this study.

Author details

[1]Nuclear Medicine Research Center, Faculty of Medicine, Mashhad University of Medical Sciences, Mashhad, Iran. [2]Pharmaceutical Research Center, Buali Research Institute, Mashhad University of Medical Sciences, Mashhad, Iran.

References

1. Khan M, Khan AU, Najeeb u R, Gilani AH. Gut and airways relaxant effects of Carum roxburghianum. J Ethnopharmacol. 2012;141:938–46.
2. Saghir MR, Sadiq S, Nayak S, Tahir MU. Hypolipidemic effect of aqueous extract of Carum carvi (black Zeera) seeds in diet induced hyperlipidemic rats. Pak J Pharm Sci. 2012;25:333–7.
3. Rezvani ME, Roohbakhsh A, Mosaddegh MH, Esmailidehaj M, Khaloobagheri F, Esmaeili H. Anticonvulsant and depressant effects of aqueous extracts of Carum copticum seeds in male rats. Epilepsy Behav. 2011;22:220–5.
4. Sadiq S, Nagi AH, Shahzad M, Zia A. The reno-protective effect of aqueous extract of Carum carvi (black zeera) seeds in streptozotocin induced diabetic nephropathy in rodents. Saudi J Kidney Dis Transpl. 2010;21:1058–65.
5. Hejazian YS, Dashti RM, Mahdavi SM, Qureshi MA. The effect of Carum Copticum extract on acetylcholine induced contraction in isolated rat's ileum. J Acupunct Meridian Stud. 2009;2:75–8.
6. Boskabady MH, Alizadeh M, Jahanbin B. Bronchodilatory effect of Carum copticum in airways of asthmatic patients. Therapie. 2007;62:23–9.
7. Dashti-Rahmatabadi MH, Hejazian SH, Morshedi A, Rafati A. The analgesic effect of Carum copticum extract and morphine on phasic pain in mice. J Ethnopharmacol. 2007;109:226–8.
8. Lemhadri A, Hajji L, Michel JB, Eddouks M. Cholesterol and triglycerides lowering activities of caraway fruits in normal and streptozotocin diabetic rats. J Ethnopharmacol. 2006;106:321–6.
9. Gilani AH, Jabeen Q, Ghayur MN, Janbaz KH, Akhtar MS. Studies on the antihypertensive, antispasmodic, bronchodilator and hepatoprotective activities of the Carum copticum seed extract. J Ethnopharmacol. 2005;98:127–35.
10. Dadkhah A, Fatemi F. Heart and kidney oxidative stress status in septic rats treated with caraway extracts. Pharm Biol. 2011;49:679–86.
11. Tran L, Hammuda M, Wood C, Xiao CW. Soy extracts suppressed iodine uptake and stimulated the production of autoimmunogen in rat thyrocytes. Exp Biol Med (Maywood). 2013;238:623–30.
12. Parmar HS, Kar A. Possible amelioration of atherogenic diet induced dyslipidemia, hypothyroidism and hyperglycemia by the peel extracts of Mangifera indica, Cucumis melo and Citrullus vulgaris fruits in rats. Biofactors. 2008;33:13–24.
13. Parmar HS, Kar A. Protective role of Mangifera indica, Cucumis melo and Citrullus vulgaris peel extracts in chemically induced hypothyroidism. Chem Biol Interact. 2009;177:254–8.
14. Parmar HS, Kar A. Antiperoxidative, antithyroidal, antihyperglycemic and cardioprotective role of Citrus sinensis peel extract in male mice. Phytother Res. 2008;22:791–5.
15. Ishikawa T, Takayanagi T, Kitajima J. Water-soluble constituents of cumin: monoterpenoid glucosides. Chem Pharm Bull (Tokyo). 2002;50:1471–8.

16. Matsumura T, Ishikawa T, Kitajima J. Water-soluble constituents of caraway: aromatic compound, aromatic compound glucoside and glucides. Phytochemistry. 2002;61:455–9.

17. Takayanagi T, Ishikawa T, Kitajima J. Sesquiterpene lactone glucosides and alkyl glycosides from the fruit of cumin. Phytochemistry. 2003;63:479–84.

18. Belhekar MN, Taur SR, Munshi RP. A study of agreement between the Naranjo algorithm and WHO-UMC criteria for causality assessment of adverse drug reactions. Indian J Pharmacol. 2014;46:117–20.

21

Statistical optimization of tretinoin-loaded penetration-enhancer vesicles (PEV) for topical delivery

Neda Bavarsad[1,2*], Abbas Akhgari[3], Somayeh Seifmanesh[2], Anayatollah Salimi[1,2] and Annahita Rezaie[4]

Abstract

Background: The aim of this study was to develop and optimize deformable liposome for topical delivery of tretinoin.

Methods: Liposomal formulations were designed based on the full factorial design and prepared by fusion method. The influence of different ratio of soy phosphatidylcholine and transcutol (independent variables) on incorporation efficiency and drug release in 15 min and 24 h (responses) from liposomal formulations was evaluated. Liposomes were characterized for their vesicle size and Differential Scanning Calorimetry (DSC) was used to investigate changes in their thermal behavior. The penetration and retention of drug was determined using mouse skin. Also skin histology study was performed.

Results: Particle size of all formulations was smaller than 20 nm. Incorporation efficiency of liposomes was 79–93 %. Formulation F7 (25:5) showed maximum drug release. Optimum formulations were selected based on the contour plots resulted by statistical equations of drug release in 15 min and 24 h. Solubility properties of transcutol led to higher skin penetration for optimum formulations compared to tretinoin cream. There was no significant difference between the amount of drug retained in the skin by applying optimum formulations and cream. Histopatological investigation suggested optimum formulations could decrease the adverse effect of tretinoin in liposome compared to conventional cream.

Conclusion: According to the results of the study, it is concluded that deformable liposome containing transcutol may be successfully used for dermal delivery of tretinoin.

Keywords: Statistical optimization, Tretinoin, Liposomal formulation, Topical delivery

Background

Tretinoin or all-trans retinoic acid in topical form is commonly used for the treatment of various skin problems like acne, photoaging and psoriasis. Furthermore, it has other functions such as sebum production, collagen synthesis and regulating growth and differentiation of epithelial cells [1]. Reduction the size and the number of comedones are considered to be the main effect of tretinoin in the treatment of acne [2]. However, it has several negative points even in topical use such as very low water solubility, skin irritation and high instability in the presence of air, light and heat. Furthermore, local irritation such as erythema, peeling and burning at the application site and increased susceptibility to sunlight are its side effects [3].

Liposomes are spherical-shaped carriers which has an internal aqueous portion surrounded by one or multiple concentric lipidic bilayers. Liposomes are used as carriers for both lipophilic and water soluble molecules. Hydrophilic substances are encapsulated in the interior aqueous portions whereas lipophilic substances are entrapped within lipid bilayers [4].

Incorporation of tretinoin in nanostructure systems such as liposomes may lead to decrease the adverse effects and protect this molecule against degradation [5–8].

* Correspondence: nbavarsad@ajums.ac.ir
[1]Nanotechnology Research Center, Ahvaz Jundishapur University of Medical Sciences, Ahvaz, Iran
[2]Department of Pharmaceutics, School of Pharmacy, Ahvaz Jundishapur University of Medical Sciences, Ahvaz, Iran
Full list of author information is available at the end of the article

Liposomes were first used as topical therapy by Mezei and Gulasekharam in 1980. The introduction of liposomes as skin drug delivery systems, initially promoted for localized effects with minimal systemic delivery. Reduction of vesicle size improves drug deposition into deeper strata. Recent advances and alteration in the composition and structure of vesicles result in vesicles with tailored properties [9].

The first generations of elastic vesicles are deformable liposomes (Transfersomes®) which consist of phospholipids and surfactant as an edge activator. Surfactant destabilizes lipid bilayers and increases deformability of the vesicles. Ethosome is another type of elastic vesicle which is composed of phospholipid, ethanol and water [10]. Recently, a novel family of liposomes which named the Penetration Enhancer-containing Vesicles (PEVs) is described for enhanced (trans)-dermal drug delivery [11]. They mainly consist of phospholipids and penetration enhancers with hydrosoluble glycols such as diethylene glycol mono ethyl ether or propylene glycol. Transient reduction of the stratum corneum barrier function and improvement in vesicular bilayer fluidity are two main functions of the PEVs [12].

The aim of this study was to prepare and evaluate deformable liposome using soy phosphatidylcholine and transcutol (Diethylene glycol monoethyl ether) for topical delivery of tretinoin. Also optimization of formulation was performed in order to obtain suitable dermal delivery system for tretinoin.

Methods
Materials
Tretinoin was purchased from Sepidaj (Iran). Soy phosphatidylcholine (phospholipon 85G®) was obtained from lipoid (Germany). Cholesterol and HEPES (4-(2-Hydroxyethyl) 1-piperazine ethanesulfonic acid) were purchased from Sigma)Germany). Diethylene glycol monoethyle ether (Transcutol®) received as a gift from Gattefosse (France). Propyl paraben, methyl paraben, propylene glycol and vitamin E were obtained from Merck (Germany). Tretinoin cream 0.05 % was purchased from the pharmacy and its base cream was provided as a gift by Iran Daru (Iran).

Animals
Female NMRI mice 7–9 weeks old were obtained from laboratory Animals Care and Breeding Center of Ahvaz Jundishapur University of Medical Sciences (Ahvaz, Iran). The experiments were conducted in full compliance with regulatory principles of ethics committee of Ahvaz Jundishapur University of Medical Sciences.

Experimental design
A full factorial 3^2 design was used for optimization procedure. The studied independent variables were amount of soy phosphatidylcholine (SPC) (X_1) and amount of transcutol (X_2) in formulation. Types and levels of the independent variables are listed in Table 1. Dependent variables (responses) were percent of incorporation efficiency (Y_1), percent of drug release in 15 min (Y_2) and percent of drug release in 24 h (Y_3). The resulted formulations are illustrated in Table 2.

Preparation of deformable liposomes
Deformable liposomes were prepared by the fusion method. Briefly, the lipid components consisted of SPC (15–20–25 % wt), transcutol (5–10–15 % wt), tretinoin) 0.05 % wt), cholesterol (2 % wt), propylene glycol (3 % wt), vitamin E (0.3 % wt), metyl paraben (0.1 % wt), and propyl paraben (0.02 % wt); these components were melted at about 75 °C. HEPES buffer (10 mM, pH 5) was heated separately and was added up to 100 % to the previously heated melted lipids, and the mixture was homogenized with a homogenizer (Ultra-Turrax IKA T25) for 5 min at 12,000 rpm and allow it to cool down to room temperature [13].

Characterization of the liposomes
Particle size measurement
The particle size of the samples were measured in triplicate by laser light scattering (Scatterscope 1, Qudix, South Korea). Samples were diluted in HEPES buffer to a suitable concentration (0.2 g formulation in 1 ml HEPES buffer).

Incorporation efficiency
Incorporation efficiency of liposomes was determined indirectly. Certain amounts of liposomal dispersions were centrifuged (VS-35SMTI, Korea) at 20,000 rpm for 25 min at 25 °C. The supernatant was collected and analyzed at 362 nm using UV spectrophotometer (Biowave II, Biochrom, England) [14]. The percent of incorporation efficiency of drug was calculated by the following formula:

Table 1 Independent variables: Types and Levels

Variables	Levels		
X_1: amount of SPC (% wt)	15	20	25
X_2: amount of transcutol (% wt)	5	10	15

Table 2 Composition of experimental formulations (runs)

Run	X_1: SPC (% wt)	X_2: transcutol (% wt)
1	15	5
2	15	10
3	15	15
4	20	5
5	20	10
6	20	15
7	25	5
8	25	10
9	25	15

$$EE\% = \left[\left(\begin{array}{l} \text{amount of initial drug} \\ - \text{amount of free drug in supernatant} \end{array} \right) \middle/ \text{amount of initial drug} \right] \times 100$$

In vitro drug release

Drug release studies were performed using dialysis membrane method. Dialysis membranes were soaked before use in distilled water for 20 h. 1 g of formulation was placed in a dialysis membrane and both ends were closed. The membrane was float in a beaker containing 150 ml phosphate buffer (pH 7.4) and methanol (2:1 v/v); and stirred at 200 rpm at 37 °C. 1 ml of receiver medium was removed at 0.25, 0.5, 0.75, 1, 1.5, 2, 4, 6, 8 and 24 h and same volume of the fresh medium was replaced. The collected samples were analyzed for their tretinoin content. The derived concentration values were corrected by using the equation (1):

$$Mt\,(n) = Vr \times Cn + Vs \times \sum Cm \qquad (1)$$

Where Mt(n) is the current cumulative mass of drug transported across the membrane at time t, n is the number (times) of sampling, Cn is the current concentration in the receiver medium, $\sum Cm$ is the summed total of the previously measured concentrations, Vr is the volume of the receiver medium, and Vs corresponds to the volume of the sample removed for analysis [15, 16].

Viscosity

Viscosity of selected formulations were measured by Brookfield viscometer (DV II + Pro, US) at 10 rpm and 25 °C using spindle 64.

In vitro skin penetration and retention

In vitro skin penetration studies were performed using jacketed Franz cells with a receiver medium of 25 ml

Phosphate buffer (pH 7.4) and methanol (2:1 v/v) at 37 °C and surface area of 4.84 cm^2. The dorsal skin of mouse was shaved with electric clippers one day before the experiment. A suitable size of full-thickness skin of mouse was cut and clamped between the donor and receiver compartment of Franz cell with the stratum corneum side facing upward. The skin samples were initially left in the Franz cells for 30 min in order to facilitate hydration. Subsequently, 1 g of the optimum formulations and tretinoin cream were placed onto the skin surface. 1 ml of receiver solution was removed at 0.25, 0.5, 0.75, 1, 1.5, 2, 4, 6 and 8 h and same volume of the fresh medium was replaced. The collected samples were analyzed for their tretinoin content. The derived concentration values were corrected according to equation (1).

For the determination of the amount of the drug retained in the skin, at the end of the experiment, the amount of the formulation remaining on the surface of the skin was collected and assayed for tretinoin. The amount of tretinoin retained in the skin was then calculated by subtracting the sum of the amount of tretinoin that remained on the surface and the amount of tretinoin that was released (penetrated through the skin) from the whole applied amount [13].

The cumulative amount of drug permeated was plotted against time. The steady-state permeation rate (J_{ss}) was calculated by divided the slop of the linear portion of the plot on the exposed surface area of the skin. Lag time was determined from the x-intercept of the linear portion of the plot [17].

Histological evaluation

For skin histological study the dorsal side of the mouse was shaved with electric clipper. The skin was cut and mounted between donor and receiver compartment of the jacketed Franz cell whit stratum corneum side facing upward. 1 g of optimum formulations and tretinoin cream were placed on the skin. After 38 h the excessive formulation and cream were removed and the skin cleaned with cotton soaked in a phosphate buffer solution (pH 7.4). The treated skins were fixed in 10 % formalin solution and embedded in paraffin wax. Then samples were cut in 5 μm thick sections by using microtome and conventionally stained with haematoxylin and eosin (H&E). Finally the samples were examined by light microscope (Olympus, BH-2, Japan) [18].

Differential scanning calorimetry (DSC)

DSC thermograms of SPC, cholesterol, transcutol and tretinoin were recorded on a differential scanning calorimeter (Mettler Toledo, DSC-1, Switzerland). Thermograms of both blank and tretinoin loaded liposomes were recorded individually. Certain amount of sample was placed in aluminum pan and scanned from 20 to 200 °C by scanning rate of 10 °C/min.

Stability study

Optimum formulations were stored at refrigerate temperature (4 °C) for 3 months. After 1 and 3 months, the particle size and drug incorporation efficiency of the formulations were measured. The results were compared with the initial size and drug incorporation efficiency of formulations [19].

Statistical analysis

All experiments were repeated three times and expressed as the mean ± standard deviation. One way analysis of variance (ANOVA) followed by multiple comparisons Tukey test was used to substantiate statistical differences between groups. Results with $P < 0.05$ were considered to be significant.

The effects of independent variables (X) on the dependent variables (Y) were modeled using a polynomial second order equation as followed:

$$Y = c + b_1X_1 + b_2X_2 + b_3X_1{}^2 + b_4X_2{}^2 + b_5X_1X_2$$

The modeling was performed using SPSS (Version 16.0) with a backward, stepwise linear regression technique and significant expressions ($P < 0.05$) were selected for the final equations. Response surface plots and contour plots resulting from equations obtained by Statgraphics version Centurion XVI.

Results and discussion

In an attempt to obtain suitable formulation containing tretinoin for dermal delivery, deformable liposomes prepared with SPC and transcutol.

Transcutol (diethylene glycol monoethylether) is a non-toxic, biocompatible with skin, penetration enhancer which is miscible in polar and non polar solvents [20]. Effect of transcutol on the lipid organizational structure of human stratum corneum was evaluated by

Table 3 Particle size (nm) and Incorporation efficiency (%) of liposomal formulations (mean ± SD, $n = 3$)

Formulation	Average size	Incorporation (%)
1	8.82 ± 0.95	85.51 ± 0.15
2	16.96 ± 3.69	80.88 ± 0.19
3	10.94 ± 1.84	79.11 ± 0.19
4	15.09 ± 4.62	89.55 ± 0.19
5	9.59 ± 2.99	91.33 ± 0.57
6	12.8 ± 1.65	89.88 ± 0.19
7	10.21 ± 1.85	93.22 ± 0.69
8	7.70 ± 2.30	93.88 ± 0.19
9	7.12 ± 0.74	89.99 ± 0.33

Moghadam et al. [21]. Their results of x-ray scattering study showed transcutol caused a slight disordering effect in the stratum corneum membrane and increasing its fluidity.

In this study the fusion method was used to prepare the topical liposomal formulations. This method is simple, efficient, and reproducible. The method is free of organic solvents like chloroform; and yields homogeneous liposomes with high incorporation efficiencies. Furthermore, liposomes prepared by fusion method showed enough viscosity that they could be applied directly on the skin without the need for the liposomal formulation to be mixed with other bases [9].

Characterization of the liposomes

Particle size

The mean particle size of the liposomal formulations was shown in Table 3. ANOVA analysis showed statistical significant differences between F2 and F1, F8, F9 ($P < 0.05$) and also, F4 and F9 ($P < 0.05$). Different concentrations of phospholipid and transcutol showed no effect on particle size of liposomal formulations.

Incorporation efficiency

The incorporation efficiency of formulations was in range of 79 to 93 % (Table 3). F8 showed maximum

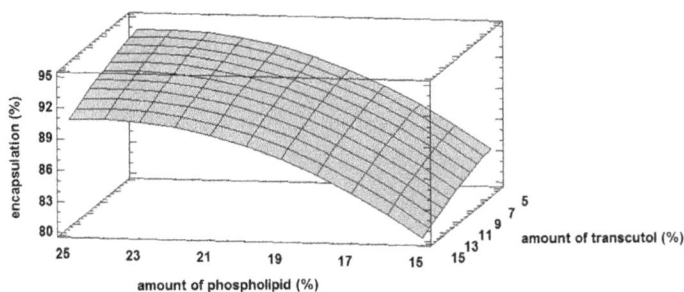

Fig. 1 Response surface plot for Y_1 response (percent of incorporation efficiency)

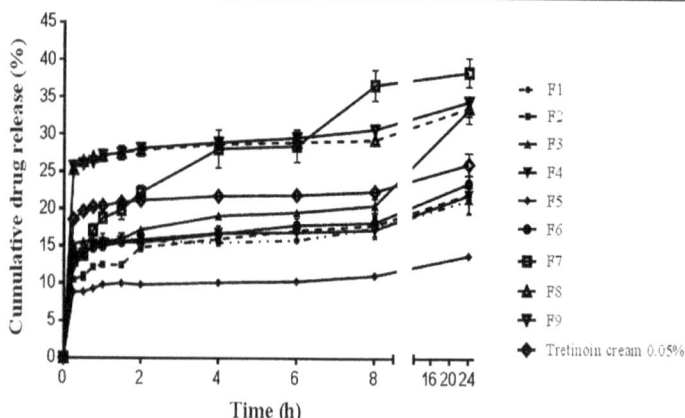

Fig. 2 Release profiles of tretinoin from various liposomal formulations and tretinoin cream

percent of incorporation. There were no statistical significant differences among F4, F6, F9 ($P > 0.05$) and also, between F7 and F8 ($P > 0.05$).

Mathematical relationships were generated between the responses and independent variables using the statistical package SPSS. The equations of the responses represent the quantitative effect of independent variables (X_1 and X_2) upon the responses (Y_1, Y_2 and Y_3). Coefficients with more than one factor represent the interaction between factors while coefficients with second order terms indicate the quadratic nature of the phenomena.

The equation of the Y_1 (percent of incorporation efficiency) is given below:

$$Y_1 = 20.560 + 6.101\,X_1 - 0.126\,X_1{}^2 - 0.016\,X_2{}^2 \qquad (2)$$

Three-dimensional response surface plot for Y_1 is shown in Fig. 1. According to the Fig. 1, incorporation efficiency was increased by increasing the amount of phospholipid, while it was slightly decreased with higher amounts of transcutol. The lipophilic nature of tretinoin may lead to incorporation of this drug between the lipid

Table 4 Analysis of variance (ANOVA) of dependent variables (percent of incorporation efficiency (Y_1) and percent of drug release in 15 min (Y_2) and 24 h (Y_3))

Source of variation	Sum of squares	Degree of freedom	Mean square	F ratio	P-value
Y_1					
Regression	604.968	3	201.656	87.409	0.000
Residuals	53.062	23	2.307		
Total	658.030	26			
$R^2 = 0.919$					
Y_2					
Regression	716.867	4	179.217	23.780	0.000
Residuals	165.800	22	7.536		
Total	882.666	26			
$R^2 = 0.812$					
Y_3					
Regression	1569.312	4	392.328	87.047	0.000
Residuals	99.156	22	4.507		
Total	1668.468	26			
$R^2 = 0.941$					

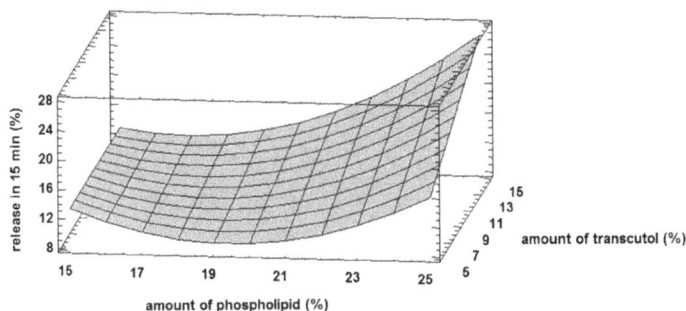

Fig. 3 Response surface plot for Y_2 Response (percent of drug release in 15 min)

bilayers. This can also explain the high incorporation efficiency of the tretinoin in liposomal formulations [22].

In vitro drug release

The release profile of tretinoin from various liposomal formulations and conventional tretinoin cream are shown in Fig. 2. In the first 2 h, drug release from F8 and F9 were significantly ($P < 0.05$) higher than other formulations, at the 4th hour no statistical significant differences were observed among F7, F8 and F9 ($P > 0.05$) and after 8 and 24 h, F7 showed maximum drug release compared with other formulations. The release pattern of tretinoin cream and all liposomal formulations except F7, showed burst release in initial times and then had a reduced rate of release [23].

The target of optimization was to obtain formulations with slow release in first 15 min and maximum release at 24 h. Therefore constraints for the Y_2 (percent of drug release in 15 min) and Y_3 (percent of drug release in 24 h) were:

$$Y_2 < 15\% \text{ and } Y_3 > 30\%$$

The equations of the responses Y_2 and Y_3 are given below:

$$Y_2 = 101.07 - 9.207\,X_1 - 1.666\,X_2 + 0.111\,X_1X_2 + 0.223\,X_1{}^2 \quad (3)$$

$$Y_3 = 149.821 - 14.491\,X_1 - 0.177\,X_1X_2 + 0.431\,X_1{}^2 + 0.194\,X_2{}^2 \quad (4)$$

Analysis of variance (ANOVA) (Table 4) demonstrated that the mathematical models generated were statistically significant and valid for each considered response.

Three-dimensional response surface plot for Y_2 and Y_3 are shown in Figs. 3 and 4. As shown in Fig. 3, drug release was decreased in 15 min by increase in the concentrations of phospholipids up to 20 %. Meanwhile, increase in the amount of phospholipid from 20 to 25 %, higher the value of drug release. Also it was shown that formulations with higher amounts of transcutol in their compositions released more elements of drug at 15 min.

According to Fig. 4, liposomes containing about 17–19 % phospholipid exhibited the lowest drug release among the formulations. However, it was increased by either lower or higher phospholipid concentrations so that drug release at 24 h from formulations composed of 25 % phospholipid (F7, F8 and F9) was maximums.

The phase transition temperature (T_m) of the lipids affected the release of liposome [24]. Phospholipids at their T_m changed from solid to liquid state. Thus the

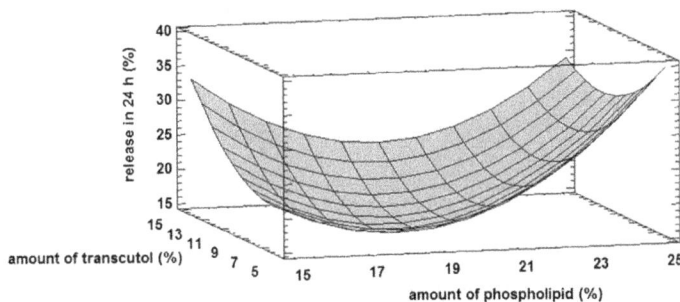

Fig. 4 Response surface plot for Y_3 Response (percent of drug release in 24 h)

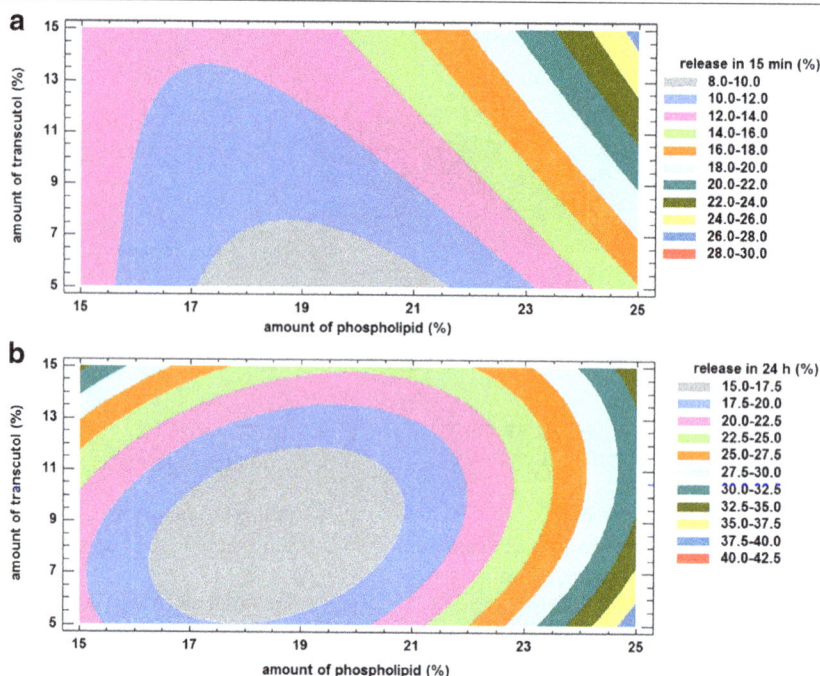

Fig. 5 Contour plots for Y_2 Response (percent of drug release in 15 min) **a** and Y_3 (percent of drug release in 24 h) **b**

permeability of liposomal membrane is increased and encapsulated drug released [25]. Chen et al. [26] prepared stealth liposome with different phosphatidylcholine and found liposome composed SPC in the presence of rat plasma showed maximum drug release which due to lower T_m of SPC.

According to contour plots of responses Y_2 and Y_3 (Fig. 5), optimized formulations were selected. The defined desirable areas of responses Y_2 and Y_3 were superimposed and the region of interest was found. The ratio of SPC: transcutol to obtained optimum formulations were 15.5:14.5, 24:7 and 25:5.

As a validation method for the process, liposomal formulations were prepared at the predicted levels of the independent variables and evaluated for percent of drug release in 15 min and 24 h. Observed and predicted responses for optimum formulations were then compared and the results were shown in Table 5.

Viscosity of F (25:5) and F (15.5:14.5) were 354.53 ± 4.51 and 266.94 ± 3.17 poise, respectively. Formulation (25:5) with the highest amount of phospholipid and lowest amount of transcutol had more viscosity compared with F (15.5:14.5). Thus Formulation (25:5) showed slower release in initial times. Fetih et al. [27] developed and evaluated liposomal gels of celecoxib and concluded that inverse relationship presented between viscosity of liposomal gels with drug diffusion rate and percent of drug released.

According to the results presented in Table 5, observed responses were close to predicted ones which confirmed that the factorial design was valid for predicting the optimum formulation.

In vitro skin penetration and retention

The skin penetration profile of F (15.5:14.5), F (24:7), F (25:5) and conventional tretinoin cream are shown in

Table 5 Observed and predicted responses (percent of drug release in 15 min (Y_2) and 24 h (Y_3)) for optimum formulations

Formulation (SPC: transcutol)	Dependent variables	Observed response	Predicted response	Residual
F (15.5:14.5)	Y_2	14.88	12.72	2.61
	Y_3	30.41	29.76	0.65
F (24:7)	Y_2	14.88	15.53	−0.65
	Y_3	33.28	30.06	3.22
F (25:5)	Y_2	12.97	15.81	- 2.84
	Y_3	38.43	39.64	- 1.21

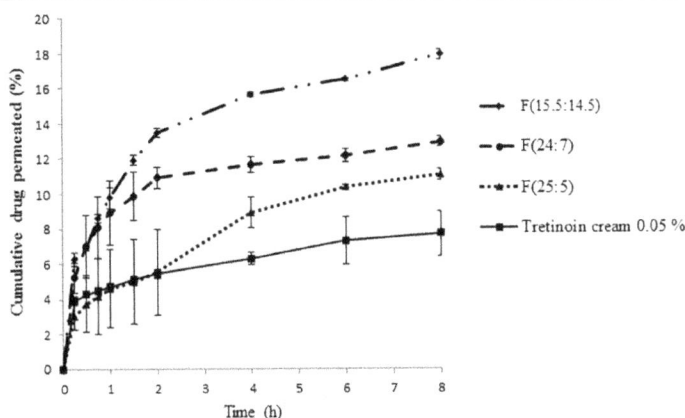

Fig. 6 In vitro permeation profiles of tretinoin from cream and optimum formulations through mice skin

Fig. 6. The penetration percent of optimum formulations was higher ($P < 0.05$) than tretinoin cream. F (15.5:14.5) showed maximum percent of penetration.

According to the Table 6, F (15.5:14.5) showed maximum flux. Formulations and cream penetrated through the skin without any lag time. The flux of F (15.5:14.5) and F (24:7) were higher than cream ($P < 0.05$), while no statistical significant differences found between F (25:5) and tretinoin cream ($P > 0.05$).

ANOVA analysis showed statistical significant differences between J_{ss} of optimum Formulations ($P < 0.05$). These results showed that by enhancement of transcutol concentration in the optimum formulations, percent of penetration and flux was increased which can be due to solubilizing properties of transcutol [28].

The percent of retained tretinoin and ratio of retained drug in the skin to penetrated drug for optimum formulations and tretinoin cream calculated and results showed in Table 6. There was no significant difference in the percent of retained tretinoin between optimum formulations and tretinoin cream ($P > 0.05$). ANOVA analysis showed that no significant difference among ratio of retention/penetration of optimum formulations ($P > 0.05$) but tretinoin cream showed higher ratio of retention/penetration than F(15.5:14.5) and F(24:7) ($P < 0.05$) that could be attributed to higher flux in formulations containing higher amount of transcutol.

Manconi et al. [29] evaluated PEVs with different penetration enhancers for dermal delivery of tretinoin. Their results showed PEVs improved cutaneous drug accumulation compared to control liposome. However, PEVs containing transcutol and labrasol had lower drug accumulated/drug permeated ratio because these vesicles increased both tretinoin deposition and flux.

Mura et al. [30] prepared PEVs with labrasol, transcutol and cineole for (trans) dermal delivery of minoxidil. They concluded that PEVs improved drug deposition into the skin when compared to the classic liposomes.

Caddeo et al. [31] developed PEVs with transcutol or propylene glycol, liposomes and ethosomes for delivered the diclofenac to the skin. Results showed PEVs containing transcutol led to higher drug accumulation in the skin compared to other carriers, diclofenac solution and voltaren. Also they found PEVs containing transcutol permeated the drug more than other vesicular formulations.

Histological evaluation

Histopathological investigation revealed that the thickness of epidermis in skin samples treated with F (15.5:14.5) (Fig. 7b) and F (25:5) (Fig. 7c) was same as untreated skin (control group) (Fig. 7a) and hyperkeratosis was increased in comparison with control group. In tretinoin cream treated skin, proliferations of keratinocytes were obvious and also hyperkeratosis was evident (Fig. 7d). Similar results obtained by Ascenso et al. [32].

Table 6 Permeation parameters, Retention (%) and ratio of retention/penetration of tretinoin from optimum formulations and cream (mean ± SD, n = 3)

Formulation	J_{ss} (µg/cm².h)	T_{lag} (h)	Retention (%)	Retention/Penetration
F(15.5:14.5)	4.71 ± 1	0	12.97 ± 2	0.72 ± 0.1
F(24:7)	3.29 ± 0.08	0	8.27 ± 1.91	0.63 ± 0.15
F(25:5)	1.05 ± 0.25	0	13.19 ± 0.71	1.18 ± 0.07
Tretinoin cream	0.88 ± 0.04	0	13.15 ± 2.77	1.72 ± 0.44

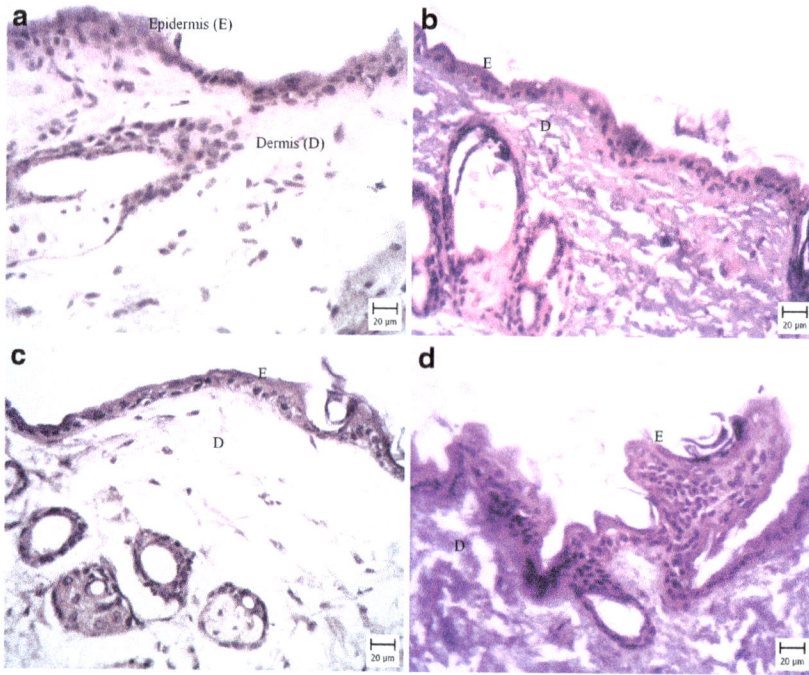

Fig. 7 Photomicrographs (20×) of hairless mice skin sections after haematoxylin and eosin staining: **a** untreated skin, **b** skin treated with F(15.5:14.5), **c** skin treated with F(25:5) and **d** skin treated with tretinoin cream 0.05 %

They evaluated in vivo skin irritation potential of tretinoin loaded ultradeformable vesicles in comparison to ketrel® and demonstrated ultradeformable vesicles caused lowest skin irritation. Their histological study showed in the skin treated with tretinoin loaded ultradeformable vesicle, hyperkeratosis was occurred and for ketrel® treated skin hyperplasia was observed.

Raza et al. [1] developed lipid-based nanocariers for dermal delivery of tretinoin and concluded these carriers were well-tolerated on mouse skin while in the skin treated with marketed product inflammation was observed.

Castro et al. [33] prepared retinoic acid loaded solid lipid nanoparticles and found this cariers considerably reduced skin irritation in rabbit and rhino mouse models when compared to marketed cream. Furthermore their histological evaluation showed in skin treated with retinoic acid loaded solid lipid nanoparticles and marketed gel epidermal thickness was increased in comparison to placebo group.

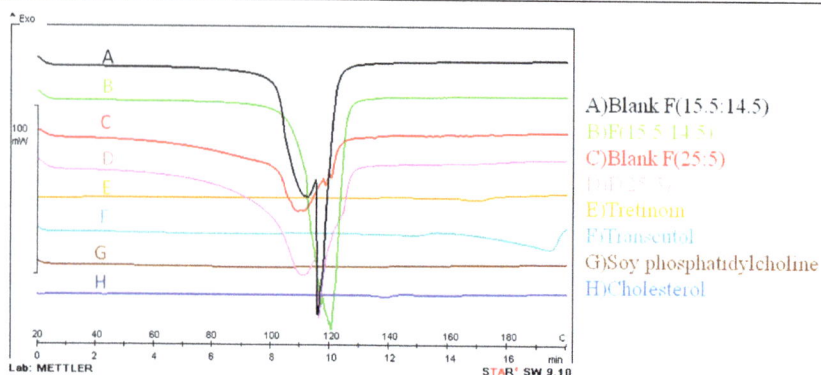

Fig. 8 DSC thermograms of **A** Blank F(15.5:14.5), **B** F(15.5:14.5), **C** Blank F(25:5), **D** F(25:5), **E** Tretinoin, **F** Transcutol, **G** Soy phosphatidylcholine, **H** Cholesterol

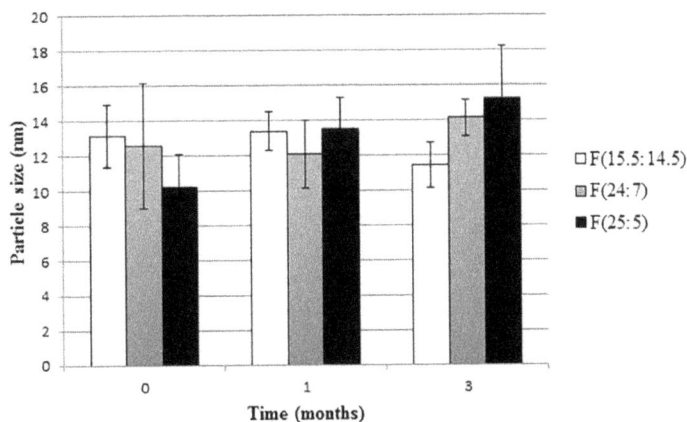

Fig. 9 Mean particle size (nm) of optimum formulations after 1 and 3 months storage at 4 °C

DSC

According to Fig. 8, DSC thermogram of tretinoin and cholesterol showed endothermic peak at 170 °C and 140 °C corresponding to their melting points, respectively [34, 35]. Transcutol thermogram showed endothermic peak about 195 °C, indicating its boiling point [36]. SPC thermogram showed a broad peak at 88 °C. In case of tretinoin loaded liposomes, the melting point of tretinoin was not observed which indicates that it is encapsulated in the liposome. The blank and tretinoin loaded liposome showed peak around 100–120 °C in their thermograms, which may be caused by evaporation of bounded water.

Stability study

The results of stability study for optimum formulations are shown in Figs. 9 and 10. Over the course of 3 months, the mean particle size of formulations did not change significantly $(P > 0.05)$. This matter could be resulted by the presence of transcutol in the formulation that may cause flexibility in vesicles [30] and cholesterol that has stabilizing effect against aggregation and fusion of the liposomes [37]. Similar results obtained by Mura et al. [38] that found particle size of PEVs with different amounts of transcutol remained constant during 3 months at 4 °C. While, particle size of liposomes without transcutol increased significantly. Incorporation efficiency of F (24:7) and F (25:5) were significantly decreased $(P < 0.05)$ after 1 and 3 months while drug loading of F (15.5:14.5) only decreased about 6 % after 3 months $(P < 0.05)$.

Chessa et al. [39] evaluated influence of PEVs with different types of penetration enhancer on (trans) dermal delivery of quercetin and concluded all PEVs promoted drug deposition in the skin.

Srisuk et al. [40] prepared deformable liposomes containing oleic acid for transepidermal delivery of

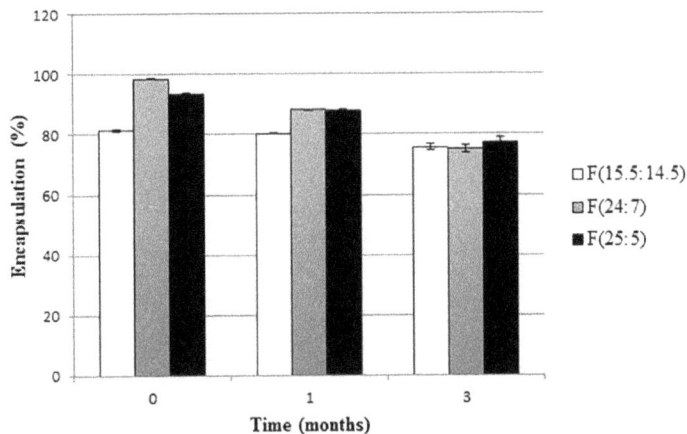

Fig. 10 Incorporation efficiency (%) of optimum formulations after 1 and 3 months storage at 4 °C

methotrexate. These vesicles showed the highest skin permeation, accumulation and flux compared to liposomes without oleic acid and methotrexate solution.

Charoenputtakun et al. [41] developed solid lipid nanoparticles, nanostructured lipid carriers and nanoemulsions containing limonene or cineol as penetration enhancer for dermal delivery of all-trans retinoic acid. They demonstrated solid lipid nanoparticles containing limonene had the highest skin permeation and flux in compression to other formulations and all-trans retinoic acid suspension.

Conclusion

PEVs are novel class of liposomes which consist of phospholipid and penetration enhancer. In this work deformable liposome containing SPC and transcutol was employed for dermal delivery of tretinoin. Particle size of all formulations was smaller than 20 nm. Liposomes showed high incorporation efficiency which may be due to lipophilic nature of tretinoin. Formulations containing 25 % phospholipid exhibited the highest drug release at 24 h while the amount of transcutol did not significantly change drug release. Drug penetrated through the skin for optimum formulations was higher than cream which can be due to solubilizing properties of transcutol. Optimum formulations compared to tretinoin cream caused milder hyperkeratosis without hyperplasia. These results suggested that deformable liposomes could gradually released tretinoin and thus decreased its adverse effects such as erythema, peeling, burning and also increased patient compliance.

Abbreviations
DSC: Differential Scanning Calorimetry; Jss: Steady-state permeation rate; PEV: Penetration-Enhancer Vesicle; SPC: Soy Phosphatidylcholine.

Competing interests
The authors declare that they have no competing interests.

Authors' contributions
Conception and Design: NB, AA, AS, AR. Acquisiotion of data: SS, AR. Analysis and interpretation of data: AA, NB, SS, AR. Drafting manuscript: NB, AA, SS. All authors read and approved the final manuscript.

Acknowledgments
This paper is issued from Pharm D thesis of Somayeh Seifmanesh and financial support was provided by a grant (N-32) from Nanotechnology Research Center of Ahvaz Jundishapur University of Medical Sciences, Ahvaz, Iran. The authors are thankful to Iran Daru for providing us base cream of tretinoin as a gift.

Author details
[1]Nanotechnology Research Center, Ahvaz Jundishapur University of Medical Sciences, Ahvaz, Iran. [2]Department of Pharmaceutics, School of Pharmacy, Ahvaz Jundishapur University of Medical Sciences, Ahvaz, Iran. [3]Targeted Drug Delivery Research Center, School of Pharmacy, Mashhad University of Medical Sciences, Mashhad, Iran. [4]Department of Pathobiology, Faculty of Veterinary Medicine, Shahid Chamran University of Ahvaz, Ahvaz, Iran.

References

1. Raza K, Singh B, Lohan S, Sharma G, Negi P, Yachha Y, Katare, O. P. Nano-lipoidal carriers of tretinoin with enhanced percutaneous absorption, photostability, biocompatibility and anti-psoriatic activity. Int J Pharm. 2013; 456:65–72. doi:10.1016/j.ijpharm.2013.08.019.
2. Brisaert M, Gabriels M, Matthijs V, Plaizier-Vercammen J. Liposomes with tretinoin: a physical and chemical evaluation. J Pharm Biomed Anal. 2001;26: 909–17.
3. Sinico C, Manconi M, Peppi M, Lai F, Valenti D, Fadda AM. Liposomes as carriers for dermal delivery of tretinoin: in vitro evaluation of drug permeation and vesicle-skin interaction. J Control Release. 2005;103:123–36. doi:10.1016/j.jconrel.2004.11.020.
4. Laouini A, Jaafar Maalej C, Limayem Blouza I, Sfar S, Charcosset C, Fessi H. Preparation, Characterization and Applications of Liposomes: State of the Art. J Colloid Sci Biotechnol. 2012;1:147–68. doi:10.1166/jcsb.2012.1020.
5. Shah KA, Date AA, Joshi MD, Patravale VB. Solid lipid nanoparticles (SLN) of tretinoin: potential in topical delivery. Int J Pharm. 2007;345:163–71. doi:10.1016/j.ijpharm.2007.05.061.
6. Ioele G, Cione E, Risoli A, Genchi G, Ragno G. Accelerated photostability study of tretinoin and isotretinoin in liposome formulations. Int J Pharm. 2005;293:251–60. doi:10.1016/j.ijpharm.2005.01.012.
7. Manconi M, Sinico C, Valenti D, Lai F, Fadda AM. Niosomes as carriers for tretinoin. III. A study into the in vitro cutaneous delivery of vesicle-incorporated tretinoin. Int J Pharm. 2006;311:11–9. doi:10.1016/j.ijpharm. 2005.11.045.
8. Anadolu RY, Sen T, Tarimci N, Birol A, Erdem C. Improved efficacy and tolerability of retinoic acid in acne vulgaris: a new topical formulation with cyclodextrin complex. J Eur Acad Dermatol Venereol. 2004;18:416–21. doi:10.1111/j.1468-3083.2004.00929.x.
9. Bavarsad N, Fazly Bazzaz BS, Khamesipour A, Jaafari MR. Colloidal, in vitro and in vivo anti-leishmanial properties of transfersomes containing paromomycin sulfate in susceptible BALB/c mice. Acta Trop. 2012;124:33–41. doi:10.1016/j.actatropica.2012.06.004.
10. Elsayed MM, Abdallah OY, Naggar VF, Khalafallah NM. Deformable liposomes and ethosomes: mechanism of enhanced skin delivery. Int J Pharm. 2006;322:60–6. doi:10.1016/j.ijpharm.2006.05.027.
11. Manconi M, Caddeo C, Sinico C, Valenti D, Mostallino MC, Biggio G, et al. Ex vivo skin delivery of diclofenac by transcutol containing liposomes and suggested mechanism of vesicle-skin interaction. Eur J Pharm Biopharm. 2011;78:27–35. doi:10.1016/j.ejpb.2010.12.010.
12. Romero EL, Morilla MJ. Highly deformable and highly fluid vesicles as potential drug delivery systems: theoretical and practical considerations. Int J Nanomedicine. 2013;8:3171–86. doi:10.2147/ijn.s33048.
13. Jaafari MR, Bavarsad N, Bazzaz BS, Samiei A, Soroush D, Ghorbani S, et al. Effect of topical liposomes containing paromomycin sulfate in the course of Leishmania major infection in susceptible BALB/c mice. Antimicrob Agents Chemother. 2009;53:2259–65. doi:10.1128/aac.01319-08.
14. Kulkamp-Guerreiro IC, Berlitz SJ, Contri RV, Alves LR, Henrique EG, Barreiros VR, et al. Influence of nanoincorporation on the sensory properties of cosmetic formulations containing lipoic acid. Int J Cosmet Sci. 2013;35:105–11. doi:10.1111/ics.12013.
15. Jafari B, Rafie F, Davaran S. Preparation and characterization of a novel smart polymeric hydrogel for drug delivery of insulin. BioImpacts. 2011;1:135–43. doi:10.5681/bi.2011.018.
16. Khan GM, Frum Y, Sarheed O, Eccleston GM, Meidan VM. Assessment of drug permeability distributions in two different model skins. Int J Pharm. 2005;303:81–7. doi:10.1016/j.ijpharm.2005.07.005.
17. Sinko PJ, Singh, Y. Martin's physical pharmacy and pharmaceutical sciences. 6ed. Philadelphia; Lippincott Williams & Wilkins; 2006.
18. Han SB, Kwon SS, Jeong YM, Yu ER, Park SN. Physical characterization and in vitro skin permeation of solid lipid nanoparticles for transdermal delivery of quercetin. Int J Cosmet Sci. 2014;36(6):588–97. doi:10.1111/ics.12160.
19. Panwar P, Pandey B, Lakhera PC, Singh KP. Preparation, characterization, and in vitro release study of albendazole-encapsulated nanosize liposomes. Int J Nanomedicine. 2010;5:101–8.
20. Mura P, Faucci MT, Bramanti G, Corti P. Evaluation of transcutol as a clonazepam transdermal permeation enhancer from hydrophilic gel formulations. Eur J Pharm Sci. 2000;9:365–72.
21. Moghadam SH, Saliaj E, Wettig SD, Dong C, Ivanova MV, Huzil JT, et al. Effect of chemical permeation enhancers on stratum corneum barrier lipid

organizational structure and interferon alpha permeability. Mol Pharm. 2013; 10:2248–60. doi:10.1021/mp300441c.

22. Awad RS, Wahed WS, Bitar Y. Evaluation the impact of preparation conditions and formulation on the accelerated stability of tretinoin loaded liposomes prepared by heating method. Int J Pharm Pharm Sci. 2015;7:171–8.

23. Tabbakhian M, Sharifian A, Shatalebi MA. Preparation and in vitro characterization of tretinoin-containing microspheres suited for dermatological preparations. Res Pharm Sci. 2008;3:31–40.

24. Aygun A, Torrey K, Kumar A, Stephenson LD. Investigation of factors affecting controlled release from photosensitive DMPC and DSPC liposomes. Appl Biochem Biotechnol. 2012;167(4):743–57. doi:10.1007/s12010-012-9724-6.

25. Chen J, Cheng D, Li J, Wang Y, Guo JX, Chen ZP, et al. Influence of lipid composition on the phase transition temperature of liposomes composed of both DPPC and HSPC. Drug Dev Ind Pharm. 2013;39(2):197–204. doi:10. 3109/03639045.2012.668912.

26. Chen J, Yan GJ, Hu RR, Gu QW, Chen ML, Gu W, et al. Improved pharmacokinetics and reduced toxicity of brucine after incorporation into stealth liposomes: role of phosphatidylcholine. Int J Nanomedicine. 2012;7: 3567–77. doi:10.2147/ijn.s32860.

27. Fetih G, Fathalla D, El-Badry M. Liposomal gels for site-specific, sustained delivery of celecoxib: in vitro and in vivo evaluation. Drug Dev Res. 2014; 75(4):257–66. doi:10.1002/ddr.21179.

28. Prasanthi D, Lakshmi PK. Effect of chemical enhancers in transdermal permeation of alfuzosin hydrochloride. ISRN Pharmaceutics. 2012;2012:1–8. doi:10.5402/2012/965280.

29. Manconi M, Sinico C, Caddeo C, Vila AO, Valenti D, Fadda AM. Penetration enhancer containing vesicles as carriers for dermal delivery of tretinoin. Int J Pharm. 2011;412:37–46. doi:10.1016/j.ijpharm.2011.03.068.

30. Mura S, Manconi M, Sinico C, Valenti D, Fadda AM. Penetration enhancer-containing vesicles (PEVs) as carriers for cutaneous delivery of minoxidil. Int J Pharm. 2009;380:72–9. doi:10.1016/j.ijpharm.2009.06.040.

31. Caddeo C, Sales OD, Valenti D, Sauri AR, Fadda AM, Manconi M. Inhibition of skin inflammation in mice by diclofenac in vesicular carriers: liposomes, ethosomes and PEVs. Int J Pharm. 2013;443:128–36. doi:10.1016/j.ijpharm. 2012.12.041.

32. Ascenso A, Salgado A, Euleterio C, Praca FG, Bentley MV, Marques HC, et al. In vitro and in vivo topical delivery studies of tretinoin-loaded ultradeformable vesicles. Eur J Pharm Biopharm. 2014;88:48–55. doi:10.1016/ j.ejpb.2014.05.002.

33. Castro GA, Oliveira CA, Mahecha GA, Ferreira LA. Comedolytic effect and reduced skin irritation of a new formulation of all-trans retinoic acid-loaded solid lipid nanoparticles for topical treatment of acne. Arch Dermatol Res. 2011;303:513–20. doi:10.1007/s00403-011-1130-3.

34. Zidan AS, Spinks C, Fortunak J, Habib M, Khan MA. Near-infrared investigations of novel anti-HIV tenofovir liposomes. AAPS J. 2010;12:202–14. doi:10.1208/s12248-010-9177-1.

35. Ascenso A, Guedes R, Bernardino R, Diogo H, Carvalho FA, Santos NC, et al. Complexation and full characterization of the tretinoin and dimethyl-beta-cyclodextrin complex. AAPS PharmSciTech. 2011;12:553–63. doi:10.1208/ s12249-011-9612-3.

36. Sullivan Jr DW, Gad SC, Julien M. A review of the nonclinical safety of Transcutol, a highly purified form of diethylene glycol monoethyl ether (DEGEE) used as a pharmaceutical excipient. Food Chem Toxicol. 2014;72: 40–50. doi:10.1016/j.fct.2014.06.028.

37. Elmeshad AN, Mortazavi SM, Mozafari MR. Formulation and characterization of nanoliposomal 5-fluorouracil for cancer nanotherapy. J Liposome Res. 2014;24:1–9. doi:10.3109/08982104.2013.810644.

38. Mura S, Manconi M, Valenti D, Sinico C, Vila AO, Fadda AM. Transcutol containing vesicles for topical delivery of minoxidil. J Drug Target. 2011;19: 189–96. doi:10.3109/1061186x.2010.483516.

39. Chessa M, Caddeo C, Valenti D, Manconi M, Sinico C, Fadda AM. Effect of Penetration Enhancer Containing Vesicles on the Percutaneous Delivery of Quercetin through New Born Pig Skin. Pharmaceutics. 2011;3:497–509. doi:10.3390/pharmaceutics3030497.

40. Srisuk P, Thongnopnua P, Raktanonchai U, Kanokpanont S. Physico-chemical characteristics of methotrexate-entrapped oleic acid-containing deformable liposomes for in vitro transepidermal delivery targeting psoriasis treatment. Int J Pharm. 2012;427:426–34. doi:10.1016/j.ijpharm.2012.01.045.

41. Charoenputtakun P, Pamornpathomkul B, Opanasopit P, Rojanarata T, Ngawhirunpat T. Terpene composited lipid nanoparticles for enhanced dermal delivery of all-trans-retinoic acids. Biol Pharm Bull. 2014;37:1139–48.

Physico-chemical characterization and pharmacological evaluation of sulfated polysaccharides from three species of Mediterranean brown algae of the genus *Cystoseira*

Hiba Hadj Ammar[1], Sirine Lajili[2], Rafik Ben Said[3], Didier Le Cerf[4], Abderrahman Bouraoui[2] and Hatem Majdoub[1*]

Abstract

Background: Seaweed polysaccharides are highly active natural substances having valuable applications. The present study was conducted to characterize the physico-chemical properties of sulphated polysaccharides from three Mediterranean brown seaweeds (*Cystoseira sedoides*, *Cystoseira compressa* and *Cystoseira crinita*) and to evaluate their anti-radical, anti-inflammatory and gastroprotective activities.

Methods: The different rates of neutral sugars, uronic acids, L-fucose and sulphate content were determined by colorimetric techniques. The different macromolecular characteristics of isolated fucoidans were identified by size exclusion chromatography equipped with a triple detection: multiangle light scattering, viscometer and differential refractive index detectors, (SEC/MALS/VD/DRI). Anti-inflammatory activity was evaluated, using the carrageenan-induced rat paw edema test in comparison to the references drugs Acetylsalicylate of Lysine and Diclofenac. The gastroprotective activity was determined using HCl/EtOH induced gastric ulcers in rats and to examine the antioxidant effect of fucoidans in the three species, the free radical scavenging activity was determined using 1,1-diphenyl-2-picrylhydrazyl.

Results: The pharmacological evaluation of the isolated fucoidans for their anti-inflammatory, and their gastroprotective effect established that these products from *C. sedoides*, *C. compressa* and *C. crinita* exhibited a significant anti-inflammatory activity at a dose of 50 mg/kg, i.p; the percentages of inhibition of the oedema were 51%, 57% and 58% respectively. And, at the same dose, these fucoidans from *C. sedoides* and *C. compressa* showed a significant decrease of the intensity of gastric mucosal damages compared to a control group by 68%, whereas, the fucoidan from *C. crinita* produced a less gastroprotective effect. Furthermore, the isolated fucoidans exhibited a radical scavenging activity.

Conclusion: The comparative study of fucoidans isolated from three species of the genus *Cystoseira* showed that they have similar chemicals properties and relatives anti-radical, anti-inflammatory and gastroprotective activities which are found to be promising.

Keywords: Fucoidans, *Cystoseiraceae*, *Cystoseira*, SEC/MALS/VS/DRI, Anti-inflammatory activity, Gastroprotective activity

* Correspondence: hatemmajdoub2002@yahoo.fr
[1]Laboratoire des Interfaces et des Matériaux Avancés (LIMA), Faculté des Sciences de Monastir, Université de Monastir, Bd. de l'environnement, 5019 Monastir, Tunisia
Full list of author information is available at the end of the article

Background

Brown seaweeds represent a rich sources of several nutraceuticals components like laminarans, fucoidans, and polyphenols. Among these, fucoidans, a sulphated polysaccharide have been the subject of much interest in recent years, mainly due to their pharmacological and biological potential with anti-viral [1], anti-cancer [2], liver protection [3], anti-inflammatory [4] and antibacterial [5] properties and it also can affect the secretion of extracellular matrix proteins [6] and activate apoptosis [7]. Several studies have attempted to determine the exact structure of fucoidans but only a few examples of regularity in the structure were found. Links, ramifications, the position of the sulphates and other sugars appear to be variables [8]. Fucoidans are generally linear, mainly composed of repeated units of fucoses sulfated at C-2 and/or C-4 with a-(1–3) and/or a-(1–4) linkages [9]. They can also contain uronic acid, optionally acetylated and other neutral sugars such as D-galactose, D-xylose, D-glucose, D-mannose. However, this chemical composition varies depending on the algal specie and it can vary even within the same species. In this paper, we will focus on a comparative study of physico-chemical and biological properties of fucoidans from three species of brown algae of the genus *Cystoseira*: *C. sedoides*, *C. compressa* and *C. crinita*. Our attention is particularly paid to this genus of algae for its abundance in the Mediterranean area and more specifically on the Tunisian coast sides. Furthermore, the only structural features of sulphated fucans from this genus of brown seaweed *Cystoseira indica* have been reported by (Mandal et al.) [10].

Methods

Sample collection

Brown seaweeds, (*C. crinita, C. compressa, and C. sedoides*) were harvested from the Mediterranean sea, from various areas of the coastal region of Monastir and Tabarka (Tunisia), in June 2007, at a depth between 1 and 3 m. These brown algae are of the family of *Cystoseiraceae*. After collection, the seaweeds were rinsed with fresh water to remove associated debris and epiphytes. The cleaned material was then air dried in the shade at 30°C. The dried samples were finally powdered and stored at − 20°C until use. Identification of specimens was carried out in the National Institute of Marine Sciences and Technologies (Salambôo, Tunisia).

Extraction of crude polysaccharides

The milled sample was soaked in Methanol-Dichloromethane (1:1) at room temperature for 48 h then filtered. This process was repeated three times. A sequential extraction of seaweed's powders was carried out with petroleum ether then acetone in a soxhlet apparatus to remove lipophilic

pigments (such as chlorophylls) and low molecular weight proteins. Depigmented dried seaweeds were treated three times with 2% aqueous solution of $CaCl_2$ during 3 hours, in order to precipitate alginates. After centrifugation, the supernatant enclosing the fucoidans was recovered and then purified by dialysis through tubing of molecular weight cut off 30 KDa and then lyophilized.

Chemical composition

Total carbohydrates were determined for all the extracted polysaccharides by the phenol – H_2SO_4 method [11] using galactose as a standard. Whereas, uronic acids were determined using carbazole method [12] and glucuronic acid as a standard. The sulphate content of the polysaccharides was determined by the turbidimetric method using sodium sulphate (Na_2SO_4) as a standard after hydrolyzing the polysaccharides in 2 M HCl at 100°C for 2 h [13]. The content of L-fucose units in fucoidans was estimated by a colorimetric assay with L-cysteine [14]. FTIR were performed in KBr pellets (1 mg polysaccharide in 100 mg KBr). The spectra were recorded on a Perkin Elmer 1600 FTIR spectrometer from 400 to 4000 cm^{-1}.

Molecular weight determination

Analysis of various samples was performed using size exclusion chromatography (SEC) equipped with a triple detection: multi-angle light scattering (MALS) (Down HELEOS II, Wyatt Technology, Ca, USA), viscometer detector (VD) (Viscostar II, Wyatt Technology, Ca, USA) and differential refractive index (DRI) (RID 10 A Shimadzu, Japan). The SEC system consists of a pump (LC10 Ai Shimadzu, Japan) at a flow rate 0.5 mL/min and two columns OHPAK SB 804 and 806 HQ.

The samples were dissolved in the eluent ($LiNO_3$ 0.1 mol/L) at 2 g/L. The dissolution was carried out by stirring at 380 rpm for 24 h at room temperature. 3 mL solutions were filtered through membrane 0.45 microns (regenerated cellulose) before injection.

The analyzes were performed by a data processing Zimm [15] "order 1" using angles from (from 34.8° to 142.8°). The corresponding value of dn/dc, in our case is about 0.15 mL/g, the typical value for a polysaccharide [16]. The Astra 6.0.1.7 software package is set to collect and extrapolate data with the aim to obtain for each elution volume the molecular weight and the gyration radius. With an integration of the peak, we calculated the number (Mn) and weight (Mw) average molecular weight and the z-average gyration radius.

The differential viscosimeter detector permits to obtain for each elution fraction the intrinsic viscosity. An integration of the peak gives the average intrinsic viscosity, which allowed us to obtain the average hydrodynamic volume (Vh) using the Einstein – Simha equation:

$$Vh = [\eta]M/\nu N_A$$

where N_A is Avogadro's number, M is the molar mass, $[\eta]$ is the intrinsic viscosity (g mL^{-1}), and ν is a conformational parameter that takes the value of 2.5 in the case of a spherical conformation.

DPPH (1,1-diphenyl-2-picrylhydrazyl) radical scavenging activity

To examine the antioxidant effect of fucoidans in the three species, the free radical scavenging activity was determined using DPPH according to the method of Kim et al. [17]. A dilution series of the extracted samples was prepared (0, 0.25, 0.5, 0.75 and 1 mg/mL). A 1 mL volume of each sample was mixed with 1 ml of 30 mmol/L DPPH-ethanol solution. The reaction mixture was then stirred vigorously for 10 seconds using the vortex. Color was allowed to develop in the dark for 30 min. The absorbance is measured at 517 nm against the blank. Radical scavenging activity is expressed as the inhibition percentage and was calculated using the following formula:

$$\text{Radical scavenging capacity(RSC, \%)} = 1 - \left[(A_{sample} - A_{sample\ blank})/A_{control} \right] \times 100.$$

Where the $A_{control}$ is the absorbance of the control (DPPH solution without sample), the A_{sample} is the absorbance of the test sample (DPPH solution plus test sample), and the $A_{sample\ blank}$ is the absorbance of the sample only (sample without DPPH solution).

Pharmacological evaluation

Animals

All experiments were performed according to the guidelines established by the European Union on Animal Care (CCE Council 86/609). Wistar rats (150 – 200 g) of both sexes purchased from Pasteur Institute (Tunis, Tunisia) were used. They were housed in groups of eight to ten animals in plastic cages at 20-25°C and maintained on a standard pellet diet with free access to water. Animals were fasted for 24 h before the experiments.

Anti-inflammatory activity

The anti-inflammatory activity of isolated fucoidans was evaluated using the carrageenan induced rat paw oedema test. Wistar rats were divided into groups of six animals and the oedema was induced by injecting 0.05 ml of 1% carrageenan subcutaneously into the subplantar region of the left hind paw [18]. Isolated fucoidans from C. crinita, C. sedoides and C. compressa (25 or 50 mg/kg) and reference drugs were administered intraperitoneally (i.p.) 30 min before the injection of carrageenan. The control group received the vehicle (Saline water 2.5 ml/kg, i.p.). The reference groups received Diclofenac (10 mg/kg, i.p) and (ASL, 300 mg/Kg, i.p.).

Measurement of paw size was done by means of volume displacement technique using Plethysmometer (Ugo Basile no. 7140) immediately before carrageenan injection and 1, 2, 3, 4 and 5 h after carrageenan injection. Percentages of inhibition in our anti-inflammatory tests were obtained for each group using the following ratio:

$$\left[(Vt-Vo)_{control} - (Vt-Vo)_{treated} \right] \times 100/(Vt-Vo)_{control}$$

Where, Vt is the average volume for each group and Vo is the average volume obtained for each group before any treatment [19].

Gastroprotective activity

The gastroprotective activity of fucoidans from three species of genus Cystoseira was studied in HCl/EtOH induced gastric ulcer [20]. Rats were divided into different groups, fasted for 24 h prior receiving an intraperitoneal injection of the isolated fucoidans (25 or 50 mg/kg). Two other groups received Ranitidine (60 mg/kg, i.p.) and Omeprazole (30 mg/kg, i.p.) as reference drugs. After 30 min, all groups were orally treated with 1 ml/100 g of 150 mM HCl/EtOH (40:60, v/v) solution for gastric ulcer induction. Animals were sacrificed 1 h after the administration of ulcerogenic agent; their stomach were excised and opened along the great curvature, washed and stretched on cork plates. The surface was examined to detect the presence of lesions and to measure their extent. The summative length of the lesions along the stomach was recorded (mm) as lesion index.

Table 1 Yields of extraction and carbohydrates analysis

		Yield* (%)	Total sugar (%)	Uronic acid (%)	Sulfate (% SO₃Na)	Fucose (%)
Fucoidans	C. sedoides	3.3	21.3	5.9	16.3	54.5
	C. compressa	3.7	13.0	9.3	16.6	61.5
	C. crinita	2.8	44.5	13.8	15.7	43.4

*Yields of extraction given in % of dry weight.

Table 2 The most diagnostic peaks in the IR spectra of extracted polysaccharides

Fucoidans			Assignment
C. compressa	C. crinita	C. sedoides	
$3421 \ cm^{-1}$	$3411 \ cm^{-1}$	$3412 \ cm^{-1}$	O-H assoc. stretching vibration
$2925 \ cm^{-1}$	$2925 \ cm^{-1}$	$2928 \ cm^{-1}$	C-H stretching vibration
$1652 \ cm^{-1}$	$1641 \ cm^{-1}$	$1639 \ cm^{-1}$	C = O stretching vibration
$1457 \ cm^{-1}$	$1441 \ cm^{-1}$	$1423 \ cm^{-1}$	asymmetrical bending vibration of CH_3
$1263 \ cm^{-1}$	$1231 \ cm^{-1}$	$1231 \ cm^{-1}$	S O stretching vibration
$1049 \ cm^{-1}$	$1050 \ cm^{-1}$	$1050 \ cm^{-1}$	C-O-C stretching vibration
$826 \ cm^{-1}$	$825 \ cm^{-1}$	$825 \ cm^{-1}$	C–O–S vibration

Statistical analysis

Results were analyzed using One Way ANOVA (Fisher LSD post hoc test) and expressed as mean ± s.e.m, using SPSS Statistics Software (SPSS for Windows software release 18.0). Difference between means of treated and control groups were considered significant at $P < 0.05$.

Results and discussion

Extraction and chemical analysis

The main concern in the isolation procedures of fucoidans was to avoid their contamination with other polysaccharides, like laminaran and especially alginic acid. The hot extraction, in the presence of $CaCl_2$ was allowed to separate the insoluble calcium alginate from the soluble fraction. This fraction is rich in fucoidan and laminaran. To eliminate this latter we had to recourse to dialysis.

The extraction yields show almost no difference between seaweed species (about 3%) (Table 1). The yields obtained were in good agreement with Rioux et al. [9] for other seaweed species (*Ascophyllum nodosum* (3.3%), *Fucus versiculosus* (4%), *Saccharina longicruris* (2.6%)).

The different colorimetric assays confirm that isolated polysaccharides are fucoidans, mainly composed by fucose (43 to 61%). The amount of sulphates was determinated for the isolated fucoidans. There was no difference found between the three species; an average of 16% was observed for all. Besides, the isolated fucoidans were moderately sulphated compared to those of *Cystoseira indica* (11.5%) [10], *Saccharina longicruris* (12%) [9], *Fucus vesiculosus* (12%) [21] and *Sargassum stenophyllum* (28%) [22].

The FTIR spectrums of the isolated polysaccharides show typical absorption bands of fucoidan. Their exact absorption peaks are given in (Table 2). The intensity of the bands at $3400–3200 \ cm^{-1}$ was assigned to the deformation of O-H. The bands between 3000 and $2925 \ cm^{-1}$ were attributed to the C-H stretching frequency and the strong absorption at approximately $1050 \ cm^{-1}$ corresponded to the C-O-C stretching frequency of the glycosidic bonds [23]. Besides, the extracted fractions showed all absorption at $1650–1620 \ cm^{-1}$, indicating the presence of uronic acid. The characteristic absorption bands of fucoidan are those who indicate the presence of sulphate (SO_4) and methyl (CH_3) groups, as fucoidan contains mainly fucose [24], which is a monosaccharide that has a methyl group attached to the C5 position. The signals at $1457–1423 \ cm^{-1}$ were attributed to the asymmetrical bending vibration of

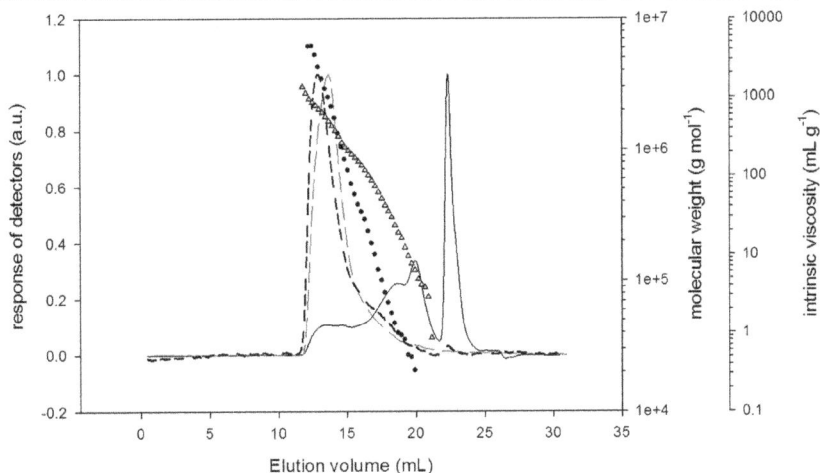

Figure 1 Elution profiles of *C. sedoides* sample with Mw and [η] distribution determined by SEC/MALS/VS/DRI in 0.1 mol L^{-1} LiNO$_3$ aqueous solution. Differential refractive index (full line), light scattering at 90° (dotted black line), specific viscosity (dotted grey line), Mw: molecular weight (black circles) and [η] intrinsic viscosity (grey triangle).

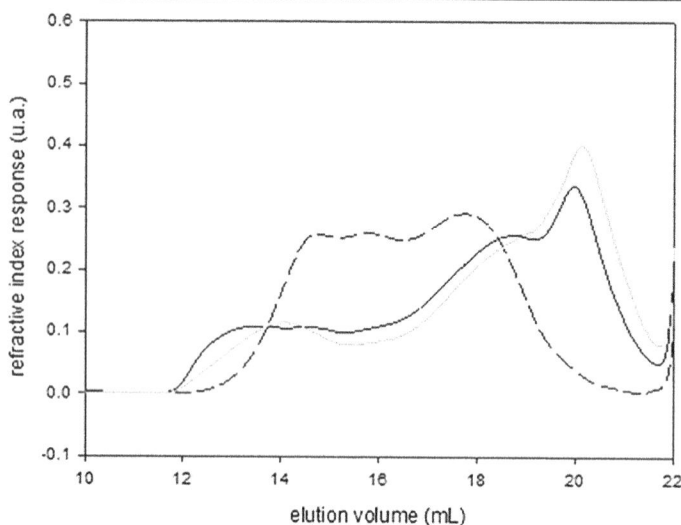

Figure 2 Elution profiles from differential refractive index of different extract determined by SEC/MALS/VS/DRI in 0.1 mol L^{-1} LiNO$_3$ **aqueous solution.** C. sedoides (full black line), C. compressa (dotted black line) and C. crinita (full grey line).

CH$_3$. The strong absorption band at 1255–1240 cm^{-1} (S = O stretching) confirms the presence of a significant amount of sulfate in the polysaccharides. The sharp band at 820 cm^{-1} (C-S-O) suggest that the majority of sulphate groups occupy positions 2 and/or 3 (equatorial positions) [25].

SEC/MALS/VD/DRI experiments were carried out in 0.1 mol/L LiNO$_3$ to determine molecular weights and size information of biopolymers studied. As an example, we have reported on (Figure 1) the elution profiles and the molecular weight and intrinsic viscosity distribution of *C. sedoides* sample. The Polysaccharides are eluted between 11 and 22 mL showing a large distribution. After 22 mL the peak obtained with refractive index detector is due to donnan effect on salt. Firstly, between 11 and 16 mL, light scattering and viscometric responses are intensive with a relative low concentration response (DRI). Consequently, *C. sedoides* have very long macromolecular chains with molecular weight up the 1 000 000 g.mol^{-1}. An other population is eluted from 16 mL to 22 mL. The DRI exhibits high intensity with low

intensity for MALS and DV detectors. The molecular weights are lower and it is no possible to obtain gyration radii due to isotropic diffusion. Nevertheless, we can estimate hydrodynamic radii all along the elution volume with viscometric data. In conclusion, SEC/MALS/VD/DRI analysis permits to obtain some characteristics of whole sample as Mn, Mw, polydispersity index (Đ) weight average (Rh) and [η].

Same analysis was made on the two other fucoidan samples. We have reported only the refractive index response for a better view of the three samples (Figure 2). *C. sedoides* and *C. crinita* are separated in the same way. They have similar molecular repartition. *C. compressa* has a shorter distribution of molecular weight with a peak between 13 and 20 mL. All results are summarized in (Table 3). The presence of very short chain in the two samples *C. sedoides* and *C. crinita* decreases drastically the Mn and consequently increases the polydispersity. In the same way, very high molecular weights obtained at the beginning of the peak (between 12 and 13 mL) influence greatly the intrinsic viscosity and

Table 3 Average macromolecular characteristics of fucoidans isolated from *C. crinita, C. compressa,* and *C. sedoides*) determined by SEC/MALS/VD/DRI (0.1 mol/L LiNO$_3$)

		Mn (g/mol)	Mw (g/mol)	Đ*	[η] (mL.g^{-1})	R$_H$ (nm)	a**
Fucoidans	C. sedoides	26 000	642 000	24	133	18	0.73
	C. compressa	114000	545 000	4.8	92	14	0.70
	C. crinita	18000	339 000	18.2	125	18	0.84

*Đ = Mw/Mn, polydispersity index.
**a: the Mark Houwink exponent.

Table 4 EC50 values of fucoidans extracted from *C. crinita*, *C. compressa*, and *C. sedoides* in radical scavenging activity

	Ascorbic acid	C. sedoides	C. compressa	C. crinita
EC50*(mg/ml)	0.13 ± 0.01	0.96 ± 0.01	0.84 ± 0.06	0.76 ± 0.04

*EC50 value: the effective concentration at which the antioxidant activity was 50%; the absorbance was 0.5 for reducing power; 1,1-diphenyl-2-picrylhydrazyl (DPPH).

average hydrodynamic diameter, which are obtained by weight average.

The knowledge of molecular weight and intrinsic viscosity for each elution volume can be used to determine the Mark-Houwink exponent. Values between 0.7-0.8 are in agreement with random coil conformation [26].

However, it's important to note that chemical composition, molecular weight and structure varies depending on the source of fucoidans, the harvest period and the extraction methods.

DPPH radical scavenging activity

DPPH is a stable radical that can directly react with anti-oxidants. It has been used extensively as a free radical to evaluate reducing substances and is a useful reagent for investigating the free radical scavenging. When the DPPH radical is scavenged by anti-oxidants through the donation of hydrogen to form a stable DPPH-H molecule, the color changes from purple to yellow. In this work, DPPH free-radical scavenging effect of each sample was calculated and the EC_{50} values were presented in (Table 4). Fucoidans from different species (*C. crinita*, *C. compressa* and *C. sedoides*) exhibited DPPH radical scavenging activity with an EC50 value of 0.76 mg/mL, 0.84 mg/mL and 0.96 mg/mL, respectively. These scavenging effects of fucoidans, were less important than

produced by the reference compound, Ascorbic acid and decreased in this order *C. crinita* > *C. compressa* > *C. sedoides*.

Anti-inflammatory activity

Carrageenan has been widely used as a noxious agent to induce experimental inflammation for the screening of compounds possessing anti-inflammatory activity. This phlogistic agent, when injected locally into the rat paw, induced a severe inflammatory reaction, discernible within 30 min [27]. Administration of fucoidans of *C. sedoides*, *C. crinita* and *C. compressa* (25 and 50 mg/kg, i.p.) produced a significant reduction of oedema throughout the period of observation in a dose-related manner. The experimental results are shown in (Table 5). All the isolated fucoidans showed significant anti-inflammatory activity; in fact treatment with sulphated polysaccharides from *C. sedoides*, *C. compressa* and *C. crinita* (at the dose of 50 mg/kg, i.p.) inhibited the formation of the oedema by 51%, 56.81% and 58.21%, respectively, 3 h after the administration of carrageenan. Results were statistically significant compared to the control and are quite similar to those observed for both the group treated with Diclofenac (10 mg/kg) and ASL (acetylsalicylic of lysine 300 mg/kg) which inhibited oedema formation by 55.07% and 56.81%, respectively. Carrageenan induced inflammation in a biphasic phenomenon [28]. The first phase of oedema is attributed to release of histamine and 5-hydroxytryptamine and the second accelerating phase of swelling is attributed to prostaglandin like substances. The knowledge of these mediators involved in different phases is important for interpreting the mode of fucoidan action. Fucoidans might have inhibited the release or actions of the various chemical mediators such as histamine, 5-HT, kinins,

Table 5 Effect of the administration of fucoïdanes isolated from *C. sedoides*, *C. compressa* and *C. crinita* and reference drugs in carrageenan induced rat paw edema

Samples		Dose (mg/kg)	Edema (mL × 10⁻²)			Edema inhibition (%)*		
			1 h	3 h	5 h	1 h	3 h	5 h
Control		-	26 ± 2.75	57.5 ± 1.51	59 ± 3.27	-	-	-
ASL (reference)		300	17.66 ± 1.63	24.83 ± 1.72	29.33 ± 1.21	32.07	56.81	50.28
Diclofenac (reference)		10	15.66 ± 5.12	25.83 ± 2.40	28.66 ± 3.61	39.76	55.07	51.42
Fucoidans	C. sedoides	25	$13.66 \pm 3.20^{***}$	$29.66 \pm 5.20^{***}$	$40.16 \pm 4.70^{***}$	47.46^{a}	48.41^{a}	31.93^{a}
		50	$10.66 \pm 4.08^{***}$	$28.16 \pm 3.38^{***}$	$41.66 \pm 1.21^{***}$	59.00^{b}	51.02^{a}	29.38^{a}
	C. compressa	25	$12.66 \pm 2.73^{***}$	$26.83 \pm 1.04^{***}$	$29.83 \pm 2.40^{***}$	51.30^{a}	53.33^{a}	49.44^{a}
		50	$11.83 \pm 4.09^{***}$	$24.83 \pm 2.48^{***}$	$28.00 \pm 2.36^{***}$	54.50^{a}	56.81^{a}	52.54^{a}
	C. crinita	25	$12.66 \pm 3.43^{***}$	$26.50 \pm 3.39^{***}$	$19.83 \pm 1.94^{***}$	51.28^{a}	54.17^{a}	66.38^{a}
		50	$13.20 \pm 2.68^{***}$	$24.16 \pm 2.56^{***}$	$28.50 \pm 2.50^{***}$	49.23^{a}	58.21^{a}	51.69^{b}

Data are expressed as mean ± s.e.m. (n = 6).
*Mean values with different superscript letters in the same row are significantly different at $p \leq 0.05$.
***$p < 0.001$.

and prostanoids known to mediate acute inflammation induced by phlogistic agents.

Gastroprotective activity

The results of gastroprotective activity of the isolated compounds from *C. compressa*, *C. sedoides* and *C. crinita* on gastric ulcer induced by HCl/ethanol solution are shown in (Table 6). Oral administration of the damaging agent to the control group clearly produced a mucosal damage characterized by multiple hemorrhage red bands of different sizes along the long axis of the glandular stomach. Pretreatment with fucoidans of *C. compressa*, *C. sedoides* and *C. crinita* (25, 50 mg/kg, i.p.) produced significant decrease in the intensity of gastric mucosal damages induced by the necrotizing agent HCl/EtOH compared with control group. Fucoidans from *C. compressa* and *C. sedoides* at the dose of 50 mg/kg produced an important protective effect against gastric mucosal lesion which is quite similar to the effect produced by the reference drug, ranitidine. The percentage of inhibition of ulcer were 68.18%, 68.51% respectively for fucoidans from *C. compressa* and *C. sedoides*. However, fucoidan from *C. crinita* showed less protection (59.90% of inhibition).

HCl-ethanol induced gastric mucosal lesions may be multifactorial, with static blood flow contributing significantly to the hemorrhagic as well as the necrotic aspects of the tissue injury [29]. The decrease in the number of lesions may be due to the reduction in the levels of gastric secretion [30]. The alteration in the acidity/volume of the gastric juice is due to the production of HCl, which may increase the permeability of the mucosal membrane [31]. Thus, the overall protection by fucoidans against HCl-ethanol induced gastric ulceration in experimental

rats suggest that it contains some anti-ulcer agents that may hasten the decomposition of free radicals generated, thereby strengthening the gastric mucosal antioxidant defense system suggesting an gastroprotective effect of fucoidans from brown algae.

Conclusion

The comparative study of fucoidans isolated from three species of the genus *Cystoseira* showed that they have similar properties regarding the percentage in sulphates, L-fucose content and their molecular weight. However this requires an advanced structural study to determine the length of the general chain and the branching of fucoidans.

These similarities are reflected on pharmacological activities; in fact the different isolated fucoidans have similar anti-radical, anti-inflammatory and gastroprotective activities which are found to be promising.

Abbreviations

ASL: Acetylsalicylic of lysine; C. sedoides: *Cystoseira sedoides*; C. compressa: *Cystoseira compressa*; C. crinita: *Cystoseira crinita*; Mn: Average molecular number; Mw: Average molecular weight; Rh: Average hydrodynamic diameter; [η]: Intrinsic viscosity; Đ: Polydispersity index.

Competing interests

The authors declare that they have no competing interests.

Authors' contributions

HM and AB were the supervisors and designed the study. HA contributes to the extraction of fucoidan from three brown algae and to the chemical study. SL carried out pharmacological activities. DL made contribution to the discussion of SEC/MALS/VD/DRI results. Identification of specimens was carried by RS. All authors read and approved the final manuscript.

Acknowledgements

We gratefully acknowledge the financial support of the Doctorale School of Materials, Devices and Microsystems of Monastir, further special thanks goes to Mr. Christophe Rihouey for the technical support regarding SEC/MALS/VD/DRI analyses.

Author details

¹Laboratoire des Interfaces et des Matériaux Avancés (LIMA), Faculté des Sciences de Monastir, Université de Monastir, Bd. de l'environnement, 5019 Monastir, Tunisia. ²Laboratoire de développement chimique, galénique et pharmacologique des médicaments, Faculté de Pharmacie de Monastir, Université de Monastir, 5000 Monastir, Tunisia. ³Institut National des Sciences et Techniques de la Mer (INSTM), Salambôo, Tunis, Tunisia. ⁴Université de la Normandie, Laboratoire Polymères Biopolymères Surfaces, UMR 6270 CNRS Université de Rouen, FRE 3101 CNRS, 76821 Mont Saint Aignan, France.

Table 6 Results of antiulcerogenic activity of fucoïdanes isolated from *C. sedoides*, *C. compressa* and *C. crinita* on gastric ulcer induced by HCl/ethanol solution

Samples		Dose (mg/kg)	Average lesion (mm)	Ulcer inhibition (%)*
Control		–	50.33 ± 5.50	–
Ranitidine (reference)		60	43.38 ± 4.35	66.96
Oméprazole (reference)		30	17.50 ± 1.38	86.67
Fucoïdans		25	$20.83 \pm 2.56^{***}$	58.57 ± 5.09^{a}
		50	$16.00 \pm 2.19^{***}$	68.19 ± 4.35^{b}
	C. sedoides	25	$22.83 \pm 3.70^{***}$	54.60 ± 7.37^{a}
		50	$15.83 \pm 4.60^{***}$	68.51 ± 5.24^{b}
	C. crinita	25	$28.33 \pm 4.09^{***}$	43.66 ± 5.13^{a}
		50	$20.17 \pm 6.17^{***}$	59.90 ± 7.26^{b}

Data are expressed as mean ± s.e.m. (n = 6).
*Mean values with different superscript letters in the same row are significantly different at $p \leq 0.05$.
***$p < 0.001$.

References

1. Hayashi K, Nakano T, Hashimoto M, Kanekiyo K, Hayashi T. Defensive effects of a fucoidan from brown alga Undaria pinnatifida against herpes simplex virus infection. Int J Immunopharmacol. 2008;8:109–16.
2. Liu JM, Bignon J, Haroun-Bouhedja F, Bittoun P, Vassy J, Fermandjian S. Inhibitory effect of fucoidan on the adhesion of adenocarcinoma cells to fibronectin. Anticancer Res. 2005;25:2129–33.
3. Saito A, Yoneda M, Yokohama S, Okada M, Haneda M, Nakamura K. Fucoidan prevents concanavalin A-induced liver injury through induction of endogenous IL-10 in mice. Hepatol Res. 2006;35:190–8.

4. Maruyamaa H, Tamauchib H, Hashimotoc M, Nakano T. Suppression of Th2 immune responses by Mekabu fucoidan from Undaria pinnatifidaSporophylls. Int Arch Allergy Immunol. 2005;137:289–94.

5. Zapopozhets TS, Besednova NN, Loenko IN. Antibacterial and immunomodulating activity of fucoidan. AntibiotKhimioter. 1995;40:9–13.

6. Moon HJ, Park KS, Ku MJ. Effect of Costaria costata Fucoidan on expression of matrix metalloproteinase-1 promoter, mRNA, and protein. J Nat Prod. 2002;72:1731–4.

7. Senthilkumar K, Manivasagan P, Venkatesan J, Kim SK. Brown seaweeds fucoidan: biological activity and apoptosis, growth signaling mechanism in cancer. Int J Biol. 2013;60:366–74.

8. Ponce NMA, Pujol CA, Damonte EB, Flores ML, Stortz CA. Fucoidans from the brown seaweed Adenocystis utricularis: extraction methods, antiviral activity and structural studies. Carbohydr Res. 2003;338:153–65.

9. Rioux LE, Turgeon SL, Beaulieu M. Characterization of polysaccharides extracted from brown seaweeds. Carbohyd Polym. 2007;69:530–7.

10. Mandal P, Mateu CG, Chattopadhyay K, Pujol CA, Damonte EB, Ray B. Structural features and antiviral activity of sulphated fucans from the brown seaweed Cystoseira indica. Antivir Chem Chemother. 2007;18:153–62.

11. Dubois M, Gilles KA, Hamilton JK, Rebers PA, Smith F. Colorometric method for determination for sugars and related substances. Anal Chem. 1956;28:350–6.

12. Bitter T, Muir HM. A modified carbazole method for uronic acid determination. Anal Biochem. 1962;4:330–4.

13. Dodgson KS, Price RG. A note on the determination of the ester sulphate content of sulphated polysaccharides. Biochem J. 1962;84:106–10.

14. Dische Z, Shettles LB. A specific color reaction of methyl pentoses and a spectrophotometric micromethod for their determination. Biol Chem. 1948;175:595–603.

15. Zimm BH. The scattering of light and the radial distribution function of high polymer solutions. J Chem Phys. 1948;16:1093–8.

16. Majdoub H, Roudesli S, Deratani A. Polysaccharides from prickly pear peel and nopals of Opuntia ficus-indica: extraction, characterization and polyelectrolyte behavior. Polym Int. 2001;50:552–60.

17. Kim JK, Noh JH, Lee S, Choi JS, Suh H, Chung HY. The first total synthesis of 2, 3, 6-tribromo-4, 5- dihydroxybenzyl methyl ether (TDB) and its antioxidant activity. Korean ChemSoc. 2002;23:661–2.

18. Winter CA, Risley EA, Nuss GW. Carrageenin-induced edema in hind paw of the rat as assay for anti-inflammatory drug. Proc Soc Exp Biol. 1962;111:544–7.

19. Lanhers MC, Fleurentin J, Dorfman P, Moitrier F, Pelt JM. Analgesic, antipyretic and Anti-inflammatory properties of Euphorbia hirta. Planta Med. 1991;57:225–31.

20. Hara N, Okabe S. Effect of gefernate on acute lesions in rats. Folia Pharmacol Jpn. 1985;85:443–8.

21. Rupérez P, Ahrazem O, Lea JA. Potential antioxidant capacity of sulfated polysaccharides from the edible marine brown seaweed Fucus vesiculosus. J Agric Food Chem. 2002;50:840–5.

22. Duarte ME, Cardoso MA, Noseda MD, Cerezo AS. Structural studies on fucoidans from the brown seaweed Sargassum stenophyllum. Carbohydr Res. 2001;333:281–93.

23. Wang Q, Song Y, He Y, Ren D, Kow F, Qiao Z, et al. Structural characterisation of algae Costaria costata fucoidan and its effects on CCl4-induced liver injury. CarbohydrPolym. 2014;107:247–54.

24. Ale MT, Maruyama H, Tamauchi H, Mikkelsen JD, Meyer AS. Fucoidan from Sargassum sp. and Fucus vesiculosus reduces cell viability of lung carcinoma and melanoma cells in vitro and activates natural killer cells in mice in vivo. Int J Biol. 2011;49:331–6.

25. Qiu X, Amarasekara A, Doctor V. Effect of oversulfation on the chemical and biological properties of fucoidan. CarbohydrPolym. 2006;63:224–8.

26. Villay A, Lakkisdefillipis F, Picton L, Lecerf D, Vial C, Michaud P. Comparison of polysaccharide degradations by dynamic High Pressure Homogenisation. Food Hydrocolloids. 2012;27:278–86.

27. Borgi W, Ghedira K, Chouchane N. An antiinflammatory and analgesic activity of Zizyphus lotus roots barks. Fitoterapia. 2007;78:16–9.

28. Vinegar R, Schreiber W, Hugo RJ. Biphasic development of carrageenin edema in rats. J Pharmacol Exp Ther. 1969;166:96–103.

29. Guth PH, Paulsen G, Nagata H. Histologic and microcirculatory changes in alcohol-induced gastric lesions in the rat: effect of prostaglandin cytoprotection. Gastroenterol. 1984;87:1083–90.

30. Wormsley K. Progress report the pathophysiology of duodenal ulceration. G Gut. 1974;15:59–64.

31. Dayton MT, Kauffman GL, Schlegel JF. Gastric bicarbonate appearance with ethanol ingestion. Mechanism and significance. Dig Dis Sci. 1983;28:449–55.

Blessings in disguise: a review of phytochemical composition and antimicrobial activity of plants belonging to the genus *Eryngium*

Sinem Aslan Erdem[1], Seyed Fazel Nabavi[2], Ilkay Erdogan Orhan[3], Maria Daglia[4], Morteza Izadi[5] and Seyed Mohammad Nabavi[2*]

Abstract

Medicinal and edible plants play a crucial role in the prevention and/or mitigation of different human diseases from ancient times to today. In folk medicine, there are different plants used for infectious disease treatment. During the past two decades, much attention has been paid to plants as novel alternative therapeutic agents for the treatment of infectious diseases due to their bioactive natural compounds such as phenol, flavonoids, tannins, etc. The genus *Eryngium* (Apiaceae) contains more than 250 flowering plant species, which are commonly used as edible and medicinal plants in different countries. In fact, some genus *Eryngium* species are used as spices and are cultivated throughout the world and others species are used for the treatment of hypertension, gastrointestinal problems, asthma, burns, fevers, diarrhea, malaria, etc. Phytochemical analysis has shown that genus *Eryngium* species are a rich source of flavonoids, tannins, saponins, and triterpenoids. Moreover, eryngial, one the most important and major compounds of genus *Eryngium* plant essential oil, possesses a significant antibacterial effect. Thus, the objective of this review is to critically review the scientific literature on the phytochemical composition and antibacterial effects of the genus *Eryngium* plants. In addition, we provide some information about traditional uses, cultivation, as well as phytochemistry.

Keywords: Antibacterial, Eryngial, *Eryngium*, Flavonoids, Saponins, Infection

Background

Infectious diseases are known as one of the most important leading causes of long and short–term morbidity and mortality worldwide [1, 2]. According to the World Health Organization, in 2011, infectious diseases were responsible for approximately 18 million deaths worldwide. In addition to the high prevalence of infectious diseases, there are some microorganisms resistant to antibiotic therapy, which lead to the increase of death rate due their ability to acquire and transmit drug resistance [2]. Nowadays, antibiotic resistance is known as one the most important and challenging health problems in the global health programs. Therefore, during the past two decades, much attention has been paid to the discovery and development of natural multi-target antimicrobial agents with high efficacy and low adverse effects [3]. Natural products are known as one of the most important and effective drugs for human disease treatment [4–6]. In addition to their efficacy, natural products are mostly non-toxic and therefore, they can be used as safe therapeutic strategies [7–9]. A plethora of scientific evidence reported that edible and medicinal plants have significant potential to synthesize antimicrobial agents as their defense mechanisms against biotic stresses such as microorganisms [10]. It has been reported that plant-derived antimicrobial compounds can be categorized into the different groups such as phenols, flavonoids, terpenoids, lectins, polypeptides, polyacetylenes as well as alkaloids [11]. In addition, in traditional medicine, many edible and medicinal plants have been widely used for the treatment of different infectious diseases [11, 12].

* Correspondence: Nabavi208@gmail.com
[2]Applied Biotechnology Research Center, Baqiyatallah University of Medical Sciences, P.O. Box 19395-5487, Tehran, Iran
Full list of author information is available at the end of the article

The genus *Eryngium* contains more than 250 flowering species worldwide [13]. Genus *Eryngium* is the largest and most complex genus in Apiaceae family [13, 14]. Some species in the genus *Eryngium* are endangered such as *E. alpinum* L., *E. aristulatum* Jeps., *E. constancei* M.Y. Sheikh, *E. cuneifolium* Small, and *e. viviparum* J. Gay [13, 14]. According to the morphological studies, the genus *Eryngium* has been classified into five subgenera, including *Eryngium* subgenus *Eryngium*, *E.* subgenus *Monocotyloidea*, *E.* subgenus *Fruticosa*, *E.* subgenus *Semiaquatica*, and *E.* subgenus *Foetida* [15, 16]. *E.* subgenus *Eryngium* is the most common one throughout Europe, Africa and Asia, while the other subgenera are widely distributed in Australia [15, 16]. However, infrageneric analysis through sequence data of chloroplast DNA trnQ-trnK 5'-exon and nuclear ribosomal DNA ITS regions showed that there are two different subgenera including *Eryngium* and *Monocotyloidea* [17–19].

Like the other members of Apiaceae family, the genus *Eryngium* plants have various culinary and/or medicinal uses (Fig. 1) [20–23]. Several species have been widely used in traditional medicine such as *E. foetidum* L., *E. caucasicum* Trautv. (syn. *Eryngium caeruleum* M. Bieb.), *E. maritimum* L., *E. planum* L., *E. dichotomum* Desf., *E. campestre* L. and *E. creticum* Lam. [24–27], whereas *E. foetidum* and *E. caucasicum* have been widely cultivated in some Asian countries such as Iran, Turkey, etc. [27, 28].

E. caucasicum is known as one the most common edible leafy vegetables in northern part of Iran and widely used in different foodstuff, pickles, etc. [28, 29]. Besides, the fruits of *E. foetidum* are known as common edible food components in Nigeria [30]. Actually, some *Eryngium* species are also used as ornamental plants [31]. A mountain of scientific evidence has shown that different species of the genus *Eryngium* possess antimicrobial effects under *in vitro* and *in vivo* conditions [32–36].

Therefore, the present paper aims to review the scientific literature on the phytochemical composition and antimicrobial activities of essential oils and extracts obtained from genus *Eryngium* species. In addition, we discuss about traditional uses, cultivation and phytochemistry of *Eryngium* species to provide a complete picture of this genus.

Materials and methods
Data sources and search strategy
Data were collected from Medline, Pubmed, Scopus, Web of Science (ISI Web of Knowledge), Science Direct, Embase, and BIOSIS Previews (from 1950 to July 20, 2015), via searching of these keywords: "*Eryngium* and phytochemistry or chemical compounds", "*Eryngium* and antibacterial", "*Eryngium* and antimicrobial", and "*Eryngium* and biological effect". We also scanned the reference list of each paper and searched Cochrane review library.

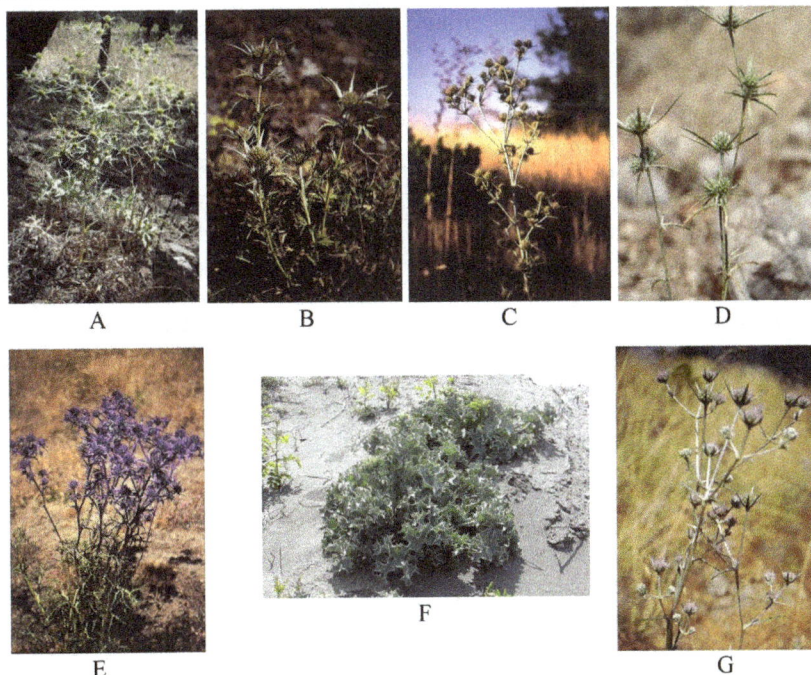

Fig. 1 Some of species from *Eryngium* genus, *Eryngium campestre L.* (**a**), *Eryngium davisii Kit Tan & Yildiz* (**b**), *Eryngium isauricum Contandr. & Quezel* (**c**), *Eryngium falcatum Delar.* (**d**), *Eryngium kotschyi Boiss.* (**e**), *Eryngium maritimum L.* (**f**), *Eryngium trisectum Wörz & H. Duman.* (**g**)

Thereafter, the bibliographies of collected data were screened for further publications. Finally, collected data were analyzed and judged by second and third authors according to the scientific standard of conduct. However, some of the references may be published after the initial search date July 2015.

Traditional uses

In traditional medicine, some of *Eryngium* species have been used for treatment of several human diseases [24–27]. It has been reported that *E. campestre* L. is widely used as antitussive, stimulant, aphrodisiac, and diuretic agent in Turkish traditional medicine [37, 38]. *E. caucasicum* is one of the most important edible plants in the northern part of Iran due to its multiple beneficial effects on human health [29, 31, 39, 40]. Moreover, *E. creticum* has been used as hypoglycemic plant in the Jordanian traditional medicine [41], while *E. elegans* Cham. & Schltdl. has been reported to be utilized as diuretic agent in the Argentinian traditional medicine [42]. Most of *Eryngium* species are also known as medicinal plants worldwide for the treatment of several human diseases such as diarrhea, gastrointestinal problems, bladder and kidney dysfunctions, and venereal diseases [24–27, 43–45]. In Chinese traditional medicine, *E. foetidum* is widely used for treatment of inflammation [24] and *E. yuccifolium* Michx. roots have been traditionally used to treat snakebites, toothache [27, 46, 47], digestive problems, diarrhea, headache, etc. [24–27, 43–45]. A large scale of evidence has pointed out to multiple pharmacological effects of the genus *Eryngium* species including antioxidant, anti-inflammatory, antihemolytic, antinociceptive effects, and protective agent against neurodegenerative deseases [25, 28, 48–50]. For instance, *Eryngium planum*, which is a rare medicinal plant, was studied to determine the effect of subchronic administration of a 70 % ethanol root extract (200 mg/kg, p.o.) on behavioral and cognitive responses in experimental animals (Wistar rats) linked with the expression levels of mRNA coding for enzymes such as acetylcholinesterase (AChE), butyrylcholinesterase (BuChE), and beta-secretase (BACE-1). At the end of the experiment, after the last dose of the *Eryngium* extract, scopolamine (SC) was administered intraperitoneally to a group of animals (treated). In the animals treated with the *Eryngium* extract, an improvement in long-term memory produced by the EP extract in both scopolamine treated and control group was registered with decreased mRNA AChE, BuChE, and BACE-1 levels, especially in the frontal cortex, suggesting the potential efficacy of this extract in this kind of pathologies [25, 28, 48–50].

This is only an example of the fact in the las decade some investigations have been carried out to demonstrate the potential pharmacological activity of *Eryngium* species extracts [51, 52].

Cultivation

Several genus *Eryngium* species have been widely used as edible plants in many countries and, consequently, mainly cultivated as an economic crop in tropical areas of the world [24, 28, 29]. In fact, numerous reports refer to the ideal and effective conditions for cultivating, harvesting as well as post-harvesting conditions of *Eryngium* species [24, 31, 53]. In the northern parts of Iran, *E. caucasicum* is one of the most important garden vegetables, which is mostly used in preparation of foodstuff, pickles, etc. [28, 29]. It has been reported that some *Eryngium* species are easily cultivated in dry, sandy, well-drained soils, and full sun [24, 31, 53]. Root cuttings are a common protocol for propagation of *Eryngium* species [24, 31, 53–55], which can also be propagated using other plant cuttings [24, 31, 53–55]. In addition, there is a close correlation between *Eryngium* species growth and fertilizer levels in the soil [24, 31, 53–55]. However, *Eryngium* species are significantly endangered by plant diseases as well as insect attacks [24, 31, 53–55].

Phytochemistry

Based on the review of the literature up to now, the aerial parts of *Eryngium* species have been reported to contain mainly saponins, flavonoids, and essential oil, while the underground parts contain triterpene saponins, monoterpene glycosides, phenolic compounds such as flavonoids and phenolic acids, coumarin derivatives, terpene aldehyde esters, acetylenes, essential oil, and oligosaccharides [56–60].

Saponins

The *Eryngium* species are the rich sources of triterpene saponins (Tables 1 and 2). Most of the saponins isolated from *Eryngium* species possess mainly hydroxylated oleanane-type aglycons such as A1-barrigenol (**1**), R1-barrigenol (**2**), or barringtogenol C (**3**) (Fig. 2). In addition to these core structures, cameliagenin A (**4**), erynginol A (**5**) and B, betulinic acid, oleanolic acid, and steganogenin (**6**) having glucose, glucuronic acid, rhamnose, xylose, galactose, and arabinose moieties have been also found in various *Eryngium* species (Fig. 2). The general saponin structures possess generally acetic, angelic, dimethylacrylic, and tiglic acid substituents, located predominantly at C21, C22 or C28 positions. On the other hand, isovaleric, *n*-butyric, and methyl butyric acids occur relatively rare substituents. Saponin glycosides found in *Eryngium* species are usually monodesmosidic saponins, where the bidesmosidic ones contain sugar groups at C3 and C28 positions [59, 61–65].

Table 1 Triterpene saponins from *Eryngium* species isolated between 1970–1978

Source	Sapogenol	Type of sapogenol	Plant part	Ref.
Eryngium planum L.	Eryngiumgenin A	A1-barrigenol	Roots	[69]
	Eryngiumgenin B	A1-barrigenol		
	Eryngiumgenin C	R1- barrigenol		
	Eryngiumgenin D	R1- barrigenol		
Eryngium planum L.	Erynginol A	Barringtogenol C	Aerial	[70]
Eryngium bromeliifolium Delar.	Oleanic acid type of sapogenols	Oleanic acid	Leaves	[66]
Eryngium planum L.	Eryngiumgenin F	Barringtogenol C	Roots	[61]
	Eryngiumgenin G	n/a		
	Eryngiumgenin H	n/a		
	Eryngiumgenin J	n/a		
	Eryngiumgenin K	R1- barrigenol		
	Eryngiumgenin L	n/a		
Eryngium bromeliifolium Delar.	Betulinic acid		Leaves	[71]
Eryngium giganteum L.	Giganteumgenin A	n/a	Leaves	[67]
	Giganteumgenin B	n/a		
	Giganteumgenin C	Oleanic acid		
	Giganteumgenin D	n/a		
	Giganteumgenin E	n/a		
	Giganteumgenin G	n/a		
	Giganteumgenin H	n/a		
	Giganteumgenin K	n/a		
	Giganteumgenin M	Barringtogenol C		
	Giganteumgenin N	R1- barrigenol		
Eryngium planum L.	Eryngiumgenin E		Roots	[72]
Eryngium bromeliifolium Delar.	Betulinic acid-3-O-β-glycoside		Leaves	[73]
Eryngium maritimum L.	Eryngiumgenin C and sapogenols with A1-barrigenol, R1-barrigenol and barringtogenol C structures		Aerial parts	[74]
Eryngium amethystinum L.	Main structure: Barringtogenol C			[68]
	R1-barrigenol			
	Erynginol A			
	A1-barrigenol			
Eryngium bromeliifolium Delar.	3-O-D-Glucopyranosyloleanolic acid–28-O-D-xsylopyranoside (Saponin F)		Leaves	[62]
Eryngium planum L.	R1-barrigenol + an acid substituent and 2 glycopyranosyl moieties		Roots	[75][a]

[a]This study was published in 1985 and it is the only study published between 1978-2002

The first phytochemical studies performed on the genus *Eryngium* starting from early 1970s were focused on their saponin content. According to the survey of the literature data published between 1970–1978 and in 1985, the identification of the isolated compounds was limited to the absolute definition of the aglycons with possible positions of sugars and acyl substituents because of inadequate chemical facilities in structure elucidation techniques [61, 66–68]. In this period, *E. planum, E. amethystinum* L., *E. giganteum* M. Bieb.,

and *E. bromeliifolium* F. Delaroche were studied in more detail. As summarized in Table 1, A1-barrigenol and R1-barrigenol-type of aglycons containing dimethylacrylic, angelic, and/or tyglic acids as the acid moieties were isolated from the roots of the *E. planum*, named as eryngiumgenine A-D [69] of which only aglycon types were identified and classified according to the R_f values. Later, compound (**5**) was isolated from the aerial parts of this species [70]. Further phytochemical studies on the same plant were continued on the leaves and

Table 2 Triterpene saponins from *Eryngium* species isolated after 2002

Source	Saponins	Plant part	Ref.
Eryngium foetidum (Linn)	O-(3)-β-D-Glucopyranosyl-(1 → 2 rham)-β-fucopyranosyl-(1 → 3 rham)-α-L-rhamnopyranosyl-(1 → 4 glu)-β-D-glucopyranosyl]-olean-12-en-23,28-diol	Aerial parts	[30]
Eryngium campestre L.	3-O-β-D-Glucopyranosyl-(1 → 2)-[α-L-rhamnopyranosyl-(1 → 4)]-β-D-glucuronopyranosyl-22-O-Angeloyl-R1-barrigenol	Roots	[59]
	3-O-β-D-Glucopyranosyl -(1 → 2)-[α-L- rhamnopyranosyl -(1 → 4)]-β-D- glucuronopyranosyl-22-O-β,β-dimethylacryloyl-A1-barrigenol		
Eryngium campestre L.	3-O-α-L- Rhamnopyranosyl -(1 → 2)-β-D- glucuronopyranosyl -22-O-β,β- dimethylacryloyl -A1-barrigenol	Roots	[63]
	3-O-α-L- rhamnopyranosyl -(1 → 2)-β-D- glucuronopyranosyl -22-O- angeloyl -R1-barrigenol		
	3-O-α-L- Rhamnopyranosyl -(1 → 2)-β-D- glucuronopyranosyl -21-O-acetyl-22-O- angeloyl -R1-barrigenol		
	3-O-α-L- Rhamnopyranosyl -(1 → 2)-β-D- glucuronopyranosyl -21-O- acetyl -22-O-β,β- dimethylacryloyl -R1-barrigenol		
	3-O-α-L- Rhamnopyranosyl -(1 → 2)-β-D- glucuronopyranosyl -22-O- angeloyl -28-O- acetyl -R1-barrigenol		
Eryngium yuccifolium Michx.	3β-[β-D-Glucopyranosyl-(1 → 2)-β-D-glucopyranosyl-(1 → 2)]-β-D-glucuronopyranosyloxy-22α-β-D-glucopyranosyloxyolean-12-ene-16α, 28-diol (Eryngioside A)	Whole plant	[64]
	3β-[β-D-Galactopyranosyl-(1 → 2)-β-D-glucopyranosyl-(1 → 2)]-β-D-glucuronopyranosyloxy-22α β-D-glucopyranosyloxyolean-12-ene-16α, 28-diol (Eryngioside B)		
	3β-[β-D-Glucopyranosyl-(1 → 2)-β-D-glucopyranosyl-(1 → 2)]-β-D-glucuronopyranosyloxy-22α β-D-glucopyranosyloxyolean-12-ene-16-oxo-28-ol (Eryngioside C)		
	3β-[β-D-Glucopyranosyl-(1 → 2)-β-D-glucopyranosyl-(1 → 2)]-β-D-glucuronopyranosyloxy-28-β-D-glucopyranosyloxyolean-12-ene-16α,22α-diol (Eryngioside D)		
	22α-Angeloyloxy-3β-[β-D-glucopyranosyl-(1 → 2)-[β-D-xylopyranosyl-(1 → 3)]-β-D- glucuronopyranosyloxyolean-12-ene-15α, 16α, 21β,28-tetrol (Eryngioside E)		
	22α-Angeloyloxy-3β-[β-D-glucopyranosyl-(1 → 2)]-[β-D-xylopyranosyl-(1 → 3)]-β-D- glucuronopyranosyloxyolean-12-ene- 16α, 21β,28-triol (Eryngioside F)		
	21β-Angeloyloxy-3β-[β-D-glucopyranosyl-(1 → 2)]-[α-L-arabinopyranosyl-(1 → 3)]-β-D- glucuronopyranosyloxyolean-12-ene-15α, 16α, 22α,28-tetrol (Eryngioside G)		
	22α-Angeloyloxy-3β-[β-D-glucopyranosyl-(1 → 2)]-[β-D-xylopyranosyl-(1 → 3)]-β-D- glucuronopyranosyloxyolean-12-ene- 15α, 16α,28-triol (Eryngioside H)		
	22α-Angeloyloxy-3β-[β-D-glucopyranosyl-(1 → 2)]-[α-L-arabinopyranosyl-(1 → 3)]-β-D- glucuronopyranosyloxyolean-12-ene- 15α, 16α,28-triol (Eryngioside I)		
	21β-Angeloyloxy-22α-acetyloxy-3β-[β-D-glucopyranosyl-(1 → 2)]-[β-D-xylopyranosyl-(1 → 3)]-β-D-glucuronopyranosyloxyolean-12-ene-15α, 16α,28-triol (Eryngioside J)		
	21β-Angeloyloxy-22α-acetyloxy-3β-[β-D-glucopyranosyl-(1 → 2)]-[β-D-xylopyranosyl-(1 → 3)]-β-D- glucuronopyranosyloxyolean-12-ene-16α,28-diol (Eryngioside K)		
	21β-Angeloyloxy-22α-acetyloxy-3β-[β-D-glucopyranosyl-(1 → 2)]-[α-L-arabinopyranosyl-(1 → 3)]-β-D- glucuronopyranosyloxyolean-12-ene-16α,28-diol (Eryngioside L)		
	Saniculasaponin III		
Eryngium yuccifolium Michx.	Eryngiosides A-L	Roots	[47]
	21 β-Acetyloxy-22 α -angeloyloxy-3 β-[β-D-glucopyranosyl-(1 → 2)]-[β-D-xylopyranosyl-(1 → 3)]-β-D-glucuronopyranosyloxyolean-12-ene-15α,16α,28-triol (Eryngioside M)		
	22α-Angeloyloxy-3β-[β-D-glucopyranosyl-(1 → 2)]-[α-L-arabinopyranosyl-(1 → 3)]-β-D- glucuronopyranosyloxyolean-12-ene-15α, 16α, 21β,28-tetrol (Eryngioside N)		

Table 2 Triterpene saponins from *Eryngium* species isolated after 2002 (*Continued*)

	Saniculasaponin II and III		
Eryngium planum L.	3-O-β-D-Glucopyranosyl-(1 → 2)-β-D-glucuronopyranosyl-21-O-acetyl-22-O-angeloyl-R1-barrigenol	Roots	[76]
	3-O-β-D-Glucopyranosyl-(1 → 2)-β-D-glucuronopyranosyl-22-O-angeloyl-A1-barrigenol		
	3-O-β-D-glucopyranosyl-(1 → 2)-β-D-glucuronopyranosyl-22-O-angeloyl-R1-barrigenol		
Eryngium kotschyi Boiss.	3-O-α-L-Rhamnopyranosyl-(1 → 4)-β-D-glucuronopyranosyl-22-O-β,β-dimethylacryloylA1-barrigenol	Roots	[65]
	3-O-α-L-Rhamnopyranosyl-(1 → 4)-β-D-glucuronopyranosyl-22-O-angeloylA1-barrigenol		
	3-O-β-D-glucopyranosyl-(1 → 2)-[β-D-glucopyranosyl-(1 → 6)]-β-D-Glucopyranosyl-21,22,28-O-triacetyl-(3β,21β,22α)-olean-12-en-16-one		
	3-O-β-D-Glucopyranosyl-(1 → 2)- glucopyranosyl-22-O-β-D- glucopyranosylsteganogenin		
	3-O-β-D-Galactopyranosyl-(1 → 2)-[α-L-arabinopyranosyl-(1 → 3)]-β-D-glucuronopyranosyl-22-O-angeloyl-A1-barrigenol		
	3-O-α-L-Rhamnopyranosyl-(1 → 4)-β-D-glucuronopyranosyloleanolic acid		

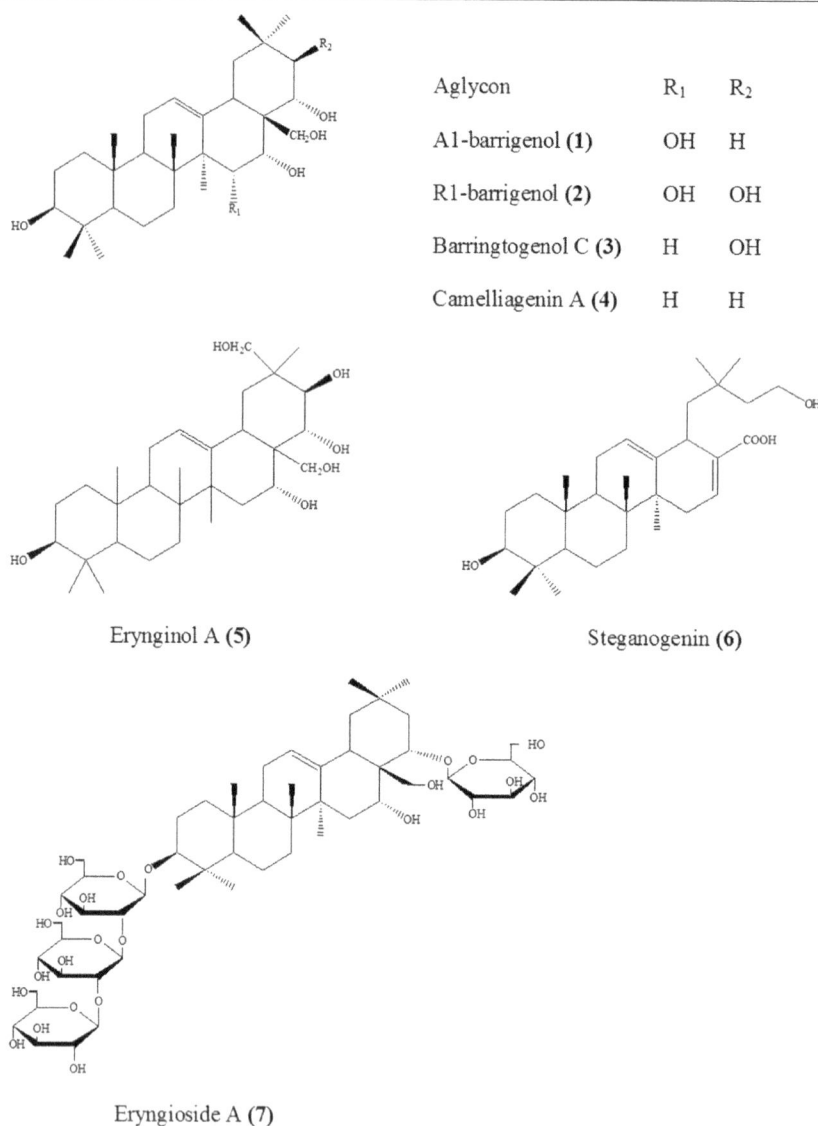

Aglycon	R$_1$	R$_2$
A1-barrigenol (1)	OH	H
R1-barrigenol (2)	OH	OH
Barringtogenol C (3)	H	OH
Camelliagenin A (4)	H	H

Erynginol A (5)

Steganogenin (6)

Eryngioside A (7)

Fig. 2 Saponin derivatives frequently found in *Eryngium* species

roots. These studies led to the isolation of a number of aglycons with (4), (3), (2) types possessing acetic, tyglic, butyric, and isovalerianic acids located at C16, C21, C22 or C28 positions [71, 72]. Isolation of saponin aglycones such as (2) and (3), and saponins bearing (2) and (3) skeletons, named as giganteumgenin A (7), B (8), C (9), D (10), E (11), G (12), H (13), K (14), M (15), and N (16) (Fig. 3), was achieved from the methanol extract of the leaves of *E. giganteum* [67]. Another phytochemical investigation on *E. amethystinum* led to isolation of the saponins with main structures in (1), (2), (3), and (5) [68]. Other sapogenols isolated from various *Eryngium* species

until 1978 are listed in Table 1 [58, 62, 72–74]. Many years later, another R1-barringtogenol derivative with an acid moiety and two glycopyranosyl moieties was reported from *E. planum* roots by Voigt et al. in 1985 [75].

Most of the scientific articles concerning saponins of the genus *Eryngium* remained limited to the identification of the sapogenol type and determination of the acid or sugar substituents. After the late 70's, publications concerning the saponins from the genus *Eryngium* have become much more detailed as giving the whole structure elucidations as a result of the developments of the techniques used for structure elucidation. For

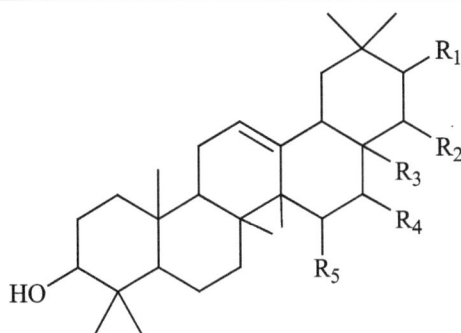

Sapogenol		R$_1$	R$_2$	R$_3$	R$_4$	R$_5$
Giganteumgenin (7)	A*	-O-Angeloyl -O-Tigloyl -O-Dimethylacryloyl	-OCOCH$_3$	-CH$_2$OCOCH$_3$	-OH	-H
Giganteumgenin (8)	B*	-O-Angeloyl -O-Tigloyl -O-Dimethylacryloyl	-OCOCH$_3$	-CH$_2$OH	-OH	-H
Giganteumgenin C (9)		-H	-H	-COOH	-H	-H
Giganteumgenin (10)	D	-OCOC$_4$H$_7$	-OCOCH$_3$	-CH$_2$OH	-OH	-OCOCH$_3$
Giganteumgenin (11)	E*	-O-Angeloyl -O-Tigloyl	-OH	-CH$_2$OH	-OH	-H
Giganteumgenin (12)	G*	-O-Angeloyl -O-Tigloyl	-OH	-CH$_2$OH	-OH	-OH
Giganteumgenin (13)	H	-OH	-OCOC$_4$H$_7$	-CH$_2$OH	-OH	-OH
Giganteumgenin (14)	K	-OH	-OCOC$_4$H$_7$	-CH$_2$OH	-OH	-OH
Giganteumgenin (15)	M	-OH	-OH	-CH$_2$OH	-OH	-H
Giganteumgenin (16)	N	-OH	-OH	-CH$_2$OH	-OH	-OH

*Mixture compound

Fig. 3 Structures of giganteumgenins A-N

instance, Anam [30] reported the full configuration of a new oleanane-type triterpene saponin structure (17) from the aerial parts of *E. foetidum* (Fig. 4). Kartal et al. [59] characterized two new triterpene saponins (18, 19) from the roots of *E. campestre* bearing A(1) and (2) types, and isolated five new triterpene saponins (20–24), one of which was (1) and the others with (2) main skeleton (Fig. 5) [63]. Another phytochemical study performed on the whole parts of *E. yuccifolium* was reported by Zhang et al. [64], who described the isolation and identification of 12 new polyhydroxylated triterpenoid saponins named as eryngiosides A-L (28–39) and two known triterpenoid saponins {21β-angeloyloxy-3β-[β-D-glucopyranosyl-(1 → 2)]-[β-D-xylopyranosyl-(1 → 3)]-β-D-glucuronopyranosyloxyolean-12-ene-15α, 16α, 22α, 28-tetrol (44) and saniculasaponin III (43)} from the same species (Fig. 6). Furthermore, the root of *E. yuccifolium*

afforded two new polyhydroxyoleanene saponins [eryngioside M (40) and N (41)], together with 15 known triterpenoid saponins (28–39; 42–44) elucidated [47].

Further studies on the roots of *E. planum* led to the isolation of two R1- and one A1-barrigenol type of triterpene saponins [76], where 3-O-β-D- glucopyranosyl-(1 → 2)-β-D-glucuronopyranosyl-21-O-acetyl-22-O-angeloyl-R1-barrigenol (25), 3-O-β-D-glucopyranosyl-(1 → 2)-β-d-glucuronopyranosyl-22-O-angeloyl-A1-barrigenol (26) and 3-O-β-D-glucopyranosyl-(1 → 2)-β-D-glucuronopyranosyl-22-O-angeloyl-R1-barrigenol (27) (Fig. 5) were also found to be present in the roots of *E. planum* [76]. Detailed phytochemical investigation on the roots of *E. kotschyi* Boiss., which is an endemic plant to Turkey, led to isolation of two known and four new triterpene saponins (45–48) (Fig. 7) [77].

Flavonoids

In an earlier study [78], isolation from *E. planum* of a new flavonol glycoside (identified as kaempferol-3-O-(6-O-β-D-glucopyranosyl)-β-D-galactopyranoside) was reported. A phytochemical study on the aerial parts of *E. campestre* led to the characterization of a new acylated flavonol named as kaempferol 3-O-β-D-(2'-Z-p-coumaroylgluco-side) **(49)** along with 10 known compounds including tiliroside **(50)**, kaempferol 3-O-β-D-glucosyde-7-O-α-L-rhamnoside **(51)**, rutin **(52)**, kaempferol **(53)**, quercetin **(54)**, isorhamnetin **(55)**, caffeic acid, chlorogenic acid, and mannitol [58] as well as luteolin 7-glucoside [79] of which some selected structures are given in Fig. 8. Using UHPLC-ESI-Q-TOF-MS technique, quantification of a number of flavonols (quercetin, kaempferol, isorhamnetin, and their derivatives) and naringenin rhamnoglucoside (a flavanone derivative) was performed in *E. bourgatii* Gouan

by Cádiz-Gurrea et al. [48]. Hawas et al. [80] isolated 11 flavonoid glycosides (including isorhamnetin 3-O-α-rhamnoside, isorhamnetin 3-O-β-galactoside, isorhamnetin 3-O-β-glucoside, isorhamnetin 3-O-β-rutinoside, myricetin 3-O-β-galactoside 4'-methylether, myricetin 3-O-β-glucoside 3'-methylether, myricetin 3-O-β-glucoside 4'-methylether, quercetin 3-O-β-glucoside, quercetin 3-O-β-glucuronide 4'-methylether, and rutoside) from the aerial parts of *E. campestre*. Then, most recently, Khalfallah et al. [36] characterized five flavonoid derivatives from the aerial parts of *E. triquetrum* Vahl. described as kaempferol 3-O-β-D-glucoside, kaempferol 3-O-[6''-O-E-p-coumaroyl]-β-D-glucopyranoside, kaempferol 3-O-[2'',6''-di–O-E-p-coumaroyl]-β-D-glucoside, kaempferol 3-O-[α-L-rhamnosyl-(6 → 1)-O-β-D-glucoside, and quercetin 3-O-[α-L-rhamnosyl-(6 → 1)-O-β-D-glucoside].

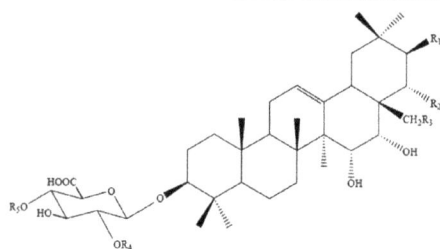

Plant Name	Compound	R_1	R_2	R_3	R_4	R_5	Ref.
E. campestre	18	OH	Angeloyl	OH	Glycose	Rhamnose	56
E. campestre	19	H	Dimethylacryloyl	OH	Glycose	Rhamnose	56
E. campestre	20	H	Dimethylacryloyl	OH	Rhamnose	H	60
E. campestre	21	OH	Angeloyl	OH	Rhamnose	H	60
E. campestre	22	Acetyl	Angeloyl	OH	Rhamnose	H	60
E. campestre	23	Acetyl	Dimethylacryloyl	OH	Rhamnose	H	60
E. campestre	24	OH	Angeloyl	Acetyl	Rhamnose	H	60
E. planum	25	Acetyl	Angeloyl	OH	Glycose	H	73
E. planum	26	H	Angeloyl	OH	Glycose	H	73
E. planum	27	OH	Angeloyl	OH	Glycose	H	73

Fig. 4 Structure of the (17) isolated from *E. foetidum*

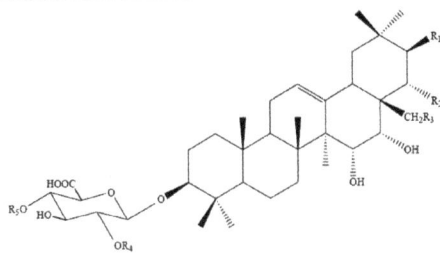

Plant Name	Compound	R_1	R_2	R_3	R_4	R_5	Ref.
E. campestre	18	OH	Angeloyl	OH	Glycose	Rhamnose	56
E. campestre	19	H	Dimethylacryloyl	OH	Glycose	Rhamnose	56
E. campestre	20	H	Dimethylacryloyl	OH	Rhamnose	H	60
E. campestre	21	OH	Angeloyl	OH	Rhamnose	H	60
E. campestre	22	Acetyl	Angeloyl	OH	Rhamnose	H	60
E. campestre	23	Acetyl	Dimethylacryloyl	OH	Rhamnose	H	60
E. campestre	24	OH	Angeloyl	Acetyl	Rhamnose	H	60
E. planum	25	Acetyl	Angeloyl	OH	Glycose	H	73
E. planum	26	H	Angeloyl	OH	Glycose	H	73
E. planum	27	OH	Angeloyl	OH	Glycose	H	73

Fig. 5 Saponins isolated from *E. campestre* and *E. planum*

Coumarin derivatives

The first coumarin derivatives isolated from *E. campestre* by Sticher & Erdelmeier [56] were agasyllin (**56**), grandivittin (**57**), aegelinol benzoate (**58**), and aegelinol (**59**) which structures are given in Fig. 9 [56]. The isolation of marmesin tiglate [also known as nodakenetin (**60**), Fig. 10] together with metetoin, a nitrogenous compound, was achieved from *E. ilicifolium* Lam. [81].

Phenolic acid derivatives

Many *Eryngium* species have been reported to contain phenolic substances. Le Claire et al. [82] characterized chlorogenic (**63**), R-(+)-rosmarinic (**61**), and *R*-(+)-3'-*O*-β-D-glucopyranosyl rosmarinic acids (**62**) in the roots of *E. alpinum* through medium pressure liquid chromatography

(MPLC) and preparative high pressure liquid chromatography (HPLC) (Fig. 11). Besides, the presence of R-(+)-rosmarinic acid and *R*-(+)-3'-*O*-β-D-glucopyranosyl rosmarinic acid was also shown in several *Eryngium* species which could be used as chemotaxanomic markers specific to this genus. Two new caffeic acid derivatives, i.e. 3,4-dihydroxyphenyl caffeate and (4-β-D-glucopyranosyloxy)-3-hydroxyphenyl caffeate, along with a new flavonoid (kaempferol-3-O-(2-O-*trans-p*-methoxycoumaroyl-6-O-*trans-p*-coumaroyl)-β-D-glucopyranoside) were isolated from the whole parts of *E. yuccifolium* in addition to following known compounds, i.e. caffeic acid and kaempferol-3-O-(2,6-di-O-*trans-p*-coumaroyl)-β-D-glucopyranoside [64]. Cádiz-Gurrea et al. [48] also revealed presence of cinnamic acid derivatives

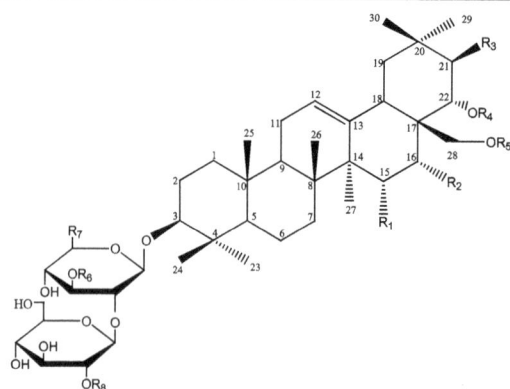

	R$_1$	R$_2$	R$_3$	R$_4$	R$_5$	R$_6$	R$_7$	R$_8$
Eryngioside A (28)	H	OH	H	Glycose	H	H	CH$_2$OH	Glycose
Eryngioside B (29)	H	OH	H	Glycose	H	H	CH$_2$OH	Galactose
Eryngioside C (30)	H	=O	H	Glycose	H	H	CH$_2$OH	Glycose
Eryngioside D (31)	H	OH	H	H	Glycose	H	CH$_2$OH	Glycose
Eryngioside E (32)	OH	OH	OH	Angeloyl	H	Xylose	COOH	H
Eryngioside F (33)	H	OH	OH	Angeloyl	H	Xylose	COOH	H
Eryngioside G (34)	OH	OH	O- Angeloyl	H	H	Arabinose	COOH	H
Eryngioside H (35)	OH	OH	H	Angeloyl	H	Xylose	COOH	H
Eryngioside I (36)	OH	OH	H	Angeloyl	H	Arabinose	COOH	H
Eryngioside J (37)	OH	OH	O- Angeloyl	Acetyl	H	Xylose	COOH	H
Eryngioside K (38)	H	OH	O- Angeloyl	Acetyl	H	Xylose	COOH	H
Eryngioside L (39)	H	OH	O- Angeloyl	Acetyl	H	Arabinose	COOH	H
Eryngioside M (40)	OH	OH	O-Acetyl	Angeloyl	H	Xylose	COOH	H
Eryngioside N (41)	OH	OH	OH	Angeloyl	H	Arabinose	COOH	H
Saniculasaponin II (42)	OH	OH	O-Acetyl	Angeloyl	H	Arabinose	COOH	H
Saniculasaponin III (43)	OH	OH	O- Angeloyl	Acetyl	H	Arabinose	COOH	H
Compound 44	OH	OH	O- Angeloyl	H	H	Xylose	COOH	H

Fig. 6 Saponins isolated from *E. yuccifolium*

(chlorogenic, rosmarinic, ferulic, caffeic acids, and their derivatives), benzoic acid derivatives (*p*-hydroxybenzoic acid glucoside, arbutin, syringic acid, glucogallin, gentisic acid, and their derivatives) and various organic acids (gluconic, citric, quinic acids, and their derivatives) in *E. bourgatii* using hyphenated advance liquid chromatographic separation techniques. On the other hand, catechin, epicatechin, chlorogenic, gallic, and rosmarinic acids were determined quantitatively in the roots of *E. palmatum* Pančić & Vis. [83]. In a similar study [60], chlorogenic, hydroxybenzoic, and caftaric acids were detected in *E. bornmuelleri* Nábĕlek along with trace amounts of caffeic, ferulic, and rosmarinic acids.

Other types of compounds

Drake and Lam [84] reported the isolation of falcarinone, a widespread acetylenic compound occurring in Apiaceae. 6-Pentyl-2-[2-oxo-butin(3)-yliden]-tetrahydropyrane from the aerial parts and roots of *E. bourgatti* and the acetylenic compounds identified as *Z* and *E* isomers of the same compound were also obtained from this species in addition to falcarinone, falcarinolone, falcarinol, and scopoletin [85]. Further phytochemical studies ensued in the characterization of two new monoterpene glycosides of the cyclohexenone type, elucidated as 3-(β-D-glucopyranosyloxymethyl)-2,4,4-trimethyl-2,5-cyclohexadien-1-one and 3-(β-D-glucopyranosyloxymethyl)-2,4,4-trimethyl-2-

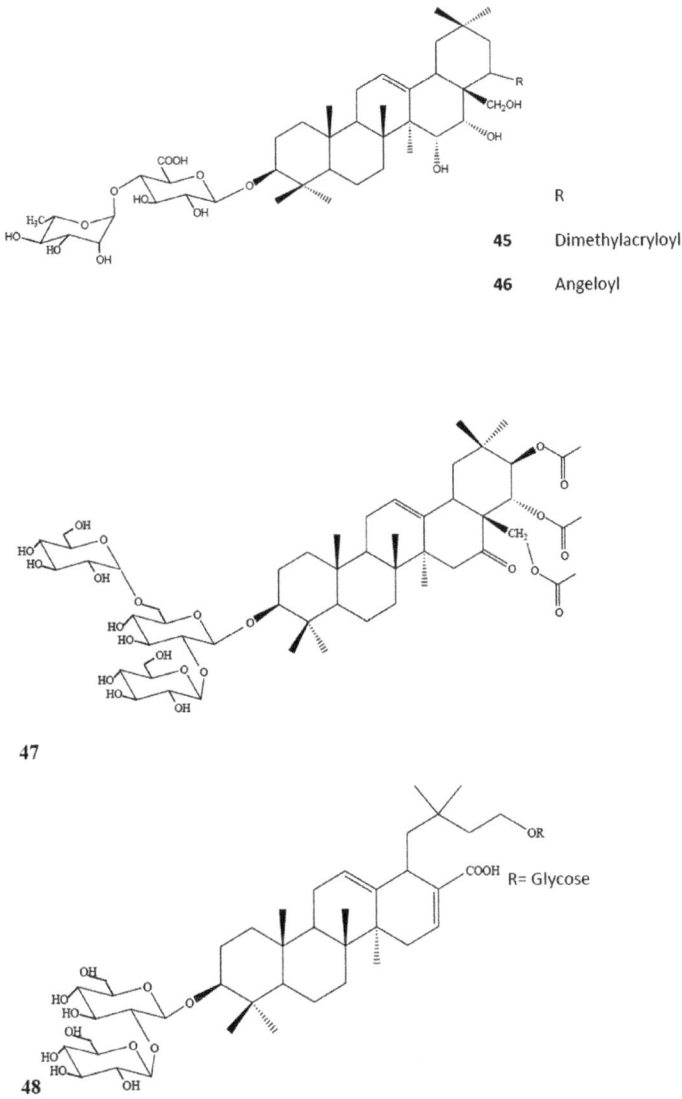

Fig. 7 Chemical structure of triterpene saponins

cyclohexen-1-one [57]. An unusual sesquiterpene whose structure was established as 1-*n*-propyl-perhydronaphtha-line   1,2,4a,5,6,7,8,8a-octahydro-4-methyl-1-propyl-naph-thalene-7-carbaldehyde was reported from the aerial parts of *E. creticum* [86], while new ester derivatives, character-ized as *cis*-chrysanthenyl hexanoate and *cis*-chrysanthenyl octanoate, were isolated from *E. planum* [87].

In order to find out the compounds possibly responsible for the anti-inflammatory activity of *E. foetidum*, compos-ition of the hexane extract from the leaves of this species was subjected to GC and GC-MS analyses [88]. Hereby, α-cholesterol, brassicasterol, campesterol, stigmasterol (as the main component, 95 %), clerosterol, β-sitosterol, Δ_5-avenasterol, $\Delta_5$24-stigmastadienol, and Δ_7-avenasterol

were detected in the extract. Muckensturm et al. [89] re-ported a phytochemical study performed on the diethyl ether extracts from *E. giganteum*, *E. variifolium* Coss., *E. planum*, and *E. maritimum*. Chromatographic separation techniques applied to the seed extract of *E. giganteum* led to the elucidation of a new *nor*-sesquiterpene hydrocarbon, i.e. 15-*nor*-α-muurolene (gigantene), and germacrene-D, *trans*-β-farnesene, 15-oxy-α-muurolene, 15-hydroxy-α-muurolene, ledol, and spatulenol. Similar studies on the seeds of the *E. planum* gave way to isolation of *cis*-chry-santhenyl acetate, while isoferulyl senecioate and 2,3,4-tri-methylbenzaldehyde were obtained from the leaves of *E. variifolium*. Nevertheless, it should be noted that the latter compound was considered as artifact by these authors. In

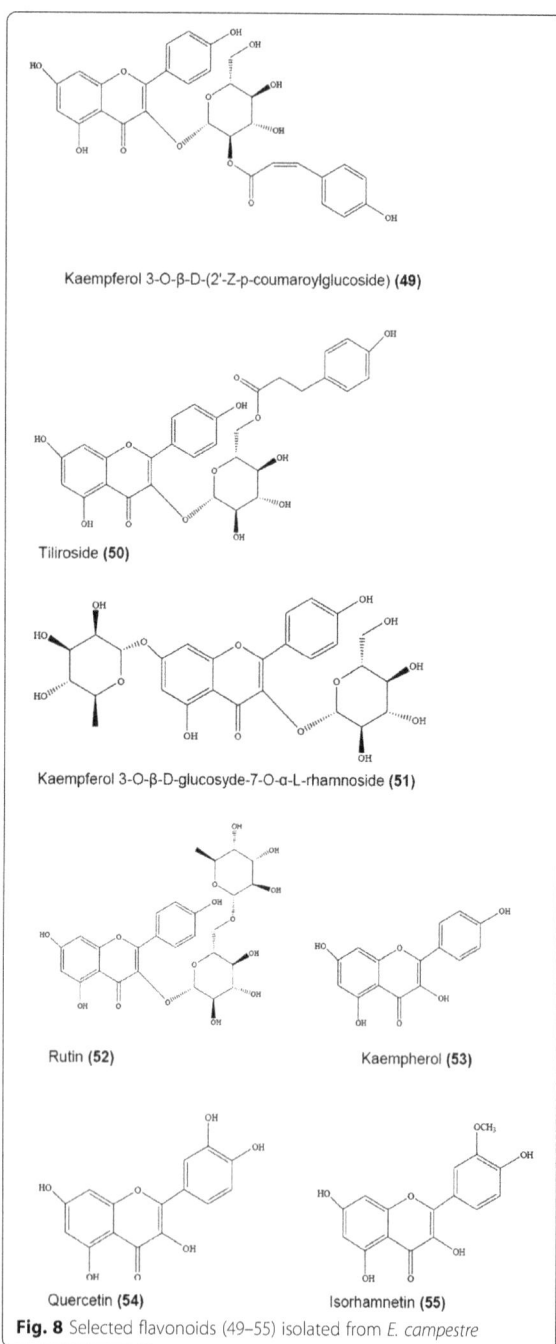

Kaempferol 3-O-β-D-(2'-Z-p-coumaroylglucoside) (49)

Tiliroside (50)

Kaempferol 3-O-β-D-glucosyde-7-O-α-L-rhamnoside (51)

Rutin (52)   Kaempherol (53)

Quercetin (54)   Isorhamnetin (55)

Fig. 8 Selected flavonoids (49–55) isolated from *E. campestre*

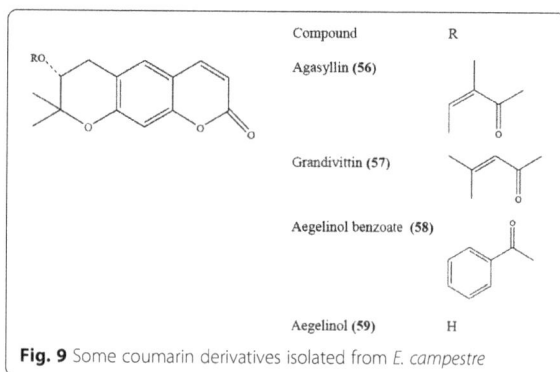

Compound	R
Agasyllin (56)	
Grandivittin (57)	
Aegelinol benzoate (58)	
Aegelinol (59)	H

Fig. 9 Some coumarin derivatives isolated from *E. campestre*

with their corresponding references in Table 3, a great interspecies variation could be easily observed. However, the most common monoterpenes analyzed in different plant parts of *Eryngium* species have been as follows; germacrene D, α-pinene, caryophyllene, muurolene, α- and β-selinene, limonene, α- and β-bisabolol, etc., whereas many hydrocarbons and some aromatics such as trimethylbenzaldehyde and dodecanal have been detected.

Antimicrobial effects of the genus *Eryngium* plants
Plants are known to produce antimicrobial substances [10], which act as plant defense mechanisms and protect them against abiotic and biotic stresses. These antimicrobial agents, which are often characterized by low adverse effects and wide spectrum activities, belong to many chemical classes such as phenolics and polyphenolics, terpenoids, alkaloids, lectins, polypeptides, and polyacetylenes [11].

Among the plants belonging to the genus *Eryngium*, some species exhibit considerable antimicrobial activity against gram-positive and gram-negative bacteria, some species of fungi and yeasts and viruses. Within this genus, the most studied species has been *E. foetidum*, which is cultivated across South Asia and Europe, Tropical Africa, and Pacific islands. As regards the antibacterial activity of *E. foetidum* extracts, the literature data are conflicting. In fact, in 2003, Alzoreky and Nakahara reported that the acetone and buffered methanol extracts obtained from *E. foetidum* leaves did not show any antibacterial activity against *Escherichia coli*, *Salmonella*

another study [90], *E. foetidum* was subjected to isolation procedures which finally afforded *trans*-2-dodecanal (eryngial) in pure form.

Essential oil
Essential oil compositions of numerous *Eryngium* species have been investigated by many researchers. As illustrated

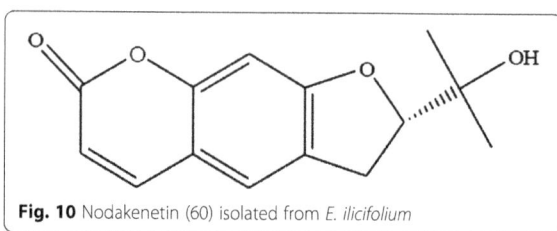

Fig. 10 Nodakenetin (60) isolated from *E. ilicifolium*

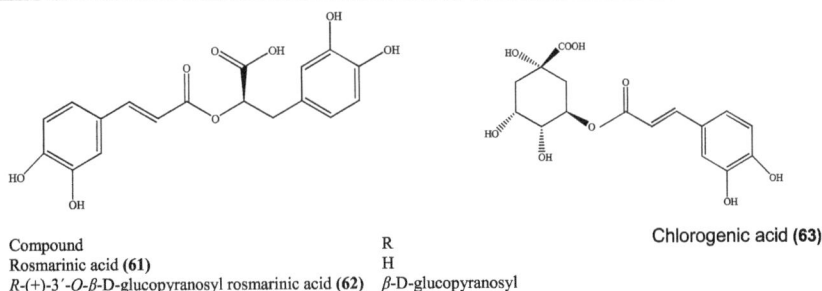

Compound | R
Rosmarinic acid (61) | H
R-(+)-3'-O-β-D-glucopyranosyl rosmarinic acid (62) | β-D-glucopyranosyl

Chlorogenic acid (63)

Fig. 11 Some phenolic acid derivatives found in *E. alpinum*

infantis, *Listeria monocytogenes* Tottori, *Staphylococcus aureus* and *Bacillus cereus* [91].

More recently, Ndip et al. showed that the methanolic extract form *E. foetidum* leaves showed moderate antibacterial activity against 6 clinical strains of *Helicobacter pylori* out of 15 tested strains, using the disk diffusion technique as antibacterial susceptibility test [92]. Besides antibacterial activity, *E. foetidum* was tested for its antiplasmodial activity, using chloroquine as positive control to evaluate the sensitivity of susceptible *Plasmodium falciparum* strains. The leaf extracts were prepared using hexane, dichloromethane, and methanol to obtain three extracts. The dried extracts were then dissolved in DMSO to give a stock solution at 10 mg/mL, used for the biological tests. The results indicated that *E. foetidum* showed low in vitro antiplasmodial activity against *P. falciparum*, with an IC50 value of 25 μg/mL [93].

Another species belonging to genus *Eryngium*, is *E. maritimum*, which is a wild perennial species growing on sand beaches in West Europe, the Mediterranean basin, and the Black Sea and has been used for its diuretic, stimulant, cystotonic, stone inhibitor, aphrodisiac, expectorant, and anthelmintic properties (http://www.botanicals.com, http://www.crescentbloom.com). The essential oil, obtained from hydrodistillation of the aerial parts, was found to contain a known sesquiterpene (muurol-9-en-15-al) and three new oxygenated sesquiterpenes with a muurolane or cadinane skeleton (4βH-cadin-9-en-15-al, 4βHmuurol-9-en-15-ol, and 4βH-cadin-9-en-15-ol), The sesquiterpenoid-rich fraction was tested in vitro using the agar diffusion method and the minimum inhibitory concentration (MIC) in the liquid phase against *L. monocytogenes* and *E.coli*. The finding revealed that the antibacterial activity of the new oxygenated sesquiterpenes against the tested bacteria, with an inhibition diameter higher than 15 mm and a MIC value lower than 90 μg/mL [94].

Another investigation on *E. maritimun* showed that the leaf hydromethanolic extract fractionated into a polar (aqueous) and apolar (chloroformic) fraction and tested using the microdilution method against food-

borne pathogens and clinical isolates, exhibited antimicrobial activity. The tested Gram-positive bacteria were *S. aureus* subsp. *aureus*, *Micrococcus luteus*, *L. monocytogenes* and *B. cereus*. The Gram-negative bacteria were two strains of *Salmonella* (*S. enterica* subsp. *arizonae* and *S. enterica* subsp. *montevideo*), three strains of *Pseudomonas* (*P. aeruginosa*, *P. fluorescens*, and *P. marginalis*), *E. coli*, and *Erwinia carotovora* subsp. *carotovora*, and a yeast (*Candida albicans*). According to the data obtained, the fractions resulted to be active against all bacteria with the exception of *L. monocytogenes*, while the most sensitive bacteria were *P. aeruginosa* and *P. fluorescens*, with MIC values of 1 and 2 μg/mL for the polar and apolar fractions, respectively [95].

The essential-oil composition and antimicrobial activity of three other species belonging to genus *Eryngium* (*E. creticum*, *E. campestre*, and *E. thorifolium*), whose infusions obtained from the aerial and root parts are commonly used in Turkish folk medicine as antitussive, diuretic, stimulant, and aphrodisiac, were studied [96]. The composition of *E. thorifolium* was found to be rich in α-pinene, a known antibacterial terpenic compound, which was present in fewer amounts in the other two species. Differently, *E. creticum* was found to be rich in hexanal, which was present in less amount in *E. thorifolium* and was not detected in *E. campestre*. Antibacterial activity of the essential oils was tested with the disc diffusion method against nine clinical strains of methicillin-resistant *S. aureus* (MRSA). The essential oil obtained from *E. thorifolium*, which caused an inhibition zone ranging from 13 to 19 mm (similar to that exhibited by vancomycin and oregano essential oil tested at 10 μL/disc and 5 μL/disc, respectively), was demonstrated to be the most active species [37]. As aforementioned, many *Eryngium* species, e.g. *E. maritimum* exerted antifungal activity against *C. albicans* and other strains. Especially, the essential oil obtained by water distillation of the aerial parts of *E. duriaei* Gay ex Boiss subsp. *juresianum* (M.Laínz) M. Laínz was tested for its antifungal activity against 13 fungi, among which there were seven dermatophyte species (*Microsporum canis* FF1,

Table 3 The major components in the essential oils of various *Eryngium* species

Plant Name	Plant part	Major components	Ref.
Eryngium alpinum L.	Aerial parts	Caryophyllene oxide (21.6 %)	[98]
		Bicyclogermacrene (11.8 %)	
		Germacrene D (10.3 %)	
Eryngium amethystinum L.	Aerial parts	β-Caryophyllene (19.7 %)	[98]
		α-Bisabolol (7.9 %)	
		2,3,6-Trimethylbenzaldehyde (7.9 %)	
	Leafy parts of the shoots	α-Pinene (11.8 %)	[99]
		2,3,6-Trimethylbenzaldehyde (24.7 %)	
		Germacrene D (31.3 %)	
	Inflorescence	α-Pinene (25.6 %)	
		2,3,6- Trimethylbenzaldehyde (22.0 %)	
		Germacrene D (14.5 %)	
	Fruit	α-Pinene (17.0 %)	
		2,3,6-Trimethylbenzaldehyde (16.9 %)	
		Germacrene D (7.6 %)	
Eryngium billardieri F. Delaroche	Aerial parts	α-Muurolene (42.0 %)	[39]
		β-Gurjunene (17.0 %)	
		δ-Cadinene (6.2 %)	
		Valencene (5.7 %)	
Eryngium bourgatii Gouan	Inflorescence	Phyllocladene (37.6 %)	[13]
		Bicyclogermacrene (15.1 %)	
	Stems & leaves	Phyllocladene (20.4 %)	
		γ-Muurolene (11.8 %)	
		(E)-Caryophyllene (10.1 %)	
	Roots	γ-Muurolene (15.4 %)	
		Phyllocladene (15.0 %)	
Eryngium bungei Boiss.	Aerial parts	Cumin alcohol (55.3 %)	[100]
		Terpinolene (14.6 %)	
		Carvacrol (8.9 %)	
		Limonene (7.5 %)	
	Aerial parts	Borneol (44.4 %)	[101]
		Isobornyl formate (14.7 %)	
		Isoborneol (9.2 %)	
		1,8-Cineol (9.1 %)	
		Camphor (7.9 %)	
Eryngium caeruleum M.B.	Aerial parts	Limonene (60.5 %)	[102]
		δ-3-Carene (13.0 %)	
	Aerial parts	Cyclobuta[1–4]dicycloocten Hexadecahydro (47.03 %)	[35]
		n-Hexadecanoic acid (11.16 %)	
		Limonene (4.23 %)	
		Cis-α-bisabolene (2.14 %)	

Table 3 The major components in the essential oils of various *Eryngium* species *(Continued)*

Eryngium campestre L.	Inflorescence	Germacrene D (30.3–40.3 %)	[103]
		β-Curcumene (0.7–22.2 %)	
		Myrcene (3.0–21.7 %)	
		(*E*)-β-Farnesene (0.1–19.0 %)	
	Stems & leaves	Germacrene D (31.1–42.4 %)	
		Myrcene (0.5–23.15 %)	
Eryngium caucasicum Trautv.	Leaves (coastal samples)	4(5)-Acetyl-1H-imidazole (63.6 %)	[104]
		Thymol (13.9 %)	
		β-Sesquiphellandrene (10.0 %)	
	Leaves (hill slope samples)	β-Sesquiphellandrene (44.3 %)	
		Limonene (20.1 %)	
		Trans-β-Farnesene (14.1 %)	
Eryngium corniculatum Lam.	Inflorescence	2,4,6-Trimethylbenzaldehyde (50.8 %)	[105]
		a-Pinene (4.0 %)	
		Crystanethylacetate (4.0 %)	
		2,4,5-Trimethylbenzaldehyde (%3.3)	
	Stems & leaves	2,4,6-Trimethylbenzaldehyde (50.0 %)	
		2,4,5-Trimethylbenzaldehyde (3.8 %)	
	Roots	2,4,6-Trimethylbenzaldehyde (29.8 %)	
		Phyllocladene isomer (13.0 %)	
		(*E*)-Nerolidol (9.4 %)	
Eryngium creticum Lam.	Flowering aerial parts	Hexanal (52.9 %)	[37]
		Heptanal (13.9 %)	
		Octane (8.95 %)	
Eryngium duriaei subsp. *juresianum* (M. Laínz) M. Laínz	Aerial parts	a-Neocallitropsene (26.0 %)	[106]
		Isocaryophyllen-14-al (16.2 %)	
		14-Hidroxy-β-caryophyllene (13.4 %)	
		Caryophyllene oxide (7.6 %)	
		E-β-Caryophyllene (6.3 %)	
Eryngium expansum F. Muell.	Aerial parts	7-*Epi*-Selinene (38.3 %)	[107]
		Cis-β-Guaiene (10.8 %)	
		2,3,6-Trimethylbenzaldehyde (8.0 %)	
Eryngium foetidum L.	Aerial parts	2,3,6-Trimethylbenzaldehyde (5.5–23.7 %)	[108]
		(E)-2-Dodecenal (15.9–37.5 %)	
		(E)-2-Tetradecenal (18.7–25.3 %)	
	Aerial parts	2,4,5-Trimethylbenzaldehyde (27.7 %)	[109]
		(*E*)-2-Dodecenal (27.5 %)	
		Carotol (8.8 %)	
		3-Dodecenal (5.2 %)	
	Aerial parts	(*E*)-2-Dodecenal (57.79–67.08 %)	[110]
		Lauraldehyde (7.04–11.53 %)	
		13-Tetradecenal (8.99–9.03 %)	
	Leaves	2,4,5-Trimethylbenzaldehyde (20.53 %)	[111]
		Hexadecanoic acid (12.05 %)	
		Carotol (9.94 %)	

Table 3 The major components in the essential oils of various *Eryngium* species *(Continued)*

	Roots	Duraldehyde (37.60–53.14 %)	[110]
		13-Tetradecenal (7.22–13.16 %)	
		(*E*)-2-Dodecenal (7.14–11.62 %)	
		Falcarinol (3.44–8.06 %)	
Eryngium glaciale Boiss.	Inflorescence	Phyllocladene isomer (43.5 %)	[112]
		(*E*)-Caryophyllene (15.2 %)	
		Valencene (11.5 %)	
	Stems & leaves	Phyllocladene isomer (41.3 %)	
	Roots	Phyllocladene isomer (49.4 %)	
		Linalool (19.1 %)	
Eryngium maritimum L.	Aerial parts	Spathulenol (18.99 %)	[77]
		Caryophyllene oxide (8.18 %)	
	Aerial parts	Germacrene D (10.4 %)	[113]
		2,4,5-Trimethylbenzaldehyde (8.3 %)	
	Roots	Germacrene D (15.9 %)	
		2,4,5-Trimethylbenzaldehyde (6.7 %)	
	Aerial parts	Germacrene D (13.7–45.9 %)	[114]
		4βH-Cadin-9-en-15-al (18.4–27.6 %)	
		4βH-Cadin-9-en-15-ol (2.2–14.3 %)	
		4βH-Muurol-9-en-15-al (4.3–9.3 %)	
Eryngium pandanifolium Cham. et Schlecht	Leaves	Bornyl acetate (20.8 %)	[107]
		β-Selinene (13.8 %)	
		α-Selinene (11.3 %)	
	Fruit	Octanal (11.5 %)	
		β-Selinene (9.2 %)	
Eryngium palmatum	Roots	Octanal (31.7 %)	[115]
		Curcumene (5.9 %)	
		2,3,6-Trimethylbenzaldehyde (5.4 %)	
Eryngium paniculatum Cav.	Inflorescence	(*E*)-Anethole (52.6 %)	[116]
		α-Pinene (19.1 %)	
Eryngium planum L.	Inflorescence	*Cis*-Chrysanthenyl acetate (43.2 %)	[117]
	Stalk leaves	Limonene (14.7 %)	
		β-Pinene (9.8 %)	
	Rosette leaves	Bornyl acetate (18.1 %)	
		Limonene (11.3 %)	
		Terpinen-4-ol (10.9 %)	
	Roots	Falcarinol (64.4 %)	
Eryngium rostratum Cav.	Stem	Spathulenol (20.0 %)	[107]
		β-Bisabolol (8.6 %)	
		Caryophyllene oxide (8.0 %)	
	Fruit	γ-Terpinene (4.5 %)	
		α-Muurolene (3.9 %)	
Eryngium rosulatum P. W. Michael ined.	Aerial parts	β-Elemene (16.0 %)	[118]
		Bicyclogermacrene (12.5 %)	
		δ-Elemene (7.0 %)	

Table 3 The major components in the essential oils of various *Eryngium* species *(Continued)*

Eryngium thorifolium Boiss.	Flowering aerial parts	(1R)-α-Pinene (58.6 %)	[37]
		Limonene (3.14 %)	
Eryngium tricuspidatum L.	Aerial parts	α-Bisabolol (32.6 %)	[34]
		α-Curcumene (6.5 %)	
Eryngium vesiculaosum Labill.	Winter leaves	β-Caryophyllene (20.3 %)	[119]
		Germacrene D (19.2 %)	
		α-Humulene (8.8 %)	
	Summer leaves	Bicyclogermacrene (22.2 %)	
		β-Caryophyllene (15.6 %)	
		Germacrene D (15.8 %)	
		α-Humulene (8.1 %)	
Eryngium yuccifolium Michaux.	Leaves	Germacrene D (18.3 %)	[120]
		Terpinolene (17.8 %)	
		Bicyclogermacrene (8.8 %)	
		α-Pinene (7.6 %)	
		β-Caryophyllene (6.2 %)	
		Falcarinol (9.6 %)	
	Stalks	Germacrene D (38.4 %)	
		γ-Amorphene (12.2 %)	
		Bicyclogermacrene (10.1 %)	
		Bicyclosesquiphellandrene (3.4 %)	
		Falcarinol (3.2 %)	
	Roots	Terpinolene (25.8 %)	
		Trans-β-Bergamotene (18.6 %)	
		Benzaldehyde 2,3,6-trimethylbenzaldehyde (13.9 %)	

Trichophyton mentagrophytes FF7, *Epidermophyton floccosum* FF9, *M. gypseum* CECT 2905, *T. rubrum* CECT 2794, *T. mentagrophytes* var interdigitale CECT 2958 and *T. verrucosum* CECT 2992), five *Candida* species (two clinical isolates from recurrent cases of vulvovaginal or oral candidosis, *C. krusei* (H9) and *C. guillermondii* MAT23, along with three reference species of *C. albicans* ATCC 10231, *C. tropicalis* ATCC 13803, and *C. parapsilosis* ATCC 90018) and a strain of *Cryptococcus neoformans* CECT 1078. Using the macrodilution broth method the MIC and Minimal Lethal Concentrations (MLC) were determined. The results disclosed that the essential oil did not possess antifungal activity against *Candida* strains, with the exception of *C. guillermondii*, which resulted to be sensitive to the antifungal activity of the oil with a MIC and MLC of 2.5 μL/mL. On the contrary, the essential oil had MIC values of 0.16–0.32 μL/mL against all the tested dermatophyte species. The essential oil was further studied to determine its chemical composition by GC-MS and the authors suggested that caryophyllene derived compounds [isocaryophyllen-14-

al (16.2 %), 14-hidroxy-β-caryophyllene (13.4 %), caryophyllene oxide (7.6 %) and *E*-β-caryophyllene (6.3 %)] are probably the responsible for the antifungal activity [97].

Finally, in 2013, the antiphytoviral activity of the essential oils obtained by water distillation of the aerial parts of *E. alpinum* and *E. amethystinum* cultivated in Croatia was described. The antiviral activity was shown in *Chenopodium quinoa* treated with the essential oils (250 ppm) prior to the inoculation of cucumber mosaic virus associated with a satellite RNA. The number of leaf local lesions, registered in the presence of the essential oils, was strongly reduced from an average value of 14.9 ± 0.8 to 3.3 ± 0.2 and 2.9 ± 0.2, for *E. alpinum* and *E. amethystinum* essential oils, respectively. The authors ascribed the antiviral activity to the occurrence of caryophyllene oxide and β-caryophyllene, which were identified as the major components of *E. alpinum* and *E. amethystinum*, respectively. Moreover, other components such as germacrene D, α-bisabolol, and γ-eudesmol, which were detected as minor oil

Table 4 Antimicrobial activity of *Eryngium* species extracts

Eryngium plant	Type of extract	Used method	Microbes	Positive control	Ref.
E. foetidum	Methanolic extract of leaves	disk diffusion technique	6 clinical strains of *Helicobacter pylori*	ns[a]	[92]
E. foetidum	hexane, dichloromethane, and methanol extracts	disk diffusion technique	*Plasmodium falciparum*	chloroquine	[93]
E. maritimum	hydrodistillation of the aerial parts	agar diffusion method and minimum inhibitory concentration (MIC)	*L. monocytogenes E. coli.*	ns[a]	[94]
E. maritimum	hydromethanolic extract of leaves	microdilution method	*S. aureus* subsp. *aureus, Micrococcus luteus, B. cereus. S. enterica* subsp. *arizonae S. enterica* subsp. *Montevideo P. aeruginosa, P. fluorescens, P. marginalis E. coli Erwinia carotovora* subsp. *carotovora, Candida albicans*	ns[a]	[95]
E. creticum, E. campestre, E. thorifolium	essential oils from aerial and root parts	disk diffusion method	9 clinical strains of methicillin-resistant *S. aureus* (MRSA)	ns[a]	[37]
E. duriaei	essential oil obtained by water distillation of the aerial parts	macrodilution broth method	*Microsporum canis* FF1, *Trichophyton mentagrophytes* FF7, *Epidermophyton floccosum* FF9, *M. gypseum* CECT 2905, *T. rubrum* CECT 2794, *T. mentagrophytes* var interdigitale CECT 2958 *T. verrucosum* CECT 2992 *Candida. guillermondii* MAT23, *Cryptococcus neoformans* CECT 1078.	ns[a]	[97]
E. alpinum, E. amethystinum	essential oils obtained by water distillation of the aerial parts	count of leaf local lesions in *Chenopodium quinoa* treated with the essential oils prior to the inoculation of virus	cucumber mosaic virus associated with a satellite RNA	ns[a]	[98]

[a]not specified

constituents, might be responsible for the inhibition of viral infection [98].

The summary of the literature data was reported in Table 4.

Conclusion

The present paper shows that essential oils and extracts obtained from various *Eryngium* species have broad range antimicrobial activity against several strains of gram-positive and gram-negative bacteria, some species of fungi and yeasts, and viruses. The findings point out to the fact that these activities can be ascribed to the presence of different phytochemicals, especially apolar compounds. However, our search at https://clinicaltrials.gov/ with keyword "*Eryngium*" accessed on February 9, 2015 showed no clinical trial regarding the beneficial effects of the genus *Eryngium* plants against different types of infection available up to date. In addition, there are only a few papers on the toxicity of the active constituents belonging to the genus *Eryngium* plants, which resulted to be cytotoxic especially at high doses. It can be suggested that more toxicity studies should be carried out prior to the clinical trials.

According to this study, we conclude that the essential oils and extracts of those *Eryngium* species that have been submitted to in vitro investigation (Table 4) should be proceeded to toxicological studies and *in vivo*

experiments as multi-target antimicrobial agents for the treatment of human infectious diseases, especially antibiotic-resistant bacterial infections. Thus, it is not quite possible to make a clear statement or comment about their clinical uses. Hence, we recommend that future studies should be performed on:

- toxicity of the *Eryngium* plant extracts and essential oil resulted to be active in in vitro experiments.
- clinical studies of the safe extracts of *Eryngium* species with in vitro activity,
- finding the exact mechanism underlying the antibacterial effects of the essential oils and extracts of members of the genus *Eryngium* and their antibacterial constituents,
- separation, isolation, and structure identification of the most antibacterial constituents of the essential oils and extracts of different members of the genus *Eryngium* and their interactions with foods as well as common synthetic antibacterial compounds,
- ascertaining the most effective and safe doses for clinical studies regarding the antibacterial effects of the essential oils and extracts of different genus *Eryngium* species against different infectious diseases.

Competing interests
The authors declare that they have no competing interests.

Authors' contributions
SMN and IEO designed the paper, SAE, MI and MD collected and selected and analyzed the literature data, SAE, SFN, SMN, IEO and MD wrote the paper. All authors participated in the analysis and interpretation of literature data, corrected the paper and approved the final manuscript.

Acknowledgement
Declared none.

Author details
[1]Department of Pharmacognosy, Faculty of Pharmacy, Ankara University, 06100 Ankara, Turkey. [2]Applied Biotechnology Research Center, Baqiyatallah University of Medical Sciences, P.O. Box 19395-5487, Tehran, Iran. [3]Department of Pharmacognosy, Faculty of Pharmacy, Gazi University, 06330 Ankara, Turkey. [4]Department of Drug Sciences, Medicinal Chemistry and Pharmaceutical Technology Section, University of Pavia, Pavia, Italy. [5]Health Research Center, Baqiyatallah University of Medical Sciences, Tehran, Iran.

References
1. World Health Organization. World health statistics 2010. WHO Press. Geneva, Switzerland. 2010.
2. Nabavi SM, Marchese A, Izadi M, Curti V, Daglia M, Nabavi SF. Plants belonging to the genus Thymus as antibacterial agents: From farm to pharmacy. Food Chem. 2015;173:339–47.
3. Högberg LD, Heddini A, Cars O. The global need for effective antibiotics: challenges and recent advances. Trends Pharmacol Sci. 2010;31(11):509–15.
4. Alinezhad H, Azimi R, Zare M, Ebrahimzadeh MA, Eslami S, Nabavi SF, et al. Antioxidant and antihemolytic activities of ethanolic extract of flowers, leaves, and stems of Hyssopus officinalis L. Var. angustifolius. Int J Food Prop. 2013;16(5):1169–78.
5. Nabavi SF, Nabavi SM, Habtemariam S, Moghaddam AH, Sureda A, Jafari M, et al. Hepatoprotective effect of gallic acid isolated from Peltiphyllum peltatum against sodium fluoride-induced oxidative stress. Ind Crops Prod. 2013;44:50–5.
6. Curti V, Capelli E, Boschi F, Nabavi SF, Bongiorno AI, Habtemariam S, et al. Modulation of human miR-17-3p expression by methyl 3-O-methyl gallate as explanation of its in vivo protective activities. Mol Nutr Food Res. 2014;58(9):1776–84.
7. Nabavi SF, Daglia M, Moghaddam AH, Habtemariam S, Nabavi SM. Curcumin and liver disease: from chemistry to medicine. Compr Rev Food Sci Food Saf. 2014;13(1):62–77.
8. Nabavi SF, Russo GL, Daglia M, Nabavi SM. Role of quercetin as an alternative for obesity treatment: you are what you eat! Food Chem. 2015;179:305–10.
9. Nabavi SF, Nabavi SM, Setzer NW, Nabavi SA, Nabavi SA, Ebrahimzadeh MA. Antioxidant and antihemolytic activity of lipid-soluble bioactive substances in avocado fruits. Fruits. 2013;68(03):185–93.
10. Daglia M. Polyphenols as antimicrobial agents. Curr Opin Biotechnol. 2012;23(2):174–81.
11. Simoes M, Bennett RN, Rosa EA. Understanding antimicrobial activities of phytochemicals against multidrug resistant bacteria and biofilms. Nat Prod Rep. 2009;26(6):746–57.
12. Cowan MM. Plant products as antimicrobial agents. Clin Microbiol Rev. 1999;12(4):564–82.
13. Palá-Paúl J, Perez-Alonso MJ, Velasco-Negueruela A, Vadaré J, Villa AM, Sanz J, et al. Essential oil composition of the different parts of Eryngium bourgatii Gouan from Spain. J Chromatogr A. 2005;1074(1):235–9.
14. Capetanos C, Saroglou V, Marin PD, Simić A, Skaltsa HD. Essential oil analysis of two endemic Eryngium species from Serbia. J Serb Chem Soc. 2007;72(10):961–5.
15. Wörz A, Diekmann H. Classification and evolution of the genus Eryngium L. (Apiaceae-Saniculoideae): results of fruit anatomical and petal morphological studies. Plant Divers Evol. 2010;128(3-4):387–408.
16. Wörz A. A new subgeneric classification of the genus Eryngium L. (Apiaceae, Saniculoideae). Bot Jahrbücher. 2005;126(2):253–9.
17. Calvino CI, Martínez SG, Downie SR. The evolutionary history of Eryngium (Apiaceae, Saniculoideae): Rapid radiations, long distance dispersals, and hybridizations. Mol Phylogenet Evol. 2008;46(3):1129–50.
18. Calviño CI, Downie SR. Circumscription and phylogeny of Apiaceae subfamily Saniculoideae based on chloroplast DNA sequences. Mol Phylogenet Evol. 2007;44(1):175–91.
19. Magee AR, van Wyk B-E, Tilney PM, van der Bank M. A Taxonomic Revision Of the South African Endemic Genus Arctopus (Apiaceae, Saniculoideae) 1. Ann Missouri Bot Garden. 2008;95(3):471–86.
20. Singh S, Singh D, Banu S, Salim K. Determination of bioactives and antioxidant activity in Eryngium foetidum L.: a traditional culinary and medicinal herb. Proc Natl Acad Sci, India Section B: Biological Sciences. 2013;83(3):453–60.
21. Ignacimuthu S, Arockiasamy S, Antonysamy M, Ravichandran P. Plant regeneration through somatic embryogenesis from mature leaf explants of Eryngium foetidum, a condiment. Plant Cell Tissue Organ Cult. 1999;56(2):131–7.
22. Shavandi MA, Haddadian Z, Ismail MHS. Eryngium foetidum L. Coriandrum sativum and Persicaria odorata L.: A review. J Asian Sci Res. 2012;2(8):410–26.
23. Singh B, Ramakrishna Y, Ngachan S. Spiny coriander (Eryngium foetidum L.): a commonly used, neglected spicing-culinary herb of Mizoram, India. Genet Resour Crop Evol. 2014;61(6):1085–90.
24. Paul J, Seaforth C, Tikasingh T. Eryngium foetidum L.: a review. Fitoterapia. 2011;82(3):302–8.
25. Kupeli E, Kartal M, Aslan S, Yesilada E. Comparative evaluation of the anti-inflammatory and antinociceptive activity of Turkish Eryngium species. J Ethnopharmacol. 2006;107(1):32–7.
26. De Natale A, Pollio A. Plants species in the folk medicine of Montecorvino Rovella (inland Campania, Italy). J Ethnopharmacol. 2007;109(2):295–303.
27. Wang P, Su Z, Yuan W, Deng G, Li S. Phytochemical constituents and pharmacological activities of Eryngium L. (Apiaceae). Pharm Crops. 2012;3:99–120.
28. Nabavi S, Nabavi S, Alinezhad H, Zare M, Azimi R. Biological activities of flavonoid-rich fraction of Eryngium caucasicum Trautv. Eur Rev Med Pharmacol Sci. 2012;16:81–7.
29. Eslami S, Ebrahimzadeh M, Moghaddam HA, Nabavi S, Jafari N, Nabavi S. Renoprotective effect of Eryngium caucasicum in gentamicin-induced nephrotoxic mice. Arch Biol Sci. 2011;63(1):157–60.
30. Anam EM. A novel triterpenoid saponin from Eryngium foetidum. Indian J Chem Section B. 2002;41(7):1500–3.
31. Khoshbakht K, Hammer K, Pistrick K. Eryngium caucasicum Trautv. cultivated as a vegetable in the Elburz Mountains (Northern Iran). Genet Resour Crop Evol. 2007;54(2):445–8.
32. Homer S, Baccus-Taylor GS, Akingbala JA, Hutchinson SD, editors. Antibacterial efficacy of Eryngium foetidum (culantro) against select food-borne pathogens: Proceedings of the West Indies Agricultural Economics Conference. 2009.
33. Türker H, Yildirim AB, Karakaş FP, Köylüoglu H. Antibacterial activities of extracts from some Turkish endemic plants on common fish pathogens. Turk J Biol. 2009;33(1):73–8.
34. Merghache D, Boucherit-Otmani Z, Merghache S, Chikhi I, Selles C, Boucherit K. Chemical composition, antibacterial, antifungal and antioxidant activities of Algerian Eryngium tricuspidatum L. essential oil. Nat Prod Res. 2014;28(11):795–807.
35. Dehghanzadeh N, Ketabchi S, Alizadeh A. Essential oil composition and antibacterial activity of Eryngium caeruleum grown wild in Iran. J Essential Oil Bearing Plants. 2014;17(3):486–92.
36. Khalfallah A, Berrehal D, Kabouche A, Kariotì A, Bilia A-R, Kabouche Z. Flavonoids, antioxidant and antibacterial activities of Eryngium triquetrum. Chem Nat Comp. 2014;50(1):130–2.
37. Çelik A, Aydınlık N, Arslan I. Phytochemical constituents and inhibitory activity towards methicillin-resistant Staphylococcus aureus strains of Eryngium species (Apiaceae). Chem Biodivers. 2011;8(3):454–9.
38. Ozcelik B, Kusmenoglu S, Turkoz S, Abbasoglu U. Antimicrobial activities of plants from the Apicaceae. Pharm Biology. 2004;42(7):526–8.
39. Sefidkon F, Dabiri M, Alamshahi A. Chemical composition of the essential oil of Eryngium billardieri F. Delaroche from Iran. J Essential Oil Res. 2004;16(1):42–3.
40. Ebrahimzadeh M, Nabavi S, Nabavi S. Antioxidant activity of leaves and inflorescence of Eryngium caucasicum Trautv at flowering stage. Pharmacogn Res. 2009;1(6):435.
41. Aburjai T, Hudaib M, Tayyem R, Yousef M, Qishawi M. Ethnopharmacological survey of medicinal herbs in Jordan, the Ajloun Heights region. J Ethnopharmacol. 2007;110(2):294–304.

42. Goleniowski ME, Bongiovanni G, Palacio L, Nuñez C, Cantero J. Medicinal plants from the "Sierra de Comechingones", Argentina. J Ethnopharmacol. 2006;107(3):324–41.

43. Redzic S. Wild medicinal plants and their usage in traditional human therapy (Southern Bosnia and Herzegovina, W. Balkan). J Med Plants Res. 2010;4(11):1003–27.

44. Morton JF. Some folk-medicine plants of Central American markets. Pharm Biol. 1977;15(4):165–92.

45. Morton JF. Caribbean and Latin American folk medicine and its influence in the United States. Pharm Biol. 1980;18(2):57–75.

46. Mathias ME. Magic, myth and medicine. Econ Bot. 1994;48(1):3–7.

47. Wang P, Yuan W, Deng G, Su Z, Li S. Triterpenoid saponins from *Eryngium yuccifolium* 'Kershaw Blue'. Phytochem Lett. 2013;6(2):306–9.

48. de la Luz C-GM, Fernández-Arroyo S, Joven J, Segura-Carretero A. Comprehensive characterization by UHPLC-ESI-Q-TOF-MS from an *Eryngium bourgatii* extract and their antioxidant and anti-inflammatory activities. Food Res Int. 2013;50(1):197–204.

49. Erdem SA, Arıhan O, Offer AM, Iskit A, Miyamoto T, Kartal M, et al. Antinociceptive activity of *Eryngium kotschyi* Boiss. root extracts. Planta Med. 2011;77(12):F66.

50. Ozarowski M, Thiem B, Mikolajczak PL, Piasecka A, Kachlicki P, Szulc M, et al. Improvement in Long-Term Memory following Chronic Administration of Eryngium planum Root Extract in Scopolamine Model: Behavioral and Molecular Study. Evid Based Complement Alternat Med. 2015;2015:145140.

51. Khalili M, Dehdar T, Hamedi F, Ebrahimzadeh M, Karami M. Antihypoxic activities of *Eryngium caucasicum*. Eur Rev Med Pharmacol Sci. 2015;19(17):3282–5.

52. Dawilai S, Muangnoi C, Praengamthanachoti P, Tuntipopipat S. Anti-inflammatory activity of bioaccessible fraction from *Eryngium foetidum* leaves. BioMed Res Int. 2013;2013:958567.

53. Mozumder S, Hossain M. Effect of seed treatment and soaking duration on germination of *Eryngium foetidum* L. seeds. Int J Hort. 2013;3:1046–51.

54. Njenga J. Production of *Eryngium*. NC Flower Growers' Bulletin. 1995;40:9–11.

55. Martin K. In vitro propagation of the herbal spice *Eryngium foetidum* L. on sucrose-added and sucrose-free medium without growth regulators and CO_2 enrichment. Sci Hort. 2004;102(2):277–82.

56. Erdelmeier C, Sticher O. Coumarin derivatives from *Eryngium campestre*. Planta Med. 1985;51(5):407–9.

57. Erdelmeier CA, Sticher O. A cyclohexenone and a cyclohexadienone glycoside from *Eryngium campestre*. Phytochemistry. 1986;25(3):741–3.

58. Hohmann J, Pall Z, Günther G, Mathe I. Flavonolacyl glycosides of the aerial parts of *Eryngium campestre*. Planta Med. 1997;63(1):96.

59. Kartal M, Mitaine-Offer A-C, Abu-Asaker M, Miyamoto T, Calis I, Wagner H, et al. Two new triterpene saponins from *Eryngium campestre*. Chem Pharm Bull. 2005;53(10):1318–20.

60. Dalar A, Türker M, Zabaras D, Konczak I. Phenolic composition, antioxidant and enzyme inhibitory activities of *Eryngium bornmuelleri* leaf. Plant Foods Hum Nutr. 2014;69(1):30–6.

61. Hiller K, Keipert M, Pfeifer S, Kraft R. The leaf sapogenin spectrum in *Eryngium planum* L. 20. Contribution on the content of several Saniculoideae. Pharmazie. 1974;29(1):54.

62. Hiller K, Nguyen K, Franke P. Isolation of 3-OD-glucopyranosyl oleanolic acid 28-OD-xylo-pyranoside from *Eryngium bromeliifolium* Delar. 29. Constituents of some Saniculoideae. Pharmazie. 1978;33(1):78–80.

63. Kartal M, Mitaine-Offer A-C, Paululat T, Abu-Asaker M, Wagner H, Mirjolet J-F, et al. Triterpene saponins from *Eryngium campestre*. J Nat Prod. 2006;69(7):1105–8.

64. Zhang Z, Li S, Ownby S, Wang P, Yuan W, Zhang W, et al. Phenolic compounds and rare polyhydroxylated triterpenoid saponins from *Eryngium yuccifolium*. Phytochemistry. 2008;69(10):2070–80.

65. Erdem SA, Mitaine-Offer AC, Miyamoto T, Kartal M, Lacaille-Dubois MA. Triterpene saponins from *Eryngium kotschyi*. Phytochemistry. 2015;110:160–5.

66. Hiller K, Thi N, Franke P. On saponin of *Eryngium bromeliifoloium* Delar. 19. Information on the components of various Saniculoideae. Pharmazie. 1973; 28(8):546.

67. Hiller K, Thi N, Döhnert H, Franke P. Isolation of new ester sapogenins from *Eryngium giganteum* MB 22. Knowledge of various Saniculoideae components. Pharmazie. 1975;30(2):105.

68. Hiller K, Nguyen K, Döhnert H, Franke P. The saponine-saponinogen spectrum in *Eryngium amethystinum* L. 27. Contribution to chemicals contained in various Saniculoidae. Pharmazie. 1977;32(3):184.

69. Hiller K, Keipert M, Pfeifer S, Tökes L, Maddox M. Structure of *Eryngium sapogenins*. 14. Information on components of some Saniculoideae. Pharmazie. 1970;25(12):769.

70. Hiller K, Keipert M, Pfeifer S, Tokes L, Nelson J. Eryninol A- A new triterpenesapogenin. 18. Knowledge of component substances of some saniculoideae. Pharmazie 1973;28(6):409–10.

71. Hiller K, Von Thi N, Lehmann G, Gründemann E. Betulinic acid—a sapogenin in *Eryngium bromeliifolium* Delar. 21. The contents of a Saniculoidea. Pharmazie. 1974;29(2):148.

72. Hiller K, Keipert M, Missbach U, Lehmann G. Eryngiurngenin E-a new ester sapogenin. 23. The contents of some Saniculoideae. Pharmazie. 1975;30(5):336.

73. Hiller K, Nguyen K, Franke P, Hintsche R. Isolation of betulic acid 3-O-beta-D glucoside, a saponin of *Eryngium bromeliifolium* Delar. 26. The contents of Saniculoideae. Pharmazie. 1976;31(12):891.

74. Hiller K, Von Mach B, Franke P. Saponins of *Eryngium maritimum* L. 25. Contents of various Saniculoideae. Pharmazie. 1976;31(1):53.

75. Voigt G, Thiel P, Hiller K, Franke P, Habisch D. Zur struktur des hauptsaponins der Wurzeln von *Eryngium planum* L.. XL: Zur Kenntnis der inhaltsstoffe einiger Saniculoideae. Pharmazie 1985;40(9):656–59.

76. Kowalczyk M, Masullo M, Thiem B, Piacente S, Stochmal A, Oleszek W. Three new triterpene saponins from roots of *Eryngium planum*. Nat Prod Res. 2014;28(9):653–60.

77. Aslan S, Kartal M. GC-MS Analysis of *Eryngium maritumum* L. volatile oil. Planta Med 2006;72(11):P_340.

78. Hiller K, Otto A, Grundemann E. Isolation of kaempferol-3-o-(6-O-beta-D-glucopyranosyl)-beta-D-galactopyranoside, a new flavonol glycoside from *Eryngium planum* I. 34. on the knowledge of the constituents of some saniculoideae. Pharmazie. 1980;35(2):113–4.

79. Kartnig T, Wolf J. Flavonoids from the aboveground parts of *Eryngium campestre*. Planta Med. 1993;59(3):285.

80. Hawas UW, El-Kassem T, Lamia A, Awad M, Hanem AA, Taie H. Anti-Alzheimer, antioxidant activities and flavonol glycosides of *Eryngium campestre* L. Curr Chem Biol. 2013;7(2):188–95.

81. Pinar M, Galan MP. Coumarins from *Eryngium ilicifolium*. J Nat Prod. 1985; 48(5):853–4.

82. Le Claire E, Schwaiger S, Banaigs B, Stuppner H, Gafner F. Distribution of a new rosmarinic acid derivative in *Eryngium alpinum* L. and other Apiaceae. J. Agric Food Chem. 2005;53(11):4367–72.

83. Marčetić MD, Petrović SD, Milenković MT, Niketić MS. Composition, antimicrobial and antioxidant activity of the extracts of Eryngium palmatum Pančić and Vis. (Apiaceae). Cent Eur J Biol. 2014;9(2):149–55.

84. Drake D, Lam J. Seseli acetylene from *Eryngium bourgatti*. Phytochemistry. 1972;11(8):2651–2.

85. Lam J, Christensen LP, Thomasen T. Acetylenes from roots of *Eryngium bourgatii*. Phytochemistry. 1992;31(8):2881–2.

86. Ayoub N, Kubeczka K-H, Nawwar M. An unique n-propyl sesquiterpene from Eryngium creticum L. (Apiaceae). Phytochemistry. 2003;58(9):674–6.

87. Korbel E, Bighelli A, Kurowska A, Kalemba D, Casanova J. New cis-chrysanthenyl esters from *Eryngium planum* L. Nat Prod Commun. 2008;3(2):113–6.

88. Garcia M, Saenz M, Gomez M, Fernandez M. Topical anti-inflammatory activity of phytosterols isolated from *Eryngium foetidum* on chronic and acute inflammation models. Phytother Res. 1999;13(1):78–80.

89. Muckensturm B, Boulanger A, Farahi M, Reduron J. Secondary metabolites from *Eryngium species*. Nat Prod Res. 2010;24(5):391–7.

90. Forbes W, Gallimore W, Mansingh A, Reese P, Robinson R. Eryngial (trans-2-dodecenal), a bioactive compound from *Eryngium foetidum*: its identification, chemical isolation, characterization and comparison with ivermectin in vitro. Parasitology. 2014;141(02):269–78.

91. Alzoreky N, Nakahara K. Antibacterial activity of extracts from some edible plants commonly consumed in Asia. Int J Food Microbiol. 2003;80(3):223–30.

92. Ndip RN, Tarkang AEM, Mbullah SM, Luma HN, Malongue A, Ndip LM, et al. In vitro anti-*Helicobacter pylori* activity of extracts of selected medicinal plants from North West Cameroon. J Ethnopharmacol. 2007;114(3):452–7.

93. Roumy V, Garcia-Pizango G, Gutierrez-Choquevilca A-L, Ruiz L, Jullian V, Winterton P, et al. Amazonian plants from Peru used by Quechua and Mestizo to treat malaria with evaluation of their activity. J Ethnopharmacol. 2007;112(3):482–9.

94. Darriet F, Bendahou M, Desjobert J-M, Costa J, Muselli A. Bicyclo [4.4.0] decane oxygenated sesquiterpenes from *Eryngium maritimum* essential oil. Planta Med. 2012;78(4):386.

95. Meot-Duros L, Le Floch G, Magné C. Radical scavenging, antioxidant and antimicrobial activities of halophytic species. J Ethnopharmacol. 2008;116(2):258–62.

96. Baytop T. Therapy with Medicinal Plants in Turkey (Past and Present). 1999;2:169.

97. Abou-Jawdah Y, Sobh H, Salameh A. Antimycotic activities of selected plant flora, growing wild in Lebanon, against phytopathogenic fungi. J Agric Food Chem. 2002;50(11):3208–13.

98. Dunkić V, Vuko E, Bezić N, Kremer D, Ruščić M. Composition and antiviral activity of the essential oils of *Eryngium alpinum* and *E. amethystinum*. Chem Biodivers. 2013;10(10):1894–902.

99. Flamini G, Tebano M, Cioni PL. Composition of the essential oils from leafy parts of the shoots, flowers and fruits of *Eryngium amethystinum* from Amiata Mount (Tuscany, Italy). Food Chem. 2008;107(2):671–4.

100. Morteza-Semnani K. Essential oil composition of *Eryngium bungei* Boiss. J Essential Oil Res. 2005;17(5):485–6.

101. Mohammadhosseini M, Mahdavi B, Akhlaghi H. Characterization and chemical composition of the volatile oils from aerial parts of *Eryngium bungei* Bioss. (Apiaceae) by using traditional hydrodistillation, microwave assisted hydrodistillation and head space solid phase microextraction methods prior to GC and GC/MS analyses: A comparative approach. J Essential Oil Bearing Plants. 2013;16(5):613–23.

102. Assadian F, Masoudi S, Nematollahi F, Rustaiyan A, Larijani K, Mazloomifar H. Volatile constituents of *Xanthogalum purpurascens* Ave-Lall., *Eryngium caeruleum* MB and *Pimpinella aurea* DC. Three Umbelliferae herbs growing in Iran. J Essential Oil Res. 2005;17(3):243–5.

103. Pala-Paul J, Usano-Alemany J, Soria AC, Perez-Alonso MJ, Brophy JJ. Essential oil composition of *Eryngium campestre* L. growing in different soil types. A preliminary study. Nat Prod Commun. 2008;3(7):1121–6.

104. Hashemabadi D, Kaviani B. Chemical constituents of essential oils extracted from the leaves and stems of *Eryngium caucasicum* Trautv. from Iran. J Essential Oil Bearing Plants. 2011;14(6):693–8.

105. Palá-Paúl J, Brophy JJ, Pérez-Alonso MJ, Usano J, Soria SC. Essential oil composition of the different parts of Eryngium corniculatum Lam. (Apiaceae) from Spain. J Chromatogr A. 2007;1175(2):289–93.

106. Cavaleiro C, Gonçalves MJ, Serra D, Santoro G, Tomi F, Bighelli A, et al. Composition of a volatile extract of *Eryngium duriaei* subsp. juresianum (M. Laínz) M. Laínz, signalised by the antifungal activity. J Pharm Biomed Anal. 2011; 54(3):619–22.

107. Brophy JJ, Goldsack RJ, Copeland LM, Palá-Paúl J. Essential oil of *Eryngium* L. species from New South Wales (Australia). J Essential Oil Res. 2003;15(6): 392–7.

108. Martins AP, Salgueiro LR, da Cunha AP, Vila R, Cañigueral S, Tomi F, et al. Essential oil composition of *Eryngium foetidum* from S. Tome e Principe. J Essential Oil Res. 2003;15(2):93–5.

109. Cardozo E, Rubio M, Rojas L, Usubillaga A. Composition of the essential oil from the leaves of *Eryngium foetidum* L. from the Venezuelan Andes. J Essential Oil Res. 2004;16(1):33–4.

110. Thi NDT, Anh TH, Thach LN. The essential oil composition of *Eryngium foetidum* L. in South Vietnam extracted by hydrodistillation under conventional heating and microwave irradiation. J Essential Oil Bearing Plants. 2008;11(2):154–61.

111. Pino JA, Rosado A, Fuentes V. Composition of the leaf oil of *Eryngium foetidum* L. from Cuba. J Essential Oil Res. 1997;9(4):467–8.

112. Palá-Paúl J, Pérez-Alonso MJ, Velasco-Negueruela A, Varadé J, Villa AM, Sanz J, et al. Analysis of the essential oil composition from the different parts of *Eryngium glaciale* Boiss. from Spain. J Chromatogr A. 2005;1094(1):179–82.

113. Maggio A, Bruno M, Formisano C, Rigano D, Senatore F. Chemical composition of the essential oils of three species of Apiaceae growing wild in Sicily: *Bonannia graeca*, *Eryngium maritimum* and *Opopanax chironium*. Nat Prod Commun. 2013;8(6):841–4.

114. Darriet F, Andreani S, De Cian MC, Costa J, Muselli A. Chemical variability and antioxidant activity of *Eryngium maritimum* L. essential oils from Corsica and Sardinia. Flav Fragr J. 2014;29(1):3–13.

115. Marcetic M, Petrovic S, Milenkovic M, Vujisic L, Tesevic V, Niketic M. Composition and antimicrobial activity of root essential oil of Balkan endemic species *Eryngium palmatum*. Chem Nat Comp. 2014;49(6):1140–2.

116. Cobos MI, Rodriguez JL, De Petre A, Spahn E, Casermeiro J, Lopez AG, et al. Composition of the essential oil of *Eryngium paniculatum* Cav. J Essential Oil Res. 2002;14(2):82–3.

117. Thiem B, Kikowska M, Kurowska A, Kalemba D. Essential oil composition of the different parts and in vitro shoot culture of *Eryngium planum* L. Molecules. 2011;16(8):7115–24.

118. Palá-Paúl J, Copeland LM, Brophy JJ, Goldsack RJ. Essential oil composition of *Eryngium rosulatum* PW Michael ined.: A new undescribed species from eastern Australia. Biochem System Ecol. 2006;34(11):796–801.

119. Palá-Paúl J, Brophy JJ, Goldsack RJ, Copeland LM, Pérez-Alonso MJ, Velasco-Negueruela A. Essential oil composition of the seasonal heterophyllous leaves of *Eryngium vesiculosum* from Australia. Austr J Bot. 2003;51(5):497–501.

120. Ayoub N, Al-Azizi M, König W, Kubeczka KH. Essential oils and a novel polyacetylene from Eryngium yuccifolium Michaux. (Apiaceae). Flav Fragr J. 2006;21(6):864–8.

Metabolic effects of newly synthesized phosphodiesterase-3 inhibitor 6-[4-(4-methylpiperidin-1-yl)-4-oxobutoxy]-4-methylquinolin-2(1H)-one on rat adipocytes

Bagher Alinejad[1], Reza Shafiee-Nick[1,2*], Hamid Sadeghian[3] and Ahmad Ghorbani[2]

Abstract

Background: Clinical use of selective PDE3 inhibitors as cardiotonic agents is limited because of their chronotropic and lipolytic side effects. In our previous work, we synthesized a new PDE3 inhibitor named MC2 (6-[4-(4-methylpiperidin-1-yl)-4-oxobutoxy]-4-methylquinolin-2(1H)-one) which produced a high positive inotropic action with a negative chronotropic effect. This work was done to evaluate the effects of MC2 on adipocytes and compare its effects with those of amrinone and cilostamide.

Methods: Preadipocytes were isolated from rat adipose tissue and differentiated to adipocyte in the presence of cilostamide, amrinone or MC2. Lipolysis and adipogenesis was evaluated by measuring glycerol level and Oil Red O staining, respectively. Adipocyte proliferation and apoptosis were determined with MTT assay and Annexin V/PI staining, respectively.

Results: Differentiation to adipocyte was induced by amrinone but not by cilostamide or MC2. Basal and isoproterenol-stimulated lipolysis significantly increased by cilostamide ($p < 0.05$). Similarly, amrinone enhanced the stimulated lipolysis ($p < 0.01$). On the other hand, MC2 significantly decreased both adipogenesis ($p < 0.05$) and stimulated lipolysis ($p < 0.001$). Also, incubation of differentiated adipocytes with MC2 caused the loss of cell viability, which was associated with the elevation in apoptotic rate ($p < 0.05$).

Conclusion: Our data indicate that selective PDE3 inhibitors produce differential effects on adipogenesis and lipolysis. MC2 has proapoptotic and antilipolytic effects on adipocytes and does not stimulate adipogenesis. Therefore, in comparison with the clinically available selective PDE3 inhibitors, MC2 has lowest metabolic side effects and might be a good candidate for treatment of congestive heart failure.

Keywords: Adipogenesis, Amrinone, Cilostamide, Lipolysis, Phosphodiesterases

Introduction

Cyclic nucleotide phosphodiesterases (PDEs) control the level of intracellular cAMP and cGMP, and hence play important roles in cellular signaling pathways. The PDEs are grouped into 11 families which differ in their physiochemical properties, substrate specificities, tissue distributions, and regulatory mechanisms [1]. Among

them PDE3 has high expression in heart, airway, liver, pancreas, and adipose tissue and involves in the regulation of cardiovascular functions, insulin secretion, and lipid metabolism [2-5]. Selective PDE3 inhibitors have vasodilatory, antithrombotic, antiproliferative, bronchodilatory, anti-inflammatory, and positive inotropic effects [6-8]. A number of PDE3 inhibitors including cilostamide, cilostazol, milirinone, and amrinone were developed to treat patients with heart failure. However, chronic treatment with these agents was associated with some life-threatening side effects, arrhythmia in particular [7-10]. Therefore, designing new PDE3 inhibitors with

* Correspondence: Shafieer@mums.ac.ir
[1]Department of Pharmacology, School of Medicine, Mashhad University of Medical Sciences, Mashhad, Iran
[2]Pharmacological Research Center of Medicinal Plants, School of Medicine, Mashhad University of Medical Sciences, Mashhad, Iran
Full list of author information is available at the end of the article

desired pharmacological properties and lesser side effects is an attractive subject.

In the previous works we synthesized novel analogs of cilostamide as selective PDE3 inhibitors and evaluated their cardiac and metabolic properties. One of the test compounds, named MC2 (6-[4-(4-methylpiperidin-1-yl)-4-oxobutoxy]-4-methylquinolin-2(1H)-one), produced a potent inotropic action without unwanted effect on basal contraction rate [11-14]. Therefore, it may be a candidate for use as a PDE inhibitor in patients with cardiovascular diseases.

However, in adipose tissue, PDE3 inhibitors increase intracellular cAMP level and thereby increases lipolysis in adipocytes and enhance adipogenesis in preadipocytes [15,16]. Dysregulation of lipid metabolism in adipose tissue may cause deleterious consequences in some pathological conditions such as diabetes mellitus, insulin resistance, fatty liver, and obesity [17-19]. Therefore, as a selective PDE3 inhibitor, MC2 is expected to produce some effects on lipid metabolism which could be a potential risk factor for clinical adverse effect.

Therefore, in the present work, we evaluated the effects of MC2 on adipose tissue functions including adipogenesis and lipolysis, and also on adipocyte viability and apoptosis. Furthermore, the effects of MC2 were compared with the effects of amrinone and cilostamide on adipose tissue.

Materials and method
Chemicals and reagents
Isoproterenol, free glycerol reagent, 4-(2-hydroxyethyl) piperazine-1-ethanesulfonic acid sodium salt (HEPES), 4, 5-Dimethylthiazol-2-yl, 2, 5-diphenyl tetrazolium (MTT), fatty acid-free bovine serum albumin (BSA), and collagenase were purchased from Sigma (USA). Dimethyl sulfoxide (DMSO) and 3-isobutyl-1-methylxanthine (IBMX) were provided from Fluka (Buchs, Switzerland). Dulbecco's modified eagle's medium (DMEM), fetal bovine serum (FBS), penicillin/streptomycin, and Annexin V/PI apoptosis kit were obtained from Invitrogen (USA). Indomethacin, dexamethasone, and insulin were kindly provided by EXIR Company (Iran).

The test compound, MC2, was synthesized based on cilostamide structure by Department of Organic Chemistry, Mashhad University of Medical Sciences (Mashhad, Iran) according to the procedure reported by Sadeghian et al. and its PDE3 inhibitory action was assessed by Bioscience Company (BPS Bioscience Inc, San Diego, United States) using PDE assay Kit as described in previous works [14,20]. Figure 1 shows the IC50 of cilostamide, amrinone, and MC2 for PDE3. All the phosphodiesterase inhibitors were dissolved in dimethyl sulfoxide (DMSO) at a final concentration of 0.1% in the medium and equal amounts of carrier were added to control groups of the cells.

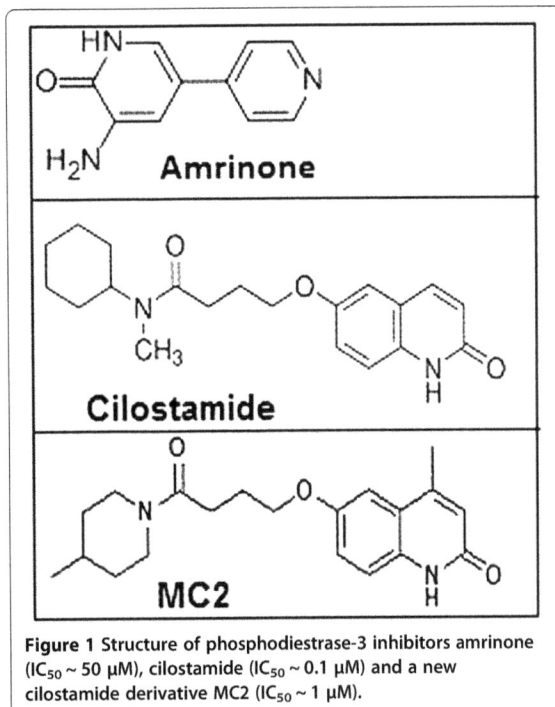

Figure 1 Structure of phosphodiestrase-3 inhibitors amrinone (IC$_{50}$ ~ 50 μM), cilostamide (IC$_{50}$ ~ 0.1 μM) and a new cilostamide derivative MC2 (IC$_{50}$ ~ 1 μM).

Animals
Adult male Wistar rats with weights of 280–300 g were obtained from Laboratory Animal House, Mashhad University of Medical School, Iran. They were housed under a 12/12 h light/dark daily cycle at 22°C and had free access to standard foods and water. All experiments were conducted in accordance with standard ethical guidelines and approved by the local ethics committee of Mashhad University of Medical Sciences.

Preadipocyte preparation and culture
The animals were sacrificed under ether anesthesia and retroperitoneal fat pads were removed immediately and placed in phosphate-buffered saline (PBS) supplemented with 100 U/ml penicillin and 100 μg/ml streptomycin in sterile condition. The tissue was minced into small pieces and incubated for 40 min in PBS containing 2 mg/ml collagenase at 37°C with mild agitation [21,22]. After centrifuging, the floated adipocytes were discarded and the stromal cells were suspended in DMEM medium supplemented with 10% fetal bovine serum, 100 U/ml penicillin and 100 μg/ml streptomycin and cultured in flask. After passage 3, the cells were seeded (at a density of 60000 cells/cm^2) in 12-well plates. On next day, adipogenesis was induced by applying "induction medium" containing DMEM supplemented with 200 nM insulin, 250 μM IBMX, 1 μM dexamethasone, 200 μM indomethacin and 3% FBS. On day 3, the cells were subsequently cultured in "maintenance medium" (induction

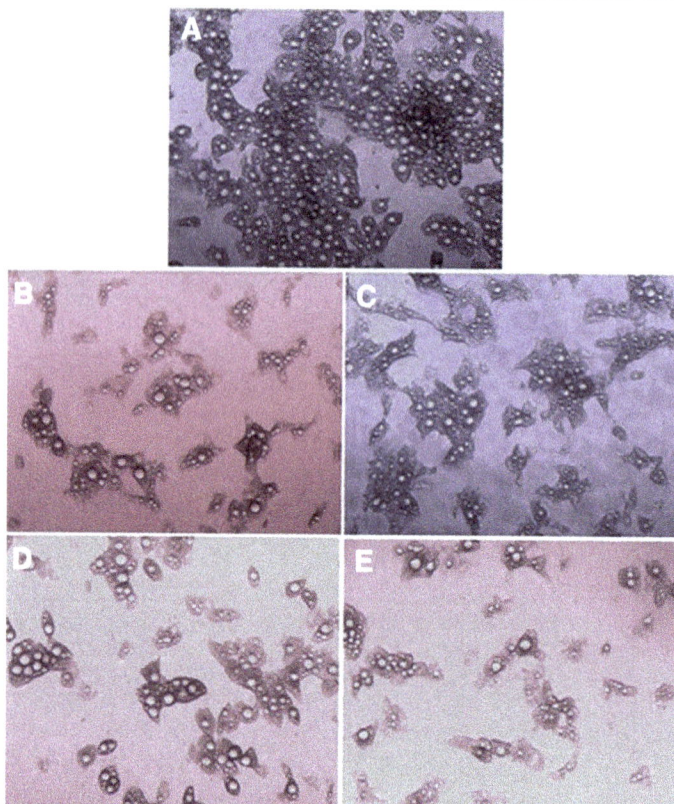

Figure 2 Differentiation of preadipocyte to adipocyte in the presence of (A) IBMX, (B) no PDE inhibitor, (C) amrinone, (D) cilostamide and (E) MC2. Adipogenesis was induced by 3 days incubation in "induction medium"; DMEM supplemented with 3% fetal bovine serum, 200 nM insulin, 250 μM of mentioned PDE inhibitors, 1 μM dexamethasone, 200 μM indomethacin. Then, the cells were subsequently cultured for 6 days in "maintenance medium" (induction medium without phosphodiestrase inhibitors and indomethacin). Magnification: ×100

medium without IBMX and indomethacin) for 9 days and the medium was changed every 3 days.

To investigate the effect of PDE inhibitors on adipogenesis, IBMX was replaced with the same concentration of amrinone, cilostamide, or MC2 in the induction medium during the first three days of incubation. The cellular triglyceride accumulation was measured as an index of the adipocyte differentiation in the presence of PDE3 inhibitors and compared with IBMX.

Oil Red O staining

Oil Red O was used to stain intracellular triglyceride droplets in differentiated adipocytes. Briefly, the cells were washed twice with PBS and fixed with 10% formalin for 30 min. After an additional washing with PBS, the cells were incubated with Oil Red O solution for 20 min [21,23]. Excess stain was removed by washing with distilled water and the stained cells were photographed. Lipid and Oil Red O were extracted using isopropyl alcohol and absorbance was measured using a spectrophotometer at a wavelength of 545 nm. The lipid content for each experimental group

is expressed relative to that of IBMX-differentiated cells (adjusted to 100%).

Determination of triglyceride

To support Oil Red O staining, the level of intracellular triglyceride (TG) was evaluated in differentiated adipocytes. Following washing the cells with PBS, intracellular TG was dissolved in 200 μl of 1% Triton X-100/PBS solution. Then, the level of TG was determined by TG assay kit (Pars azma, Co., Ltd., Iran). The protein concentrations were also measured by Bio-Rad protein assay dye reagent (Bio-Rad Laboratories, Inc.). Then the level of TG was normalized to cellular protein content of each treatment group [24]. The TG/protein content (mg/mg) was expressed as percentage compared to IBMX treated group as a control.

Cell proliferation assay

To investigate the effects of the PDE inhibitors on adipocyte proliferation, preadipocytes were seeded (10^4 cell/well) in flat-bottomed 96-well culture plates. After differentiation, adipocytes were incubated with amrinone, cilostamide and

MC2 at the various concentrations (10, 100 and 500 μM) for 6, 12 and 24 h. After completion of the treatment, the cells were incubated with MTT solution for 3 h at 37°C. The supernatants were aspirated, DMSO was added to each well, and the plates were agitated to dissolve the crystal product [25-27]. Absorbance was measured at 545 nm (630 nm as a reference) using a StatFAX303 plate reader.

Annexin V/PI double staining analysis

To detect the apoptosis induced by PDE inhibitors, Annexin V/PI double staining and flow cytometry analysis were used [28]. After adipocyte differentiation in 12-well plates, the cells were exposed to 10, 100 and 500 μM of MC2 for 24 h. After treatment, the cells were washed twice with cold PBS and resuspended in 100 μl binding buffer at a concentration of 1×10^6 cells/ml. Then, 5 μl Annexin V-FITC and 10 μl PI (1 mg/ml) were added to these cells according to manufacturer's instructions. Finally, the cells were analyzed with a FACScalibur flow cytometer (Becton Dickinson) and the distribution of normal, apoptotic and necrotic cells was calculated using WinMDI 2.7 software.

Lipolysis assay

The differentiated adipocytes (cultured in 12-well culture plates) were pre-incubated with serum-free DMEM for 3 h and then bathed with 1 ml Krebs-Ringer bicarbonate buffer containing 5.5 mM glucose, 25 mM HEPES and 2% (w/v) bovine serum albumin. The cells were left untreated (basal lipolysis) or treated with iso-proterenol (stimulated lipolysis) and incubated in the absence or presence of PDE inhibitors at 37°C in a humidified chamber under constant shaking for 2 h. Glycerol release in the medium was measured as index of lipolysis using the free glycerol determination kit [29,30].

Statistical analysis

The results are presented as the mean ± standard error. The values were compared using the one-way analysis of variances followed by Dunnett's post hoc test. The results were considered to be statistically significant, if the p-value was less than 0.05.

Results

Effect of PDE inhibitors on adipogenesis

The absence of IBMX in culture medium significantly decreased preadipocyte differentiation to adipocyte comparing to the control medium containing IBMX. Also, the level of adipogenesis in cilostamide and MC2 containing medium was lower than that of control medium. However, the effect of amrinone on preadipocyte differentiation was more than cilostamide and MC2, close to that of IBMX (Figure 2).

Oil Red O staining showed that in the presence of cilostamide and MC2 the level of lipid droplet accumulation was $69 \pm 6\%$ and $46 \pm 4\%$, respectively, which was significantly lower than control medium containing IBMX ($100 \pm 4\%$, $p < 0.01$-$p < 0.001$) (Figure 3A). These findings were confirmed by measurement of intracellular TG in the differentiated adipocytes. As shown in Figure 3B, the level of intracellular TG in the presence of cilostamide (78 ± 6, $P < 0.05$) and MC2 (43 ± 5, $P < 0.001$) was lower than that of IBMX treated cells (100 ± 10).

Effect of PDE inhibitors on adipocyte proliferation

Incubation of differentiated adipocytes with 10–500 μM of cilostamide, 10–500 μM of amrinoe and 10–100 μM

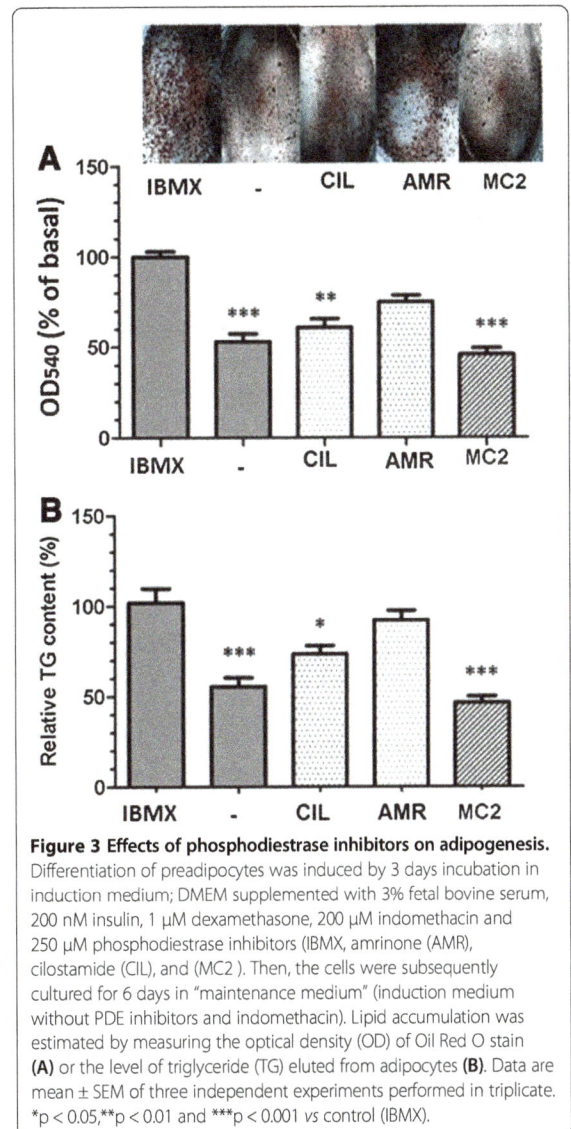

Figure 3 Effects of phosphodiestrase inhibitors on adipogenesis.
Differentiation of preadipocytes was induced by 3 days incubation in induction medium; DMEM supplemented with 3% fetal bovine serum, 200 nM insulin, 1 μM dexamethasone, 200 μM indomethacin and 250 μM phosphodiestrase inhibitors (IBMX, amrinone (AMR), cilostamide (CIL), and (MC2). Then, the cells were subsequently cultured for 6 days in "maintenance medium" (induction medium without PDE inhibitors and indomethacin). Lipid accumulation was estimated by measuring the optical density (OD) of Oil Red O stain **(A)** or the level of triglyceride (TG) eluted from adipocytes **(B)**. Data are mean ± SEM of three independent experiments performed in triplicate. *$p < 0.05$,**$p < 0.01$ and ***$p < 0.001$ *vs* control (IBMX).

of MC2 had no effect on their proliferation after 6, 12 and 24 h (Figure 4). MC2 at 500 μM significantly decreased proliferation of differentiated adipocyte to 86 ± 6 (p < 0.05), 82 ± 3 (p < 0.01) and 79 ± 6 (p < 0.01) after 6, 12 and 24 h, respectively.

Effect of MC2 on adipocyte apoptosis

Figure 5A shows the results of bivariate Annexin V/PI flow cytometry of differentiated adipocyte after 24 h incubation with MC2. The lower left quadrant of the histograms shows the viable cells, which exclude PI and are negative for FITC-Annexin V binding. The upper right quadrant represents the early apoptotic cells, which are PI negative and Annexin V positive, indicating integrity of the cytoplasmic membrane. The lower right quadrant represents the non-viable necrotic and late-stage apoptotic cells, which are positive for Annexin V binding and PI uptake. As shown in Figure 5B, incubation of differentiated adipocytes with MC2 caused the loss of cell viability at concentrations of 100 μM (p < 0.05) and 500 μM (p < 0.05). This effect was associated with the elevation in the number of apoptotic (concentrations of 10 and 100 μM, p < 0.05) and necrotic (concentrations of 500 μM, p < 0.01) cells.

Effect of PDE inhibitors on lipolysis

The differentiated adipocytes were incubated with different concentrations of PDE inhibitors and glycerol release was measured as index of lipolysis. Amrinone at 100 μM

significantly increased isoproterenol-induced (but not basal) lipolysis (p < 0.05). Cilostamide at concentration of 100 μM significantly increased basal lipolysis from 100 ± 7% to 334 ± 24% (p < 0.001) and also enhanced stimulated lipolysis from 375 ± 48% to 668 ± 34% (p < 0.01) (Figure 6A). At the concentration of 10 and 100 μM, basal lipolysis was not changed by MC2. However, it significantly decreased isoproterenol-induced lipolysis from 374 ± 48 to 225 ± 27% (p < 0.01) at 100 μM (Figure 6B).

Discussion

The PDEs play an important role in endocrine and cardiovascular functions, cell proliferation, cell differentiation, inflammation, and oxidative stress. Therapeutic application of PDE inhibitors, therefore, ranges from heart failure to pulmonary diseases to erectile dysfunction [31,32]. However, clinical application of these agents is limited because of their side effects, such as arrhythmia, impaired insulin secretion, and alterations in lipid metabolism [4,7]. Therefore, synthesis of new PDE3 inhibitors with desired pharmacological properties and lesser side effects is of great interest. In our previous work, we synthesized MC2 as a new cilostamide derivative and showed that it has inotropic action without unwanted effect on contraction rate [11,13]. In the present work, to assess the effect of synthesized compound on lipid metabolism, we investigated its effects on adipose tissue functions. Our data showed that MC2 unlike

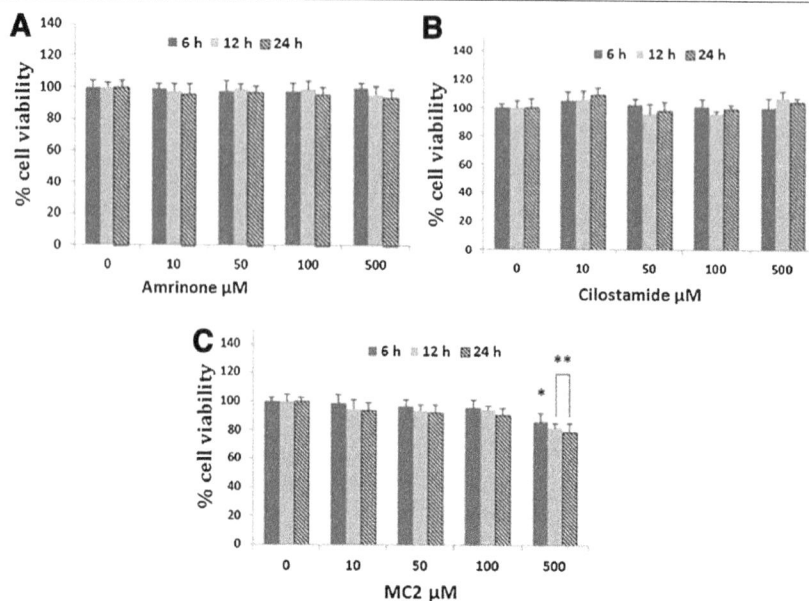

Figure 4 Effects of phosphodiestrase inhibitors on viability of differentiated adipocytes. The cells were incubated with various concentrations of amrinone (**A**), cilostamide (**B**) and MC2 (**C**) for 6, 12 or 24 h. Cell viability was detected using MTT colorimetric assay. Values are mean ± SEM (n = 9). *p < 0.05 and **p < 0.01 vs control cells (0 μM).

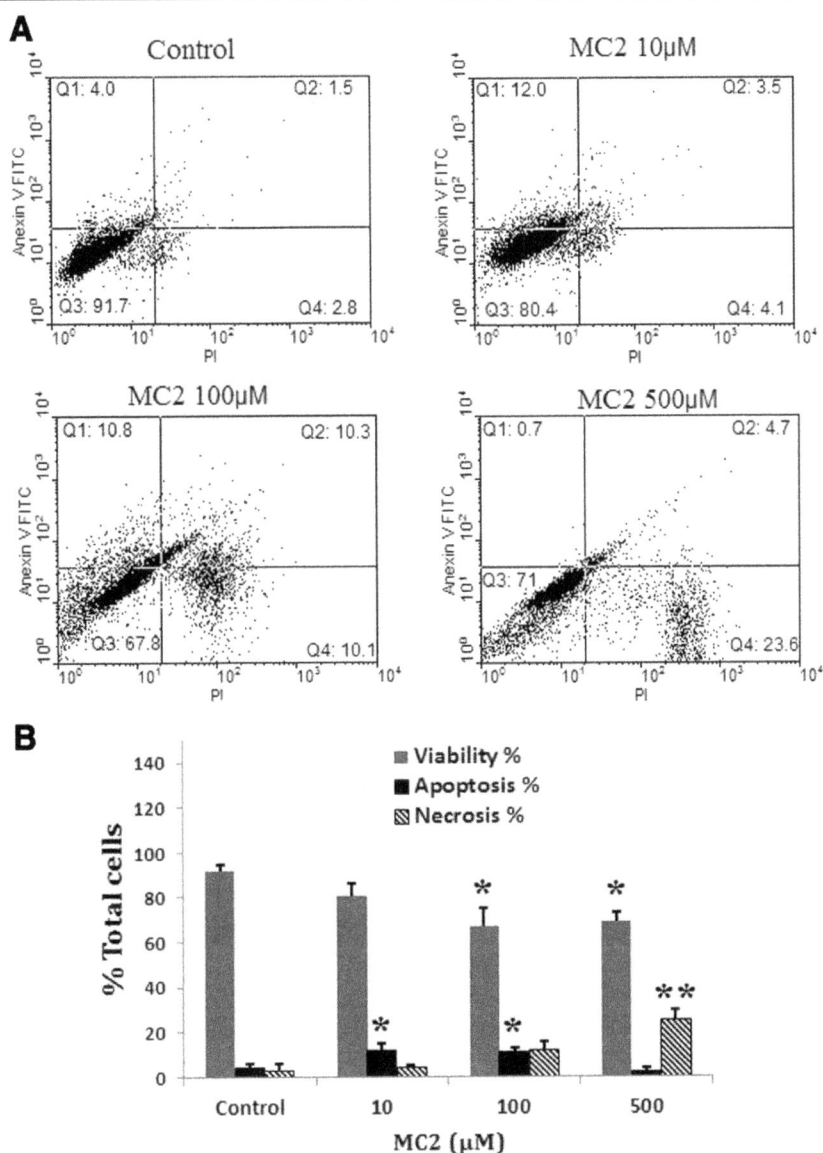

Figure 5 Effect of MC2 on apoptosis of adipocyte. (A) Detection of apoptosis and necrosis assessed with annexin-V-FITC and PI staining. The cells were treated with the indicated concentration of MC2 for 24 h. **(B)** Column bar graph of mean cell florescence for Annexin V-/PI- (Viable cells), Annexin V+/PI- (apoptotic cells), Annexin V+/PI+ (necrotic cells). Data are mean ± SEM of three experiments. *p < 0.05 and **p < 0.01 *vs* control.

other PDE3 inhibitors does not increase adipogenesis and lipolysis and even has antilipolytic effect.

In agreement with previous reports, in our study the PDE3 inhibitors amrinone and cilostamide potentiated both basal and catecholamine (isoproterenol)-stimulated glycerol release from adipocyte [33]. However, MC2 not only did not increase lipolysis, but inhibited catecholamine-induced glycerol release. Previously, in an *in-vitro* study we showed that MC2 increases liver glycogen storage in

rat and mouse which was different from those of other PDE inhibitors [12]. These effects of MC2 cannot be explained with its PDE3 inhibitory action because PDE inhibitors enhance lipolysis via elevation of intracellular cAMP [2].

In our previous studies we found that different PDE3 inhibitors produce differential cardiac and metabolic effects. All of test compounds produced positive inotropic effect but with different efficacies, which were not

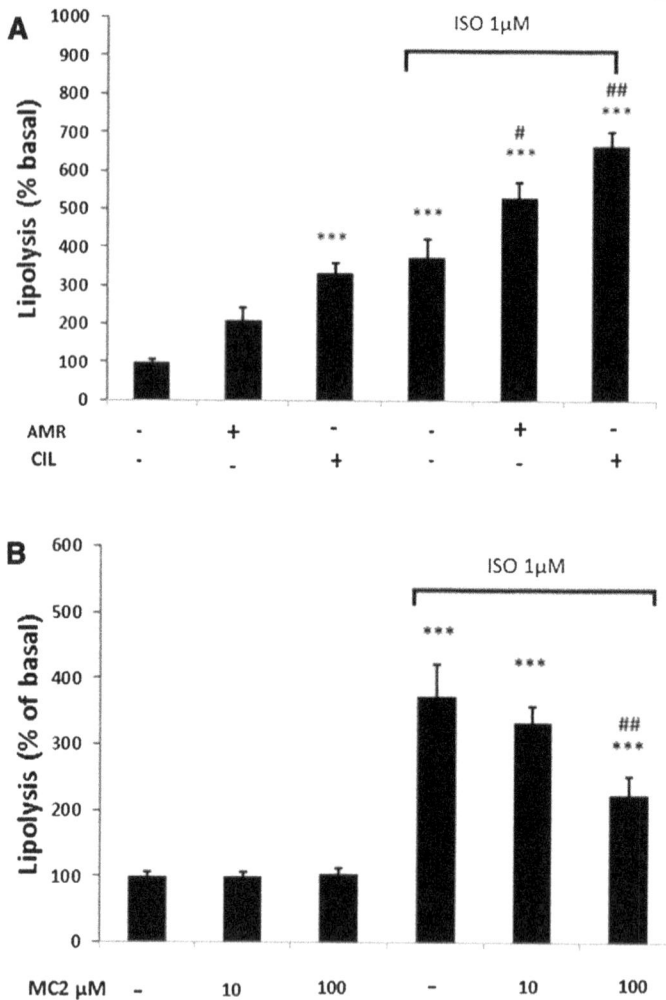

Figure 6 Effects of phosphodiestrase inhibitors on basal and isoproterenol (ISO)-induced lipolysis. Differentiated adipocytes were incubated with 100 μM amrinone (AMR), 100 μM cilostamide (CIL) (A) or indicated concentration of MC2 (B) for 120 min. Glycerol release in the culture media was assayed as lipolysis indicator. Data are mean ± SEM of three experiments. *P < 0.05 and ***P < 0.001 vs Control; #p < 0.05 and ##p < 0.01 vs ISO treated cells.

correlated with their IC_{50} of PDE3 inhibition. Also, they modified atrial contraction rates differently and some of which produced a negative chronotropic effect in spite of having a high positive inotropic effects [11]. Also, in rat hyperglycemic clamp model MC2 increased insulin secretion similar to the other tested PDE inhibitors, but opposite to others it increased the level of glycogen in the liver [12]. These effects implicate that a cAMP-independent signaling pathways may be involved in the biological effects of PDE inhibitors which is manifested by MC2 and may mediate its antilipolytic effect.

In patients with poorly controlled diabetes, deficiency of insulin in conjunction with catecholamine- and glucagon-stimulated lipolysis enhances fatty acid delivery to liver which may lead to ketoacidosis and even death [19]. It is reasonable to conclude that MC2 can decrease the risk of ketoacidosis through inhibition of lipolysis in diabetic patients who are candidate to PDE inhibitor therapy due to cardiovascular diseases.

Consistent with previous reports on the role of PDE inhibitors in adipogenesis [16,34], we found that deprivation of differentiation medium from IBMX attenuated adipogenesis. Neither cilostamide nor MC2 could restore the level of adipocyte differentiation to that of IBMX treated group. It has been revealed that PDEs exist in two forms: soluble (cytosolic) and particulate (membrane-associated) [35]. It is generally accepted that inhibition of soluble but not particulate PDE activity is responsible for IBMX-stimulated differentiation of pre-adipocytes [36]. Therefore, inhibition of PDE3 which predominately exist in the form of particulate cannot mimic the role of IBMX in adipocyte differentiation. On the other hand, similar to what happens in the heart and kidney [37], amrinone, in high concentration may inhibit soluble PDE and therefore could induce adipocyte differentiation approximately to the level induced by IBMX.

The mass of adipose tissue is determined by size and number of adipocytes. The size of adipocytes is reduced by lipolysis and increased by lipogenesis [38,39]. Number of adipocytes is directly related to the rate of adipogenesis and inversely related to the rate of apoptosis. Results of Annexin V/PI and MTT assays showed that MC2 increases adipocyte apoptosis. However, this effect was produced at high concentrations which reduced cell viability and proliferation. Since MC2 cannot increase adipogenesis, its potential proapoptotic effect may reduce total adipocytes number in fat tissue. However, antilipolytic effect of MC2 may prevent severe alteration in the mass of adipose tissue. Future works are needed to address long term effect of MC2 on fat mass.

In conclusion, our data showed that different types of PDE3 inhibitors induce different effects on lipolysis and adipogenesis. Here we introduced MC2 as a new PDE3 inhibitor with potential proapoptotic and antilipolytic effects on adipocytes and without stimulatory action on adipogenesis. These effects of MC2 implicate that, in comparison with amrinone or milrinone, this drug may have lowest metabolic side effect and might be a good candidate for treatment of congestive heart failure.

Competing interests
The authors declare that they have no competing interests.

Authors' contributions
RS-N and AG designed and supervised the study. RSN and HS designed and synthesized the test compounds. BA and AG collected data and wrote the first draft of the manuscript. BA performed the statistical analysis and managed the literature searches. All authors read and approved the final manuscript.

Acknowledgments
This work was a part of the Ph.D. thesis of one of the authors (Bagher Alinejad) and supported by a grant from Research Council of Mashhad University of Medical Sciences, Mashhad, Iran.

Author details
[1]Department of Pharmacology, School of Medicine, Mashhad University of Medical Sciences, Mashhad, Iran. [2]Pharmacological Research Center of Medicinal Plants, School of Medicine, Mashhad University of Medical Sciences, Mashhad, Iran. [3]Department of laboratory Sciences, School of Paramedical Sciences, Mashhad University of Medical Sciences, Mashhad, Iran.

References
1. Francis SH, Turko IV, Corbin JD. Cyclic nucleotide phosphodiesterases: relating structure and function. Prog Nucleic Acid Res Mol Biol. 2001;65:1–52.
2. Snyder BP, Esselstyn JM, Loughney K, Wolda SL, Florio VA. The role of cyclic nucleotide phosphodiesterases in the regulation of adipocyte lipolysis. J Lipid Res. 2005;46:494–503.
3. Palmer D, Maurice DH. Dual expression and differential regulation of phosphodiesterase 3A and phosphodiesterase 3B in human vascular smooth muscle: implications for phosphodiesterase 3 inhibition in human cardiovascular tissues. Mol Pharmacol. 2000;58:247–52.
4. Degerman E, Ahmad F, Chung YW, Guirguis E, Omar B, Stenson L, et al. From PDE3B to the regulation of energy homeostasis. Curr Opin Pharmacol. 2011;11:676–82.
5. Liu H, Maurice DH. Expression of cyclic GMP-inhibited phosphodiesterases 3A and 3B (PDE3A and PDE3B) in rat tissues: Differential subcellular localization and regulated expression by cyclic AMP. Br J Pharmacol. 1998;125:1501–10.
6. Hall IP. Isoenzyme selective phosphodiesterase inhibitors: potential clinical uses. Br J Clin Pharmacol. 1993;35:1–7.
7. Movsesian M, Wever-Pinzon O, Vandeput F. PDE3 inhibition in dilated cardiomyopathy. Curr Opin Pharmacol. 2011;11:707–13.
8. Boswell-Smith V, Spina D, Page CP. Phosphodiesterase inhibitors. Br J Pharmacol. 2006;147:S252–7.
9. Curfman GD. Inotropic therapy for heart failure-an unfulfilled promise. New Engl J Med. 1991;325:1509–60.
10. Smith AH, Owen J, Borgman KY, Fish FA, Kannankeril PJ. Relation of milrinone after surgery for congenital heart disease to significant postoperative tachyarrhythmias. Am J Cardiol. 2011;108:1620–4.
11. Hosseini A, Shafiee-Nick R, Parsaee H, Sadeghian H. Inotropic and chronotropic effects of new cilostamide derivatives on isolated rat atria. Iran J Physiol Pharmacol. 2011;15:341–50.
12. Hosseini A, Shafiee-Nick R, Pour Ali Behzad N, Sadeghian H. Differential metabolic effects of novel cilostamide analogs, methyl carbostiryl derivatives, in mouse and hyperglycemic rat. Iran J Basic Med Sci. 2012;15:916–25.
13. Mansouri SM, Shafiee-Nick R, Parsaee H, Seyedi SM, Saberi MR, Sadeghian H. Inotropic and chronotropic effects of 6-hydroxy-4-methylquinolin-2(1H)-one derivatives in isolated rat atria. Iran Biomed J. 2008;12:77–84.
14. Sadeghian H, Seyedi SM, Saberi MR, Nick RS, Hosseini A, Bakavoli M, et al. Design, synthesis and pharmacological evaluation of 6-hydroxy-4-methylquinolin-2 (1H)-one derivatives as inotropic agents. J Enzyme Inhib Med Chem. 2008;24:918–29.
15. Chaves VE, Frasson D, Kawashita NH. Several agents and pathways regulate lipolysis in adipocytes. Biochimie. 2011;93:1631–40.
16. Jia B, Madsen L, Petersen RK, Techer N, Kopperud R. Activation of Protein kinase A and exchange protein directly activated by cAMP promotes adipocyte differentiation of human mesenchymal stem cells. PLoS One. 2012;7:e34114.
17. Arner P, Langin D. Lipolysis in lipid turnover, cancer cachexia, and obesity-induced insulin resistance. Trends Endocrinol Metab. 2014;25:255–62.
18. Fabbrini E, Mohammed BS, Magkos F, Korenblat KM, Patterson BW, Klein S. Alterations in adipose tissue and hepatic lipid kinetics in obese men and women with nonalcoholic fatty liver disease. Gastroenterology. 2008;134:424–31.
19. Perilli G, Saraceni C, Daniels MN, Ahmad A. Diabetic ketoacidosis: a review and update. Curr Emerg Hosp Med Rep. 2013;1:10–7.
20. Degerman E, Belfrage P, Newman AH, Rice KC, Manganiello VC. Purification of the putative hormone-sensitive cyclic AMP phosphodiesterase from rat adipose tissue using a derivative of cilostamide as a novel affinity ligand. J Biol Chem. 1987;262:5797–807.
21. Ghorbani A, Hadjzadeh MR, Rajaei Z, Zendehbad SB. Effects of fenugreek seeds on adipogenesis and lipolysis in normal and diabetic rat. Pakistan J Biol Sci. 2014;17:523–8.
22. Ghorbani A, Feizpour A, Hashemzahi M, Gholami L, Hosseini M, Soukhtanloo M, et al. The effect of adipose derived stromal cells on oxidative stress level, lung emphysema and white blood cells of guinea pigs model of chronic obstructive pulmonary disease. DARU J Pharm Sci. 2014;22:26.

23. Ghorbani A, Jalali SA, Varedi M. Isolation of adipose tissue mesenchymal stem cells without tissue destruction: a non-enzymatic method. Tissue Cell. 2014;46:54–8.
24. Okazaki H, Igarashi M, Nishi M, Tajima M, Sekiya M, Okazaki S, et al. Identification of a novel member of the carboxylesterase family that hydrolyzes triacylglycerol: a potential role in adipocyte lipolysis. Diabetes. 2006;55:2091–7.
25. Mortazavian SM, Ghorbani A. Antiproliferative effect of viola tricolor on neuroblastoma cells in vitro. Aust J Herbal Med. 2012;24:93–6.
26. Mortazavian SM, Ghorbani A, Hesari TG. Effect of hydro-alcoholic extract of *Viola tricolor* and its fractions on proliferation of uterine cervix carcinoma cells. Iranian J Obstet Gynecol Infertility. 2012;15:9–16.
27. Forouzanfar F, Goli AA, Assadpour E, Ghorbani A, Sadeghnia HR. Protective effect of *Punica granatum* L. against serum/glucose deprivation-induced PC12 cells injury. Evid Based Complement Alternat Med. 2013;2013:716730.
28. Vermes I, Haanen C, Steffens-Nakken H, Reutelingsperger C. A novel assay for apoptosis flow cytometric detection of phosphatidylserine expression on early apoptotic cells using fluorescein labelled annexin V. J Immunol Methods. 1995;184:39–51.
29. Ghorbani A, Abedinzade M. Comparison of *in vitro* and *in situ* methods for studying lipolysis. ISRN Endocrinol. 2013;2013:205385.
30. Ghorbani A, Omrani GH, Hadjzadeh MR, Varedi M. Proinsulin C-peptide inhibits lipolysis in diabetic rat adipose tissue through phosphodiestrase-3B enzyme. Horm Metab Res. 2013;45:221–5.
31. Lugnier C. PDE inhibitors: a new approach to treat metabolic syndrome? Curr Opin Pharmacol. 2011;11:698–706.
32. Rajiv M, Vinod K. Phosphodiesterase inhibitors and their role in therapeutics. J Res Med Educ Ethics. 2013;3:115–23.
33. Ghorbani A, Omrani GH, Hadjzadeh MR, Varedi M. Effects of rat C-peptide-II on lipolysis and glucose consumption in cultured rat adipose tissue. Exp Clin Endocrinol Diabetes. 2011;119:343–7.
34. Jeon YH, Heo YS, Kim CM, Hyun YL, Lee TG. Phosphodiesterase: overview of protein structures, potential therapeutic applications and recent progress in drug development. Cell Mol Life Sci. 2005;62:1198–220.
35. Elks ML, Manganiello VC. A role for soluble cAMP phosphodiesterases in differentiation of 3 T3-L1 adipocytes. J Cell Physiol. 1985;124:191–8.
36. Sun L, Nicholson AC, Hajjar DP, Gotto Jr AM, Han J. Adipogenic differentiating agents regulate expression of fatty acid binding protein and CD36 in the J744 macrophage cell line. J Lipid Res. 2003;44:1877–86.
37. Ghosh R, Sawant O, Ganpathy P, Pitre S, Kadam V. Phosphodiesterase inhibitors: their role and implications. 2009;1:1148-1160
38. Rayalam S, Della-Fera MA, Baile CA. Phytochemicals and regulation of the adipocyte life cycle. J Nutr Biochem. 2008;19:717–26.
39. Ghorbani A, Varedi M, Hadjzadeh MR, Omrani GH. Type-1 diabetes induces depot-specific alterations in adipocyte diameter and mass of adipose tissues in the rat. Exp Clin Endocrinol Diabetes. 2010;118:442–8.

Does pharmacist-supervised intervention through pharmaceutical care program influence direct healthcare cost burden of newly diagnosed diabetics in a tertiary care teaching hospital in Nepal: a non-clinical randomised controlled trial approach

Dinesh Kumar Upadhyay[1], Mohamed Izham Mohamed Ibrahim[2], Pranaya Mishra[3], Vijay M. Alurkar[4] and Mukhtar Ansari[5*]

Abstract

Background: Cost is a vital component for people with chronic diseases as treatment is expected to be long or even lifelong in some diseases. Pharmacist contributions in decreasing the healthcare cost burden of chronic patients are not well described due to lack of sufficient evidences worldwide. In developing countries like Nepal, the estimation of direct healthcare cost burden among newly diagnosed diabetics is still a challenge for healthcare professionals, and pharmacist role in patient care is still theoretical and practically non-existent. This study reports the impact of pharmacist-supervised intervention through pharmaceutical care program on direct healthcare costs burden of newly diagnosed diabetics in Nepal through a non-clinical randomised controlled trial approach.

Methods: An interventional, pre-post non-clinical randomised controlled study was conducted among randomly distributed 162 [control ($n = 54$), test 1 ($n = 54$) and test 2 ($n = 54$) groups] newly diagnosed diabetics by a consecutive sampling method for 18 months. Direct healthcare costs (direct medical and non-medical costs) from patients perspective was estimated by 'bottom up' approach to identify their out-of-pocket expenses (1USD = NPR 73.38) before and after intervention at the baseline, 3, 6, 9 and 12 months follow-ups. Test groups' patients were nourished with pharmaceutical care intervention while control group patients only received care from physician/ nurses. Non-parametric tests i.e. Friedman test, Mann–Whitney U test and Wilcoxon signed rank test were used to find the differences in direct healthcare costs among the groups before and after the intervention ($p \leq 0.05$).

Results: Friedman test identified significant differences in direct healthcare cost of test 1 ($p < 0.001$) and test 2 ($p < 0.001$) groups patients. However, Mann–Whitney U test justified significant differences in direct healthcare cost between control group and test 1 group, and test 2 group patients at 6-months ($p = 0.009$, $p = 0.010$ respectively), 9-months ($p = 0.005$, $p = 0.001$ respectively) and 12-months ($p < 0.001$, $p < 0.001$ respectively).

(Continued on next page)

* Correspondence: mukhtaransari@hotmail.com
[5]Department of Pharmacy and Pharmacology, National Medical College, Birgunj, Nepal
Full list of author information is available at the end of the article

(Continued from previous page)

Conclusion: Pharmacist supervised intervention through pharmaceutical care program significantly decreased direct healthcare costs of diabetics in test groups compared to control group and hence describes pharmacist's contribution in minimizing direct healthcare cost burden of patients.

Keywords: Diabetes mellitus, Healthcare costs, Intervention, Nepal, Pharmacists, Pharmaceutical care, Randomised controlled trial

Background

Cost is a vital component for people with chronic diseases as treatment is expected to be long, even life-long in many cases. Pharmacist contributions in decreasing the healthcare cost burden of chronic patients are not well described due to lack of sufficient evidences worldwide. Direct healthcare costs (DHCs) are the "actual monetary expenditure used in treating or coping with a disease" [1]. In a broader sense, the direct healthcare cost is the expenditure spent for detection, treatment, rehabilitation and care of a disease [2]. Distinguishing the definition of cost from price, "cost is a function of the inputs (labour, consumable goods, depreciation, etc.) required to produce a particular service" while "price is a function of what is paid in the market place" [3]. Due to the chronic nature of diabetes, it is associated with a substantial impact on the healthcare cost of patients[2]with the largest proportion attributed to treatment cost among other components of direct cost of diabetes [1, 4]. The global estimation of direct healthcare expenditure for people with diabetes is about USD 153 billion per year [5].

In Nepal, where healthcare services are poor [6] and not streamlined, people have difficulty in accessing the healthcare services most of the time. Furthermore, in absence of government and private healthcare insurance coverage, patients pay from their pocket to avail the acquired healthcare services, which increase their out-of-pocket expenses and make the treatment unaffordable to them. This result in a delay in disease diagnosis and early episodes of complications that may lead to frequent hospitalization and increased prescription cost with subsequent effects on other components of the direct cost domain [7]. Pharmacist role in patient care is still theoretical and practically non-existent in Nepal resulting in huge healthcare cost burden on patients. This study reports the impact of pharmacist-supervised intervention through pharmaceutical care program on direct healthcare costs of newly diagnosed diabetics in Nepal.

Methods
Study design

An interventional, pre-post non-clinical randomised controlled trial among the control group (CG), test 1 group (T1G) and test 2 group (T2G) with three treatment arms was conducted to explore the impact of pharmacist-supervised pharmaceutical care intervention on direct healthcare cost of newly diagnosed diabetics at the Manipal Teaching Hospital, Pokhara, Nepal for 18 months (July 2010 to December 2011). The study was approved by the Research and Ethics Committee of Manipal Teaching Hospital, Nepal [8].

Study population

Newly diagnosed type 1 and type 2 diabetes mellitus patients of aged 16 years and above were selected. Pregnant women, mentally incompetent patients, patients not willing to participate and did not come at their first follow-up were excluded from the study. Written consent was taken from patients participating in the study. However, in case of minors, parental consent was sought and obtained.

Sample and sampling technique

Sample size was calculated by using a finite population correction formula [9]. Diabetes prevalence of 9 % was taken as the calculation factor from previous studies [10, 11]. The Z value was set at 1.96, with a 95 % of confidence interval and 5 % as margin of error. The calculated sample size was 125 patients. A drop-outs margin of 30 % was taken from previous studies [12, 13] and added to the sample to achieve the final targeted sample size of 162 patients. The targeted sample was achieved by a consecutive sampling method (based on time capsule frame) over 6 months duration (July 2010 to December 2010) [14]. The randomisation of 162 patients was done by 1:1:1 in three parallel groups [CG ($n = 54$), T1G ($n = 54$) and T2G ($n = 54$)] without disturbing the sequence of randomisation [15]. Ten patients (CG = 4; T1G = 3 and T2G = 3) did not complete their first assessment follow-up (3-months) and therefore, further study was carried out with 152 patients [CG ($n = 50$), T1G ($n = 51$) and T2G ($n = 51$)] [8].

Study tools

Study tools were prepared in the Nepali language due to language fluency and barriers to the English language among most of the patients visiting the hospital. Socio-demography form was used to collect the patients' demographic characteristics. Direct healthcare costs documentation form was used to analyse the cost incurred by the patients in diabetes management during study period. Diabetes information booklet, diabetes complication chart and diabetic food chart were educational materials to improve the patients' awareness about diabetes and its management. A diabetic kit (including glass tubings, chart of human anatomy with circulatory system, daily medication calendar and calendar of anti-diabetic medicines) was made especially for T2G (PC + Diabetic kit group) patients to explain about anatomical and physiological relationship of diabetes and its impact on physiological system. The intention to use diabetic kit only in T2G patients was to identify whether an extra demonstration of diabetic kit would increase patient's understanding about diabetes and assist them for better disease control. This extra initiative might bring remarkable differences in direct healthcare cost burden of patients between T1G and T2G [8].

Estimation of direct medical and non-medical costs of patients

The direct healthcare costs estimation (direct medical and non-medical costs) from the patient's perspective was done by a 'bottom up' approach [16] to calculate their out-of-pocket expenses in managing their diabetes during the study period (12-months). The 'bottom-up' approach is based on the cost of individual units of service provided. The 'bottom-up' approach in fact starts from a selected subpopulation with the actual disease and all the costs associated with the disease is collected and extrapolated to the national level [17].

Patient's direct healthcare costs were estimated before and after pharmacist-supervised pharmaceutical care intervention at the baseline and 3, 6, 9 and 12 months' follow-ups respectively. Direct healthcare costs incurred by patients at baseline and each follow-up are the total sum of direct medical and non-medical costs. Direct medical costs comprised of various cost-variables including patient registration cost, cost for emergency care, lab investigation cost, drug(s) cost and cost of hospitalization and in-patient care. However, direct non-medical costs include transportation cost, meal cost on the way to hospital [1, 18] and dietary management cost during investigation in hospital. Information related to direct medicals cost was taken from patient's medical record (bills and prescriptions, etc.) and hospital rate lists for different services.

To calculate direct medical costs on patient is multiplying the number of each service/care provided by the unit cost of each service/care. For laboratory investigations, the number of laboratory tests performed was multiplied by the unit cost of each test. However, the calculation of drug cost(s) was done by multiplying the number of dose by the unit price of the drug and the resulting total costs was then multiplied by duration of therapy to obtain the total drug costs. However, direct non-medical cost estimation was done on the basis of information collected from patients and their relatives with regard to transportation cost, meal cost on the way to hospital (to and fro) and dietary management cost on each visit to the hospital.

Patients were asked to maintain a copy of all the bills and prescriptions related to their treatment to ensure the maximum accuracy of cost estimation. The calculation of DHCs at each follow-up covered direct medical and non-medical costs of patient between the two follow-ups (e.g. direct healthcare costs at 3-months will be the sum of direct medical and non-medical costs between baseline and 3-months period and so on). All the information related to direct healthcare costs were documented in a pre-designed direct healthcare cost documentation form.

Pharmacist intervention among diabetes patients

Pharmacist had made an attempt to minimize direct healthcare cost burden of diabetics by improving their understanding about diabetes. Pharmacist led intervention was done among the patients of test groups (T1G and T2G). Education and counselling about different aspects of diabetes and its management and, the correct use of antidiabetic medications were the important information covered by the pharmacist during the intervention. Patients from the test groups received the information about meaning of diabetes, its types, sign and symptoms, reasons for high blood glucose, risk factors of diabetes, different short term and long term complications of diabetes and role of pharmacological (anti-diabetic medication) and non-pharmacological (lifestyle modification, diet and exercise) measures in management of diabetes from pharmacist. Besides this, test groups patients were also taught about how to administer insulin by using insulin pen or insulin syringe (if insulin was prescribed in therapy) and trained regarding the use of glucometer for self-monitoring of blood glucose (SMBG) at home. Medication envelopes were used to dispense the prescribed medication (s) to the patients.

In addition to it, the test 2 group patients received the demonstration of diabetic kit components such as glass tubing's showing the change in the viscosity pattern of blood among diabetic and non-diabetic patients and the impact of increased sugar on the blood flow in different organ system with emphasis of blood coagulation and obstruction in blood flow in blood vessels in diabetes. Chart of human anatomy with circulator system was described to make the patients aware to locate the different organ system in the body and the supply of blood to these organs via blood vessels. Special focus was given to those organs which are mainly affected in diabetes i.e. cardiac system, renal system, eye and brain. They were also explained about the location of pancreas and its role in diabetes. Daily medication calendar and anti-diabetic medicine calendar were used to enhance the patients' knowledge and compliance about the use of anti-diabetic medication in diabetes management [8].

Statistical analysis

The direct healthcare costs of patients from three groups were calculated at the baseline, 3, 6, 9 and 12 months' follow-ups. Data was entered in SPSS version 16 and descriptive analysis was done as required for data analysis. Data was skewed ($p < 0.05$) on Kolmogorov-Smirnov test. Non-parametric tests i.e. Friedman test, Mann–Whitney U test were used to find out the differences between dependent and independent variables within and between the groups before and after the interventions respectively. The Wilcoxon signed rank test was used for pre- and post-comparison within the groups. Post hoc analysis with Wilcoxon signed rank test was used to find out in which follow-up the significant differences actually occurred in the group at a new p-value of ≤ 0.005 after Bonferroni adjustment. A significance level of $p \leq 0.05$ was used in all analyses.

Results

Socio-demography of patients

The study enrolled 162 patients. The mean age (in years) of the patients was 49.14 ± 12.56. Males were greater in number ($n = 106$, 65.43 %). The median monthly income and inter-quartile range of the patients was Nepali rupees (NPR) 10,000 [(9,000)-(16,000)] (1USD = 73.38 NPR). About 40.7 % patients were unemployed, 25.9 % businessman, 18.5 % employed, 13.6 % pensioner and 1.2 % students in the study. The study found 30.9 % patients either primary educated or secondary educated and, only 24 % and 14.2 % patients were non-educated and tertiary educated respectively. There were no significant differences in education level and health related knowledge among the patients of three groups at baseline. There were 92 % patients of non-vegetarian food habits. Nearly 42.6 % and 57.4 % patients never had alcohol and smoking habits respectively. Type 2 diabetics were found more ($n = 156$, 96.3 %) in the study [8].

Geometric changes in direct medical and non-medical costs of CG, T1G and T2G patients at the baseline and follow-ups

Descriptive analysis was done to calculate direct medical and non-medical costs burden on diabetics and results are presented in mean ± sd and median (IQR) cost. The chief contributors of direct medical and non-medical costs of the control and test groups' patients were cost of investigation, drug(s) costs, patient registration cost, and transportation cost, dietary management cost

respectively. Pharmacist-provided intervention reduced direct medical and non-medical cost burden on patients in test groups with greater reduction in anti-diabetic treatment cost in subsequent follow-ups (Table 1).

Direct healthcare costs (direct medical + non-medical costs) of CG, T1G and T2G patients at baseline and follow-ups

The median direct medical costs, the median direct non-medical costs and the total median direct healthcare costs of CG, T1G and T2G patients at the baseline and follow-ups are mentioned in Table 2. The reduction in cost variables attributed to increased cost of patients could be achieved by successive counselling and diabetes education related to diabetes care from the pharmacist, which ultimately affected the direct medical and non-medical costs of patients resulting in a substantial reduction in total direct healthcare cost of patients in both test groups compared to control group in their follow-ups (Table 2).

Direct healthcare costs comparison of patients at the baseline and follow-ups within test groups (T1G and T2G)

Friedman test identified the significant differences in DHCs of test 1 group ($p < 0.001$) and test 2 group ($p < 0.001$) patients due to pharmaceutical care intervention (Table 3).

However, it was difficult to explore from Friedman test where the actual significant differences occurred in each group on different occasions, which was resolved by using post-hoc analysis with the Wilcoxon signed rank test after Bonferroni adjustment applied (Table 4).

Comparison of direct healthcare costs between test groups (T1G and T2G), and CG and test groups' patients

Although there were differences in median direct healthcare costs between the test groups (T1G and T2G) over time but differences were not statistically significant at Mann–Whitney U-test. Moreover, the significant differences in direct healthcare cost between CG and T1G, and T2G were noted at 6-months ($p = 0.009$, $p = 0.010$ respectively), 9-months ($p = 0.005$, $p = 0.001$ respectively) and 12-months ($p < 0.001$, $p < 0.001$ respectively) (Table 5).

Discussion

Diabetes is a very costly illness that creates a major impact on patient's direct healthcare costs (out-of-pocket expenses) [19]. The trend of increasing burden on patients' out-of-pocket expenses is due to lack of patients' focus on disease management in absence of their disease awareness and self-care practices.

The major contribution in total median direct healthcare costs of patients was attributed to median direct

Table 1 Geometric changes in direct medical and non-medical costs of CG, T1G, and T2G patients at the baseline and follow-ups[a]

Direct medical cost

Cost variables	Groups[b]	Baseline Mean cost ± sd	Baseline Median cost (IQR)	3-months (1st FU) Mean cost ± sd	3-months (1st FU) Median cost (IQR)	6-months (2nd FU) Mean cost ± sd	6-months (2nd FU) Median cost (IQR)	9-months (3rd FU) Mean cost ± sd	9-months (3rd FU) Median cost (IQR)	12-months (4th FU) Mean cost ± sd	12-months (4th FU) Median cost (IQR)
Patient registration	CG	30.00 ± .00	30 (30)-(30)	76.20 ± 29.82	60 (60)-(90)	94.80 ± 22.15	90 (90)-(120)	81.00 ± 34.41	90 (60)-(97.50)	90.60 ± 22.26	90 (90)-(90)
	T1G	30.00 ± .00	30 (30)-(30)	102.94 ± 20.12	90 (90)-(120)	66.47 ± 19.26	60 (60)-(90)	50.58 ± 20.33	60 (30)-(60)	49.41 ± 20.63	60 (30)-(60)
	T2G	30.00 ± .00	30 (30)-(30)	69.41 ± 23.61	60 (60)-(90)	67.05 ± 22.28	60 (60)-(90)	53.52 ± 20.18	60 (30)-(60)	41.17 ± 17.96	30 (30)-(60)
Emergency care (if any)	CG T1G T2G	0	0	0	0	0	0	0	0	0	0
Hospitalization and in-patient care (if any)	CG	51.12 ± 264.08	0 (0)-(0)	0	0	16.00 ± 113.13	0 (0)-(0)	0	0	0	0
	T1G	27.48 ± 139.55	0 (0)-(0)	0	0	0		0		0	
	T2G	19.44 ± 142.88	0 (0)-(0)	0	0	0		0		0	
Investigations	CG	406.20 ± 222.35	350 (313.25)-(430)	464.60 ± 92.45	450 (400)-(542.50)	462.88 ± 89.96	450 (440)-(492.50)	445.46 ± 104.63	400 (400)-(455)	459.50 ± 114.59	450 (400)-(500)
	T1G	413.29 ± 161.34	350 (340-460)	474.90 ± 88.20	455 (450)-(500)	425.92 ± 72.33	405 (400)-(450)	398.07 ± 72.60	400 (355)-(405)	385.05 ± 56.29	355 (350)-(400)
	T2G	399.75 ± 116.60	350 (340)-(405)	435.49 ± 91.76	400 (400)-(450)	417.90 ± 82.49	400 (390)-(450)	398.68 ± 53.69	400 (355)-(405)	367.35 ± 34.19	350 (350)-(400)
Drug (s) cost[c] — ADD	CG	211.40 ± 226.82	109 (45)-(304.75)	1080.00 ± 869.36	870 (560)-(1236.50)	869.48 ± 435.99	880 (584)-(995)	755.86 ± 302.69	760 (560)-(978.50)	661.28 ± 294.93	650 (495)-(884.70)
AntiHTN	CG	50.14 ± 101.61	0 (0)-(77)	148.66 ± 366.41	0 (0)-(182)	250.34 ± 398.26	0 (0)-(650)	248.00 ± 310.34	0 (0)-(560)	253.58 ± 306.02	0 (0)-(540.75)
Others	CG	132.12 ± 496.84	0 (0)-(73.50)	157.16 ± 541.23	0 (0)-(13.50)	182.06 ± 358.23	0 (0)-(91.75)	164.52 ± 389.07	0 (0)-(67.75)	154.90 ± 390.06	0 (0)-(54)
ADD	T1G	216.75 ± 274.08	141 (47)-(316)	993.19 ± 838.77	761 (288)-(1544)	790.49 ± 840.25	480 (0)-(1222)	665.27 ± 538.23	508 (284)-(929)	436.21 ± 534.41	254 (48)-(692)
AntiHTN	T1G	33.11 ± 76.89	0 (0)-(6.25)	169.15 ± 353.51	0 (0)-(222)	166.39 ± 389.02	0 (0)-(0)	114.62 ± 234.93	0 (0)-(0)	84.64 ± 195.71	0 (0)-(0)
Others	T1G	82.85 ± 153.45	0 (0)-(110.75)	250.76 ± 720.28	0 (0)-(0)	172.31 ± 579.29	0 (0)-(0)	148.54 ± 506.22	0 (0)-(0)	121.29 ± 360.94	0 (0)-(0)
ADD	T2G	158.42 ± 186.14	83.50 (20.50)-(212)	1035.80 ± 669.29	1015 (480)-(1500)	754.33 ± 856.70	350 (48)-(1269)	579.00 ± 798.76	367 (139)-(750)	315.47 ± 470.88	157 (0)-(413)
AntiHTN	T2G	33.48 ± 90.07	0 (0)-(0)	178.00 ± 309.62	0 (0)-(215)	121.29 ± 218.61	0 (0)-(277)	91.45 ± 210.78	0 (0)-(0)	73.07 ± 180.94	0 (0)-(0)
Others	T2G	64.70 ± 207.71	0 (0)-(0)	192.66 ± 509.89	0 (0)-(0)	151.86 ± 386.75	0 (0)-(54)	154.07 ± 536.24	0 (0)-(0)	112.96 ± 379.02	0 (0)-(0)

Table 1 Geometric changes in direct medical and non-medical costs of CG, T1G, and T2G patients at the baseline and follow-ups[a] (Continued)

Direct non-medical cost

Cost variables	Groups[b]	Baseline		3-months (1st FU)		6-months (2nd FU)		9-months (3rd FU)		12-months (4th FU)	
		Mean cost ± sd	Median cost (IQR)	Mean cost ± sd	Median cost (IQR)	Mean cost ± sd	Median cost (IQR)	Mean cost ± sd	Median cost (IQR)	Mean cost ± sd	Median cost (IQR)
Transport (round trips)	CG	166.53 ± 314.99	54 (30)-(162.50)	233.36 ± 196.70	155 (87.50)-(312.50)	112.34 ± 53.20	120 (69)-(150)	101.60 ± 49.29	100 (70)-(140)	125.32 ± 71.84	120 (78.75)-(165)
	T1G	110.38 ± 277.22	30 (24)-(85)	108.62 ± 62.76	100 (80)-(150)	117.54 ± 98.23	80 (50)-(160)	109.80 ± 100.45	80 (40)-(150)	108.33 ± 95.28	80 (48)-(120)
	T2G	100.09 ± 176.45	40 (28.75)-(70)	116.82 ± 64.04	120 (60)-(200)	117.39 ± 77.31	100 (60)-(160)	113.07 ± 113.07	80 (48)-(120)	117.98 ± 154.49	80 (40)-(108)
Meal on the way to hospital (round trip, if any)	CG	1.85 ± 13.60	0 (0)-(0)	11.70 ± 29.06	0 (0)-(0)	6.24 ± 22.65	0 (0)-(0)	8.60 ± 24.05	0 (0)-(0)	7.10 ± 21.33	0 (0)-(0)
	T1G	3.70 ± 27.21	0 (0)-(0)	8.56 ± 27.75	0 (0)-(0)	6.54 ± 18.77	0 (0)-(0)	5.86 ± 20.77	0 (0)-(0)	3.54 ± 10.07	0 (0)-(0)
	T2G	2.22 ± 16.32	0 (0)-(0)	7.05 ± 20.20	0 (0)-(0)	3.88 ± 11.20	0 (0)-(0)	7.01 ± 23.35	0 (0)-(0)	7.25 ± 23.18	0 (0)-(0)
Dietary management during investigation	CG	137.37 ± 293.93	60 (50)-(100)	147.00 ± 44.82	150 (120)-(200)	183.20 ± 100.21	180 (140)-(200)	157.50 ± 52.37	160 (120)-(200)	172.00 ± 30.10	170 (150)-(200)
	T1G	111.12 ± 191.28	60 (60)-(80)	142.15 ± 34.13	150 (120)-(160)	123.03 ± 47.46	120 (80)-(150)	111.07 ± 59.27	90 (80)-(120)	114.31 ± 47.17	100 (80)-(150)
	T2G	86.66 ± 145.06	60 (50)-(60)	162.64 ± 60.69	160 (120)-(200)	142.54 ± 57.37	140 (100)-(180)	131.07 ± 52.18	120 (100)-(150)	103.03 ± 44.83	100 (60)-(130)

a = costs were calculated in Nepali rupees (NPR) [Exchange rate: 1 USD = NPR 73.38]
b = CG = control group, T1G = test 1 group, T2G = test 2 group
c = ADD = antidiabetic drug, AntiHTN = antihypertensive, others = Lipid lowering agents, Anti anginal drugs, Vitamin B complex, Antibiotic, Proton pump inhibitors, Antihistaminic, Antiplatelet agent

Table 2 Total direct healthcare costs (direct medical and non-medical costs) of CG, T1G and T2G patients at the baseline and follow-ups

Follow-ups	Groups[b]	Direct medical costs[a]		Direct non-medical costs[a]		Total direct healthcare costs (Direct medical + non-medical costs)[a]	
		Mean cost ± sd	Median cost (IQR)	Mean cost ± sd	Median cost (IQR)	Mean cost ± sd	Median cost (IQR)
Baseline	CG	881.01 ± 1024.31	657 (445)-(879)	305.75 ± 557.60	129 (90)-(232)	1186.77 ± 1444.30	861 (583.75)-(1104.25)
	T1G	803.50 ± 455.06	737 (468)-(944.50)	225.22 ± 379.79	92.50 (80)-(200)	1028.72 ± 667.85	914 (615)-(1144)
	T2G	705.81 ± 450.93	567.50 (429)-(838)	188.98 ± 310.18	99 (80)-(150)	894.79 ± 660.23	712 (525.75)-(986.25)
3-months	CG	1926.62 ± 1226.31	1714.50 (1234.75)-(2176.25)	392.06 ± 211.27	320 (243.75)-(492.50)	2318.68 ± 1247.24	2057.50 (1645)-(2527.75)
	T1G	1990.96 ± 1180.94	1769 (1100)-(2452)	259.35 ± 80.69	240 (200)-(300)	2250.31 ± 1179.84	2071 (1350)-(2802)
	T2G	1911.37 ± 1003.66	1733 (1146)-(2358)	286.52 ± 111.37	300 (198)-(360)	2197.90 ± 1043.56	2062 (1384)-(2673)
6-months	CG	1875.56 ± 918.03	1712.50 (1235.50)-(2459)	301.78 ± 144.03	305 (218)-(360)	2177.34 ± 998.34	2080 (1467.25)-(2761.25)
	T1G	1621.58 ± 1220.84	1037 (738)-(2142)	247.13 ± 129.06	200 (150)-(310)	1868.72 ± 1217.24	1410 (925)-(2327)
	T2G	1512.45 ± 981.02	1309 (690)-(2020)	263.82 ± 119.56	255 (178)-(330)	1776.27 ± 1029.89	1543 (913)-(2263)
9-months	CG	1694.84 ± 730.40	1609.50 (1192.50)-(2098.25)	267.70 ± 90.34	275 (200)-(320)	1962.54 ± 767.27	1894.50 (1376.25)-(2378.50)
	T1G	1377.11 ± 723.19	1219 (753)-(1739)	226.74 ± 160.15	160 (128)-(320)	1603.86 ± 758.96	1374 (1104)-(1888)
	T2G	1276.74 ± 935.41	947 (631)-(1586)	251.17 ± 169.73	200 (148)-(300)	1527.92 ± 951.75	1260 (925)-(2144)
12-months	CG	1568.86 ± 565.84	1548 (1122.75)-(1866.75)	304.42 ± 92.58	307.50 (225)-(362.50)	1873.28 ± 587.99	1851.50 (1437.25)-(2272.25)
	T1G	1076.62 ± 726.61	768 (500)-(1488)	226.19 ± 126.02	184 (140)-(252)	1302.82 ± 771.70	1020 (660)-(1833)
	T2G	910.03 ± 650.91	620 (460)-(1116)	228.27 ± 193.20	180 (100)-(240)	1138.31 ± 682.27	900 (597)-(1455)

[a] = costs were calculated in NPR [Exchange rate: 1 USD = NPR 73.38]

[b] = CG = control group, T1G = test 1 group, T2G = test 2 group

Table 3 Direct healthcare costs comparison of patients at the baseline and follow-ups within test groups (T1G and T2G)

Groups	T1G (PC group)	T2G (PC + Diabetic kit group)
Follow-ups	Median cost (IQR)	Median cost (IQR)
Baseline	914 (615)-(1144)	712 (525.75)-(986.25)
3-months (1st FU)	2071 (1350)-(2802)	2062 (1384)-(2673)
6-months (2nd FU)	1410 (925)-(2327)	1543 (913)-(2263)
9-months (3rd FU)	1374 (1104)-(1888)	1260 (925)-(2144)
12-months (4th FU)	1020 (660)-(1833)	900 (597)-(1455)
p-value*	**<0.001****	**<0.001****

*Friedman test applied
**Difference was significant at $p \le 0.05$ level (2-tailed)

medical costs. The direct medical costs of patients in present study were greatly occupied with investigation costs followed by drug costs at baseline [5]. It was estimated that the total median direct healthcare costs of individual group at baseline was occupied by slightly more than half of median direct medical costs, which was further occupied by nearly one third of total median medication cost in each group. This is higher than the observation made from a study conducted in Italy [4]. Similarly, the dietary management costs and transportation costs were the main contributing components of direct non-medical costs at baseline in the present study.

Patients must be alert and proactive in managing their diabetes to avoid the co-morbidities that may cause significant out-of-pocket expenses of patients due to increased medical and medication costs related to diabetes and co-morbid conditions [19]. The out-of-pocket expenses of patients can be minimised by improving their health related outcomes. Pharmacist being an important member of healthcare team can provide a good support to patient in improving their health related outcomes

and hence minimizing their out-of-pocket expenses. It is already evident from Asheville project in which authors demonstrated the impact of pharmaceutical care on economic outcomes in diabetes management [20]. There was significant increase in out-of-pocket expenses of patients in three groups at 3 months due to increase direct medical costs. The sudden increase in patients' out-of-pocket expenses was due to the high degree of glycaemia that required frequent patient visits to the hospital during the first 3 months of the initiation phase of treatment to get the physician's consultation. This subsequently increased the costs of other components of direct medical and non-medical domains with major impact on drug costs, investigation cost, registration cost, transportation cost and dietary management cost. Together, this amplified the median direct healthcare costs of patients in the three groups at 3 months. A rise in out-of-pocket expenses may decrease or prevent the health-seeking behavior of the patients and prevent them from medication procurement [21].

Pharmacist led intervention reduced direct healthcare costs burden of patients significantly in test groups at 6, 9 and 12 months' follow-ups compared to control group when tested by Mann–Whitney U-test. Similarly, few studies from USA also described a reduction in total direct medical costs and per patient direct healthcare cost due to pharmacist led intervention through pharmaceutical care program [20, 22, 23]. The major reduction was calculated in direct medical cost components such as investigation cost and prescription cost of patients [24]. This reduction could be due to improvement in glycaemic symptoms of patients that reduces their drug prescription and frequency of investigations. Moreover, a Colombian study also highlighted the reduction in medical cost of those patients who were under the care of pharmacist compared to control group patients [25].

Table 4 Differences in direct healthcare costs of patients in both test groups (T1G and T2G) over time

Follow-ups	T1G (PC group)		T2G (PC + Diabetic kit group)	
	Z- value	p-value*	Z-value	p-value*
Baseline + 3-months	-5.352	**<0.001****	-5.676	**<0.001****
Baseline + 6-months	-4.396	**<0.001****	-5.015	**<0.001****
Baseline + 9-months	-4.134	**<0.001****	-4.898	**<0.001****
Baseline + 12-months	-2.132	0.033	-2.531	0.010
3-months + 6-months	-1.978	0.048	-2.235	0.025
3-months + 9-months	-4.134	**<0.001****	-3.674	**<0.001****
3-months + 12-months	-4.387	**<0.001****	-5.408	**<0.001****
6-months + 9-months	-1.322	0.186	-1.429	0.153
6-months + 12-months	-2.690	**0.005****	-3.890	**<0.001****
9-months + 12-months	-2.090	0.037	-4.218	**<0.001****

* Wilcoxon signed rank test for paired data
**Difference was significant at $p \le 0.005$ level (2-tailed) after Bonferroni adjustment applied

Table 5 Comparison of direct healthcare costs between test groups (T1G and T2G) and, CG and test groups patients

Follow-ups	Baseline	3-months (1st FU)	6-months (2nd FU)	9-months (3rd FU)	12-months (4th FU)
Groups	Median cost (IQR)	Median cost (IQR)	Median cost (IQR)	Median cost (IQR)	Median cost (IQR)
T1G	914 (615)-(1144)	2071 (1350)-(2802)	1410 (925)-(2327)	1374 (1104)-(1888)	1020 (660)-(1833)
T2G	712 (525.75)-(986.25)	2062 (1384)-(2673)	1543 (913)-(2263)	1260 (925)-(2144)	900 (597)-(1455)
p-value*	0.057	0.917	0.870	0.254	0.174
CG	861 (583.75)-(1104.25)	2057.50 (1645)-(2527.75)	2080 (1467.25)-(2761.25)	1894.50 (1376.25)-(2378.50)	1851.50 (1437.25)-(2272.25)
T1G	914 (615)-(1144)	2071 (1350)-(2802)	1410 (925)-(2327)	1374 (1104)-(1888)	1020 (660)-(1833)
p-value*	0.463	0.642	**0.009****	**0.005****	**<0.001****
CG	861 (583.75)-(1104.25)	2057.50 (1645)-(2527.75)	2080 (1467.25)-(2761.25)	1894.50 (1376.25)-(2378.50)	1851.50 (1437.25)-(2272.25)
T2G	712 (525.75)-(986.25)	2062 (1384)-(2673)	1543 (913)-(2263)	1260 (925)-(2144)	900 (597)-(1455)
p-value*	0.260	0.405	**0.010****	**0.001****	**<0.001****

* Mann–Whitney U test
**Difference was significant at $p \leq 0.05$ level (2-tailed)

The median DHCs of patients in test groups decreased significantly compared to control group due to reduction in their median direct medical costs at 12 month follow-up. Although, there were differences in median DHCs (in Nepali rupees) of patients in both test groups throughout the study period but it was not significant at any of the follow-ups. The insignificant decrease in median direct healthcare costs of patients in control group compared to test groups could be due to the doctor/nurse provided care. The additional out-of-pocket expenses on patients in the absence of government and private health-insurance coverage[1] demands an urgent need of various healthcare schemes(e.g. health-insurance coverage) for the patients in developing countries like Nepal in order to protect their domestic budget, that may lead to improvement in their medication adherence and decrease the risk of chronic complications.

Limitations of the study

Diabetes patients were selected from only one hospital of the Kaski district in western Nepal and hence the study findings may not be able to generalize to the entire diabetic population of the country. The study estimated the reduction in treatment costs but fail to analyse the decrease in number of drug (s) per prescription of patient after the intervention. Similarly, the decrease in number of patient visits to the hospital was also not accounted. Furthermore, cost of pharmacist services was not taken into account in present study as there was no such cost taken by the hospital from the patient where study was conducted.

Conclusion

Direct healthcare costs of patients were mainly attributed to direct medical costs but contribution of transportation cost and dietary management cost cannot be ignored in direct non-medical cost. Pharmacist-provided intervention significantly decreased the direct healthcare costs of patients in test groups during their follow-ups with a greater reduction in drug costs and investigation costs. However, reduction in direct healthcare costs among control group patients was insignificant. The reduction in the direct healthcare costs of patients indicates the benefits of pharmacist-provided counselling and consultation through pharmaceutical care program in diabetes patient care and hence indicates pharmacist role and contribution in healthcare system.

Competing interests
The author(s) declare that they have no competing interests associated with this study.

Authors' contributions
DK conceptualized the research study, synthesized, analysed and interpreted data and wrote the manuscript. MI helped in designing the study, supervised the study. PM and MA translated the educational materials into Nepali language and assisted in literature review. VM and MA helped in collecting the data in hospital and assisted in analysis of data. MI, PM, VM and MA critically reviewed, revised and edited the manuscript as well. All authors read and approved the final version of manuscript for the publication.

Author details
[1]Faculty of Pharmacy, Asian Institute of Medicine, Science and Technology University, Jalan Bedong-Semeling, 08100 Bedong, Kedah, Malaysia. [2]Social and Administrative Pharmacy, College of Pharmacy, Qatar University, 2713 Doha, Qatar. [3]Department of Pharmacology, American University of the Caribbean School of Medicine, 1 University Drive at Jordan Road, Cupecoy, St. Maarten, Netherlands Antilles. [4]Department of Medicine, Manipal College of Medical Sciences and Manipal Teaching Hospital, Phulbari-11, Pokhara, Nepal. [5]Department of Pharmacy and Pharmacology, National Medical College, Birgunj, Nepal.

References
1. Grover S, Avasthi A, Bhansali A, Chakrabarti S, Kulhara P. Cost of ambulatory care of diabetes mellitus: a study from north India. Postgrad Med J. 2005;81:391–95.
2. Tharkar S, Devarajan A, Kumpatla S, Viswanathan V. The socioeconomics of diabetes from a developing country: a population based cost of illness study. Diabetes Res Clin Pract. 2010;89:334–40.
3. Javitt JC, Chiang YP. Economic impact of diabetes. In: Harris M, editor. Diabetes in America. 2 ed. Washington D C: National Institute of Diabetes and Digestive and Kidney Diseases, NIH Publication; 1995. p. 1468.

4. Bruno G, Karaghiosoff L, Merletti F, Costa G, DeMaria M, Panero F, et al. The impact of diabetes on prescription drug costs: the population-based Turin study. Diabetologia. 2008;51:795–01.

5. Khowaja LA, Khuwaja AK, Cosgrove P. Cost of diabetes care in out-patient clinics of Karachi, Pakistan. BMC Health Serv Res. 2007;7:189.

6. Karki P, Baral N, Lamsal M, Rijal S, Koner BC, Dhungel S, et al. Prevalence of non-insulin dependent diabetes mellitus in urban areas of eastern Nepal: a hospital based study. Southeast Asian J Trop Med Public Health. 2000;31:163–66.

7. Narayan KMV, Zhang P, Williams D, Engelgau M, Imperatore G, Kanaya A, et al. How should developing countries manage diabetes? Can Med Assoc J. 2006;175:733.

8. Upadhyay DK, Mohamed Ibrahim MI, Mishra P, Alurkar VM. A non-clinical randomised controlled trial to assess the impact of pharmaceutical care intervention on satisfaction level of newly diagnosed diabetes mellitus patients in a tertiary care teaching hospital in Nepal. BMC Health Serv Res. 2015;15:57. doi:10.1186/s12913-015-0715-5.

9. Daniel WW. Biostatistics: a foundation for analysis in the health sciences. New York: John Wiley & Sons; 1999.

10. Singh D, Bhattarai M. High prevalence of diabetes and impaired fasting glycaemia in urban Nepal. Diabet Med. 2003;20:170–71.

11. Ono K, Limbu YR, Rai SK, Kurokawa M, Yanagida J, Rai G, et al. The prevalence of type 2 diabetes mellitus and impaired fasting glucose in semi-urban population of Nepal. Nepal Med Coll J. 2007;9:154–56.

12. Graber AL, Davidson P, Brown AW, McRae JR, Woolridge K. Dropout and relapse during diabetes care. Diabetes Care. 1992;15:1477–83.

13. Mourao AOM, Ferreira WR, Martins MAP, Reis AMM, Carrillo MRG, Guimaraes AG, et al. Pharmaceutical care program for type 2 diabetes patients in Brazil: a randomised controlled trial. Int J Clin Pharm. 2013;35:79–86.

14. Hjelm K, Mufunda E. Zimbabwean diabetics' beliefs about health and illness: an interview study. BMC Int Health Hum Rights. 2010;10:7.

15. Hopewell S, Dutton S, Yu LM, Chan AW, Altman DG. The quality of reports of randomised trials in 2000 and 2006: comparative study of articles indexed in PubMed. BMJ. 2010;340:c723.

16. Javanbakht M, Baradaran HR, Mashayekhi A, Haghdoost AA, Khamseh ME, Kharazmi E, et al. Cost-of-illness analysis of type 2 diabetes mellitus in Iran. PLoS One. 2011;6:e26864.

17. Henriksson F, Agardh CD, Berne C, Bolinder J, Lonnqvist F, Stenstrom P, et al. Direct medical costs for patients with type 2 diabetes in Sweden. J Intern Med. 2000;248:387–96.

18. Sarker AR, Islam Z, Khan IA, Saha A, Chowdhury F, Khan AI, et al. Cost of illness for cholera in a high risk urban areas in Bangladesh: an analysis from household perspective. BMC Infect Dis. 2013;13:518.

19. Rodbard HW, Green AJ, Fox KM, Grandy S. Impact of type 2 diabetes mellitus on prescription medication burden and out-of-pocket healthcare expenses. Diabetes Res Clin Pract. 2010;87:360–65.

20. Cranor CW, Bunting BA, Christensen DB. The Asheville Project: long-term clinical and economic outcomes of a community pharmacy diabetes care program. J Am Pharm Assoc. 2003;43:173–84.

21. Fox KM, Grandy S. Out-of-pocket expenses and healthcare resource utilization among individuals with or at risk of diabetes mellitus. Curr Med Res Opin. 2008;24:3323–29.

22. Garrett DG, Bluml BM. Patient self-management program for diabetes: first-year clinical, humanistic, and economic outcomes. J Am Pharm Assoc. 2005;45:130–37.

23. Monte SV, Slazak EM, Albanese NP, Adelman M, Rao G, Paladino JA. Clinical and economic impact of a diabetes clinical pharmacy service program in a university and primary care–based collaboration model. J Am Pharm Assoc. 2009;49:200–08.

24. Borges APS, Guidoni CM, Freitas O, Pereira LRL. Economic evaluation of outpatients with type 2 diabetes mellitus assisted by a pharmaceutical care service. Arq Bras Endocrinol Metabol. 2011;55:686–91.

25. Machado-Alba JE, Torres-Rodríguez S, Vallejos-Narváez A. Effectiveness the pharmaceutical care in diabetic patients. Colomb Med. 2011;42:72–80.

Permissions

List of Contributors

Ishtiyaq A Najar, Manoj K Tikoo, Gurdarshan Singh, Subhash C Sharma and Rakesh K Johri
PK/PD and Toxicology Division, CSIR-Indian Institute of Integrative Medicine, Canal Road, Jammu, India

Mahendra K Verma, Rajneesh An and Ravi K Khajuria
Analytical Chemistry Division (Instrumentation), CSIR-Indian Institute of Integrative Medicine, Canal Road, Jammu, India

Devinder K Gupta
Biorganic Chemistry Division, CSIR-Indian Institute of Integrative Medicine, Canal Road, Jammu, India

Vahid Kiarostami and Razieh Mohammadian
Department of Chemistry, North Tehran Branch, Islamic Azad University, P.O. Box 1913674711, Tehran, Iran

Hoda Lavasani and Mohamad-Reza Rouini
Biopharmaceutics and Pharmacokinetics Division, Department of Pharmaceutics, Faculty of Pharmacy, Tehran University of Medical Sciences, Tehran, Iran

Mehri Ghazaghi
Department of Applied Chemistry, Faculty of Science, Semnan University, Semnan, Iran

Mohammad K Mohammadi
Faculty of sciences, Ahvaz Branch, Islamic Azad University, Ahvaz, Iran.

Omidreza Firuzi and Mehdi Khoshneviszadeh
Medicinal and Natural Products Chemistry Research Center, Shiraz, University of Medical Sciences, PO Box 3288–71345, Shiraz, Iran

Ramin Miri
Medicinal and Natural Products Chemistry Research Center, Shiraz, University of Medical Sciences, PO Box 3288–71345, Shiraz, Iran. Departments of Medicinal Chemistry, School of Pharmacy, Shiraz University of Medical Sciences, Shiraz, Iran

Nima Razzaghi-Asl
Departments of Medicinal Chemistry, School of Pharmacy, Shiraz University of Medical Sciences, Shiraz, Iran

Saghi Sepehri
Departments of Medicinal Chemistry, Faculty of Pharmacy, Isfahan University of Medical Sciences, Isfahan, Iran

Hossein Khalili and Farzaneh Dastan
Department of Clinical Pharmacy, Faculty of Pharmacy, Tehran University of Medical Sciences, Tehran 1417614411, Iran

Seyed Ali Dehghan Manshadi
Department of Infectious Diseases, Faculty of Medicine, Tehran University of Medical Sciences, Tehran, Iran

Ali Almasirad and Mohammad Javad Assarzadeh
Department of Medicinal Chemistry, Pharmaceutical Sciences Branch, Islamic Azad University, Tehran, Iran

Zahra Mousavi
Department of Toxicology and Pharmacology, Pharmaceutical Sciences Branch, Islamic Azad University, Tehran, Iran

Abbas Shafiee and Mohammad Tajik
Department of Medicinal Chemistry, Faculty of Pharmacy and Pharmaceutical Sciences Research Center, Tehran University of MedicalnSciences, Tehran, Iran

Mohsen Zeeb, Parisa Tayebi Jamil, Ali Berenjian and Mohamad Reza Talei Bavil Olyai
Department of Applied Chemistry, Faculty of science, Islamic Azad University, South Tehran Branch, Tehran, Iran

Mohammad Reza Ganjali
Center of Excellence in Electrochemistry, Faculty of Chemistry, University of Tehran, Tehran, Iran

Vahideh Sadat Motamedshariaty and Sara Amel Farzad
Pharmaceutical Research Center, School of Pharmacy, Mashhad University of Medical Sciences, Mashhad, Iran

Marjan Nassiri-Asl
Cellular and Molecular Research Centre, Department of Pharmacology, School of Medicine, Qazvin University of Medical Sciences, Qazvin, Iran

Hossein Hosseinzadeh
Pharmacodynamics and Toxicological Department, Pharmaceutical Research Center, School of Pharmacy, Mashhad University of Medical Sciences, Mashhad, Iran

Akram Jamshidzadeh
Pharmaceutical Sciences Research Center, Shiraz University of Medical Sciences, Shiraz, Iran
Department of Pharmacology and Toxicology, Faculty of pharmacy, Shiraz University of Medical Sciences, Shiraz, Iran

Fatemeh Vahedi and Asma Najibi
Department of Pharmacology and Toxicology, Faculty of pharmacy, Shiraz University of Medical Sciences, Shiraz, Iran

Hassan Seradj
International Branch, Shiraz University of Medical Sciences, Shiraz, Iran

Hassan Seradj
Department of Pharmacognosy, Faculty of Pharmacy, Shiraz University of Medical Sciences, Shiraz, Iran

Gholamreza Dehghanzadeh
Food and Drug Control Laboratory, Shiraz University of Medical Sciences, Shiraz, Iran

Nahid Kabiri and Seyed Reza Fatemi Tabatabaie
Department of Physiology, Faculty of Veterinary Medicine, Shahid Chamran University of Ahvaz, Ahvaz, Iran

Mohammad Reza Tabandeh
Department of Biochemistry and Molecular Biology, Faculty of Veterinary Medicine, Shahid Chamran University of Ahvaz, Ahvaz, Iran

Darshana S Jain, Rajani B Athawale and Shruti S Shrikhande
Department of Pharmaceutics, C.U. Shah College of Pharmacy, SNDT Women's University, Juhu Tara Road, Santacruz (West), Mumbai 400 049, India

Amrita N Bajaj
SVKM's Dr. Bhanuben Nanavati College of Pharmacy, Vileparle, Mumbai 400 056, India

Peeyush N Goel, Yuvraj Nikam and Rajiv P Gude
Gude Lab, Advanced Centre for Treatment, Research & Education in Cancer (ACTREC), Tata Memorial Centre, Kharghar, Navi Mumbai 410 210, India

Hoda Lavasani, Behjat Sheikholeslami, Yalda H Ardakani and Lida Hakemi
Biopharmaceutics and Pharmacokinetics Division, Department of Pharmaceutics, Faculty of Pharmacy, Tehran University of Medical Sciences, 14155-6451, Tehran, Iran

Mohammad-Reza Rouini
Biopharmaceutics and Pharmacokinetics Division, Department of Pharmaceutics, Faculty of Pharmacy, Tehran University of Medical Sciences, 14155-6451, Tehran, Iran
Pharmaceutical Sciences Research Centre, Faculty of Pharmacy, Tehran University of Medical Sciences, 14155-6451, Tehran, Iran

Mohammad Abdollahi
Department of Pharmacology and Toxicology, Faculty of Pharmacy, Tehran University of Medical Sciences, 14155-6451, Tehran, Iran Pharmaceutical Sciences Research Centre, Faculty of Pharmacy, Tehran University of Medical Sciences, 14155-6451, Tehran, Iran

Balaram Gajra and Chintan Dalwadi
Department of Pharmaceutics & Pharmaceutical Technology, Ramanbhai Patel College of Pharmacy, Charotar University of Science and Technology, CHARUSAT Campus, Changa 388 421, Gujarat, India

Ravi Patel
Department of Pharmaceutics, Indian Institute of Technology, Banaras Hindu University (IIT-BHU), Varanasi 221 005, UP, India

Saeed Hosseini and Bagher Larijani
Endocrinology and Metabolism Research Center, Endocrinology and Metabolism Clinical Sciences Institute, Tehran University of Medical Sciences, Tehran, Iran

Hasan Fallah Huseini
Pharmacology and Applied Medicine Department of Medicinal Plants Research Center, Institute of Medicinal Plants, ACECR, Karaj, Iran

Kazem Mohammad and Kazem Mohammad
Department of Epidemiology and Biostatistics, Tehran University of Medical Sciences, School of Public Health, Tehran, Iran

Alireza Najmizadeh
Karaj Diabetes Society, Alborz, Karaj, Iran

Leila Jamshidi
Department of Nutrition, Tehran University of Medical Sciences, School of Public Health, Tehran, Iran

Negar Mohammadhosseini, Najmeh Edraki, Alireza Foroumadi and Abbas Shafiee
Department of Medicinal Chemistry, Faculty of Pharmacy and Pharmaceutical Sciences Research Center, Tehran University of Medical Sciences, Tehran 14176, Iran

Farideh Siavoshi and Parastoo Saniee
Department of Microbiology, Faculty of Sciences, University of Tehran, P.O. Box: 14155–6455, Tehran, Iran

Ameneh Ghamaripour and Hassan Aryapour
Department of Biology, Faculty of Science, Golestan University, Gorgan, Iran

Farzaneh Afshar
Department of Chemistry, Science and Research Branch, Islamic Azad University, Arak, Iran

Parichehreh Yaghmaei and, Katia Azarfar
Department of Biology, Science and Research Branch, Islamic Azad University, Tehran, Iran

Mehrooz Dezfulian
Department of Microbiology, College of Science, Islamic Azad University, Karaj Branch, Karaj, Iran

Azadeh Ebrahim-Habibi
Biosensor Research Center, Endocrinology and Metabolism Molecular-Cellular Sciences Institute, Tehran University of Medical Sciences, Tehran, Iran
Endocrinology and Metabolism Research Center, Endocrinology and Metabolism Clinical Sciences Institute, Tehran University of Medical Sciences, North Kargar Avenue, 1411413137
Tehran, Iran

Mohammad Reza Nabatchian and Hamid Shahriari
Department of Industrial Engineering, K.N. Toosi University of Technology, No 7, Pardis St., Mollasadra Ave., Tehran, Iran

Mona Shahriari
Department of Dermatology, University of Connecticut Health Center, Farmington, CT, USA

Zahra Shokri and Mehdi Ardjmand
Department of Chemical Engineering, Islamic Azad University-Tehran South Branch, Tehran, Iran

Mohammad Reza Fazeli
Probiotic Research Laboratory, Department of Drug and Food Control, Pharmaceutical Sciences Research Center, Faculty ofPharmacy, Tehran University of Medical Sciences, Tehran, Iran

Seyyed Mohammad Mousavi
Biotechnology Group, Chemical Engineering Department, Tarbiat Modares University, Tehran, Iran

Kambiz Gilani
Aerosol Research Laboratory, Department of Pharmaceutics, Faculty of Pharmacy, Tehran University of Medical Sciences, Tehran, Iran

Sureerat Buahorm
Program in Biotechnology, Faculty of Science, Chulalongkorn University, 254 Phayathai Road, Bangkok 10330, Thailand

Songchan Puthong
Institute of Biotechnology and Genetic Engineering, Chulalongkorn University, 254 Phayathai Road, Bangkok 10330, Thailand

Tanapat Palaga
Department of Microbiology, Faculty of Science, Chulalongkorn University, 254 Phayathai Road, Bangkok 10330, Thailand

Kriengsak Lirdprapamongkol and Jisnuson Svasti
Laboratory of Biochemistry, Chulabhorn Research Institute, Vipawadee Rangsit Highway, Bangkok 10210, Thailand

Preecha Phuwapraisirisan
Department of Chemistry, Faculty of Science, Chulalongkorn University, 254 Phayathai Road, Bangkok 10330, Thailand

Chanpen Chanchao
Department of Biology, Faculty of Science, Chulalongkorn University, 254 Phayathai Road, Bangkok 10330, Thailand

Hassan Hashemi, Mohammad Amin Seyedian, Mohammad Miraftab, Hooman Bahrmandy and Araz Sabzevari
Noor Ophthalmology Research Center, Noor Eye Hospital, No. 96 Esfandiar Blvd., Vali'asr Ave, Tehran, Iran

Soheila Asgari
Department of Epidemiology and Biostatistics, School of Public Health, Tehran University of Medical Sciences, International Campus (TUMS-IC), Tehran, Iran

Seyede Maryam Naghibi, Narjess Ayati and Seyed Rasoul Zakavi
Nuclear Medicine Research Center, Faculty of Medicine, Mashhad University of Medical Sciences, Mashhad, Iran

Mohamad Ramezani
Pharmaceutical Research Center, Buali Research Institute, Mashhad University of Medical Sciences, Mashhad, Iran

Neda Bavarsad and Anayatollah Salimi
Nanotechnology Research Center, Ahvaz Jundishapur University of Medical Sciences, Ahvaz, Iran
Department of Pharmaceutics, School of Pharmacy, Ahvaz Jundishapur University of Medical Sciences, Ahvaz, Iran

Somayeh Seifmanesh
Department of Pharmaceutics, School of Pharmacy, Ahvaz Jundishapur University of Medical Sciences, Ahvaz, Iran

Abbas Akhgari
Targeted Drug Delivery Research Center, School of Pharmacy, Mashhad University of Medical Sciences, Mashhad, Iran

Annahita Rezaie
Department of Pathobiology, Faculty of Veterinary Medicine, Shahid Chamran University of Ahvaz, Ahvaz, Iran

Hiba Hadj Ammar and Hatem Majdoub
Laboratoire des Interfaces et des Matériaux Avancés (LIMA), Faculté des Sciences de Monastir, Université de Monastir, Bd. de l'environnement, 5019 Monastir, Tunisia

Sirine Lajili and Abderrahman Bouraoui
Laboratoire de développement chimique, galénique et pharmacologique des médicaments, Faculté de Pharmacie de Monastir, Université de Monastir, 5000 Monastir, Tunisia

Rafik Ben Said
Institut National des Sciences et Techniques de la Mer (INSTM), Salambôo, Tunis, Tunisia

Didier Le Cerf
Université de la Normandie, Laboratoire Polymères Biopolymères Surfaces, UMR 6270 CNRS Université de Rouen, FRE 3101 CNRS, 76821 Mont Saint Aignan, France

Sinem Aslan Erdem
Department of Pharmacognosy, Faculty of Pharmacy, Ankara University, 06100 Ankara, Turkey

Seyed Mohammad Nabavi and Seyed Fazel Nabavi
Applied Biotechnology Research Center, Baqiyatallah University of Medical Sciences, P.O. Box 19395-5487, Tehran, Iran

Ilkay Erdogan Orhan
Department of Pharmacognosy, Faculty of Pharmacy, Gazi University, 06330 Ankara, Turkey

Maria Daglia
Department of Drug Sciences, Medicinal Chemistry and Pharmaceutical Technology Section, University of Pavia, Pavia, Italy

Morteza Izadi
Health Research Center, Baqiyatallah University of Medical Sciences, Tehran, Iran

Bagher Alinejad
Department of Pharmacology, School of Medicine, Mashhad University of Medical Sciences, Mashhad, Iran

Reza Shafiee-Nick
Department of Pharmacology, School of Medicine, Mashhad University of Medical Sciences, Mashhad, Iran
Pharmacological Research Center of Medicinal Plants, School of Medicine, Mashhad University of Medical Sciences, Mashhad, Iran

Ahmad Ghorbani
Pharmacological Research Center of Medicinal Plants, School of Medicine, Mashhad University of Medical Sciences, Mashhad, Iran

Hamid Sadeghian
Department of laboratory Sciences, School of Paramedical Sciences, Mashhad University of Medical Sciences, Mashhad, Iran

Dinesh Kumar Upadhyay
Faculty of Pharmacy, Asian Institute of Medicine, Science and Technology University, Jalan Bedong-Semeling, 08100 Bedong, Kedah, Malaysia

Mohamed Izham Mohamed Ibrahim
Social and Administrative Pharmacy, College of Pharmacy, Qatar University, 2713 Doha, Qatar

Pranaya Mishra
Department of Pharmacology, American University of the Caribbean School of Medicine, 1 University Drive at Jordan Road, Cupecoy, St. Maarten, Netherlands Antilles

Vijay M. Alurkar
Department of Medicine, Manipal College of Medical Sciences and Manipal Teaching Hospital, Phulbari-11, Pokhara, Nepal

Mukhtar Ansari
Department of Pharmacy and Pharmacology, National Medical College, Birgunj, Nepal

Index

A

Acenaphtho Derivatives, 18-19, 22-25, 27-28

Acquired Immunodeficiency Syndrome, 29

Acrylamide-induced Neurotoxicity, 51, 53, 55, 57

Adipogenesis, 210-213, 215-217

Amitriptyline Adsorption, 62

þÿ Amyloid-² Plaque Accumulation, 121, 123, 125

Analgesic, 33, 35-40, 91, 164, 166, 187

Anti-helicobacter Pylori Activity, 112

Anti-inflammatory Activities, 33, 35, 37, 39-40, 208

Antibacterial, 111, 113, 116, 119, 149, 157, 187-188, 200-201, 206-208

Antitumor Agents, 18-19, 28

Apis Mellifera, 148-149, 151, 153, 155-157

Aqueous Extract, 107-109, 111

B

Behavioural Index, 53-55

Beta Amyloid, 120, 125

Bifidobacterium Bifidum, 139-141, 143, 145, 147

Binary Solvents, 11, 13, 15, 17

Biological Samples, 10, 17, 41-43, 48

Body Mass Index (bmi), 71

Box-behnken Design, 92-93, 106

Breast Cancer Cells, 8, 82, 106, 148

C

Cellular Morphology, 79, 81

Chemotherapeutic Agent, 148

Chromatograms, 3, 5, 15-16

Confocal Microscopy, 74, 76, 92, 105

Cytoprotective Effects, 49

Cytotoxic Activity, 18-19, 21, 23, 25, 27, 156-157

Cytotoxic Potential, 75, 77, 79, 81

D

Demethoxycurcumin (dmc), 3

Desirability Function, 127, 133, 147

Diabetic Patients, 83, 107, 109-110, 221, 228

Diabetic Rats, 17, 83, 85-91, 110-111, 157

D (continued)

Dispersive Liquid-liquid Microextraction, 10-11, 17, 48

Doxepin Adsorption, 59, 61, 63

Drug Loading, 92, 94, 99

Drug Release, 80, 95, 99-100, 105-106, 127-130, 133-135, 168-170, 172-174, 178

E

Effects of Pioglitazone, 65, 67, 69, 71, 73

Effects of Rutin, 49, 51, 53, 55-57

Eliminate Xenobiotics, 83

Entrapment Efficiency, 92, 94-95, 98-99, 104-105

Ethyl Acetate, 10-11, 13-16, 121

F

Fetal Bovine Serum (fbs), 21

G

Gene Expression, 64-67, 69, 71-72, 120-121, 123-125, 149, 151, 157

Genus Eryngium, 188-190, 194, 200-201, 206-207

Glioblastoma Multiforme, 158

H

Healthcare Costs, 219-222, 225-227

Hearing Loss, 29-32

Hepatic Biotransformation, 83

Human Immunodeficiency Virus, 29

Hypoglycemic Effect, 107, 109, 111

Hypothyroidism, 164-167

J

Juglans Regia Leaves, 109, 111

K

Keratoconus, 159-163

L

Limit Of Detection (lod), 41

Liposomal Formulation, 168, 171

Liquid Microextraction, 10-11, 13, 15, 17, 42, 48

Liquid Phase Microextraction, 10, 41, 43

Liver Enzymes, 85, 107, 109

M

Mathematical Model, 127, 129, 133, 135

Medicinal Plants, 107, 110, 188, 190, 208, 210

Molecular Docking Studies, 23

N

Nitrofuran, 112-113, 115-119

Nitrothiophen, 112-114, 117

Non Ulcerogenic, 33

O

Oligonucleotides, 18

Optimization of Itraconazole, 92-93, 95, 97, 99, 101, 103, 105

Osiris Property Explorer (ope), 37

P

P21 Upregulation, 148

Parameter Design, 130

Passive Avoidance Learning, 120

Pharmaceutical Formulations, 41, 43, 47, 159

Pharmacokinetic Changes of Tramadol, 17, 85, 87, 89, 91

Pharmacokinetic Study, 8

Phosphodiesterases, 210, 217-218

Piroxicam (pxm), 41

Plga Nanoparticles, 74-77, 79-81

Polycystic Ovary Syndrome (pco), 64, 72

Polydispersity Index, 75, 184, 186

Polymerase Chain Reaction, 66

Polymeric Lipid Hybrid Nanoparticles, 92-93, 95, 97, 99, 101, 103, 105

Q

Quantitative Analysis, 41, 43, 45, 47, 158

R

Response Surface Methodology, 139, 141, 147

S

Seaweed Polysaccharides, 180

Sensorineural Hearing Loss, 30-32

Silymarin Effect, 120-121, 123, 125

Sodium Polystyrene Sulfonate, 58-59, 61-63

Sodium Polystyrene Sulfonate (sps), 62

Spray Drying, 139-147

Statistical Optimization, 168-169, 171, 173, 175, 177, 179

Stopped-flow Injection Spectrofluorimetry, 41, 43

Streuli Pharma, 159, 161-162

T

Temozolomide, 74-75, 77, 79, 81-82

Time-oriented Quality Characteristic, 127

Tramadol, 10-17, 83-87, 89-91

U

Uplc-qtof-ms Method, 3, 5, 7, 9

Z

Zeta Potential, 75, 79-80, 92, 95, 100

www.ingramcontent.com/pod-product-compliance
Lightning Source LLC
Chambersburg PA
CBHW061939190326
41458CB00009B/2777